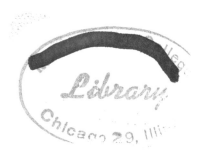
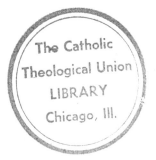

ADOLESCENCE

PSYCHOLOGY,
PSYCHOPATHOLOGY,
AND
PSYCHOTHERAPY

DEREK MILLER, M.D.

ADOLESCENCE

PSYCHOLOGY,
PSYCHOPATHOLOGY,
AND
PSYCHOTHERAPY

Jason Aronson, New York

Copyright © 1974 by Jason Aronson, Inc.

Library of Congress Cataloging in Publication Data

Miller, Derek.
  Adolescence: psychology, psychopathology, psychotherapy.

  Includes bibliographical references.
  1. Adolescent psychiatry.   2. Adolescent psychology.
I. Title. [DNLM: 1. Adolescent psychiatry.
2. Adolescent psychology. WS462 M647p 1974]
RJ503.M55   616.8'9   73-81211
ISBN 0-87668-101-1

Manufactured in the United States of America

To my children
who allege this book should
be dedicated to them

Contents

Introduction

A real need today is to understand how the development of personality in adolescents is modified by the world in which they live and how far the reverse is also true. Without this comprehension, adequate assistance for emotionally maladjusted youth is unlikely. Although it is too easy to blame all the ills of the young on society, it is equally facile to see the failures of social processes as they affect any one person, as the result of a projection of inner disturbance. A healthy mind requires a healthy body, but it also needs a society that makes it possible for developmental needs to be met without excessive difficulty.

All too often books about youth designed for experts in the field have a language that makes them incomprehensible both to other workers with a slightly different expertise and to the lay public. I have attempted to write a book that keeps technical jargon to a minimum but that will be useful to everyone who is seriously involved in the care of youth. It is unclear why a teacher cannot read the same book as a family practitioner, why a parent cannot get value from a work that is also useful to a psychiatrist.

A book cannot be a substitute for knowledge acquired in day-to-day living, but it is hoped that this one will enlarge the understanding of readers and offer practical guidelines as to what might be done to help the young people of our society. A distant uncomprehending relationship between parent and adolescent, home and school, teacher and taught, family practitioner and young patient, becomes menacing for the future of society.

The most common complaints of the young are that they feel lost, helpless, or empty. Alternately, they project their despair, see only the corruption of society and seek a solution in alternate lifestyles, unfortunately often more drug intoxicated than any middle-age, mildly alcoholic establishment figure whom they claim to despise. Some accept a degree of alienation and with that lead a reasonably full life. Few are able to use their potential as human beings.

The emotional development of children and adolescents does not just depend on a stable nuclear family. At all stages of development other significant groups are important—the extended family, peer groups, and extraparental adults (Miller, 1970). Up to adolescence a developmental order of importance would put the nuclear family first in Western society; after puberty a peer group and extraparental adults are at least as important, if not more so. In recent decades important sections of the framework of society against which young people might grow, in particular the large family group and extended social networks, have often been lost.

The organization of the school system from grade school upwards often interferes with a stable peer group. The skill with which society, parents, and school approach the young can improve. Teachers may be the only nonparental adults who are potentially available to relate to children. The organization within which teachers and pupils work needs to be modified to make such relationships more possible. Teachers particularly need to understand how to help adolescents to mature, although this understanding is necessary for all who work with youth.

Emotional illness and personal maladjustment in adolescence can neither be treated nor properly understood unless the helping adults of society understand something of the maturational processes of the young, how these are influenced by social systems, and what is then normal behavior. Apart from being knowledgeable about the effects, in particular, of the social environment of the schools and, in general, of the world at large on the behavior of youth, such helping adults also need to understand their relationship with adolescents, their families, and their community.

No society can ever provide enough technically trained people to assist through special treatment techniques those adolescents who become disturbed. Community mental health organizations often attempt to handle this problem by assuming that the lay public automatically has a vast fund of expertise. A particular problem exists for minority groups in that they, too, are offered magic solutions. If, for example, a school is offered black teachers, counselors, and courses in black history, the assumption is often made that this in some way will magically improve the lot of the black minority and lead to them being treated with dignity. However, the staff, black and white, usually perpetuate the system in which all children are treated as inferior; after all, separate staff toilets, lounges, and cafeterias carry an important institutional message about segregation. The staff may inferentially preach the virtues of an integrated society; but the social segregation is similar to that fought against by civil rights workers in the 1950s. Traditional techniques of relating to children may be supported by distant school administrations, which, to the outside observer, often appear more interested in perpetuating their own power than in being concerned with the education of children.

Social organizations concerned with youth need to be assisted to change their style so that people can be helped to reach not only academic and physical but also emotional and imaginative potential. Schools, besides helping their pupils to be prepared to earn a living, should help them build capacities for human and personal relations.

Prevention of maladjustment has always been an appropriate mental health goal. With the assumption that parents are almost totally responsible for the maturation of their children, much technical expertise has been offered to them. On the other hand, sociologists, architects, educational planners, and politicians, who often have little awareness of the needs of individuals, perpetrate social changes that take little note of these. As a result, in rearing children and adolescents in an increasingly disturbed and disruptive society, the family has to help individuals mature. It should expect help from social systems that still have the capacity for constructive change; it often does not get this.

The achievement of a less fearful and more adult society will be possible only if the difficulties associated with social change are faced. Unfortunately, society finds change very difficult. There are at least two reasons for this. The social organization of society tends to separate power from responsibility, and an awareness of a need for change is slow to percolate to society's upper levels. There is also a psychological resistance to change in both individuals and society; the older either is, the more this is likely to be true. Like a disturbed individual, the institutions of society often continue to repeat the same actions, although the conflicts that lead to their appearance are long since buried in the past.

In individuals, identity can constantly be modified. If important social systems are offered constructive change techniques, it should be possible to help the maturation of the young. Change agents, whatever their basic professional role, whether they work with individuals or groups, need to be aware of what is produced by the social organizations with which they work. This book looks at the production of young people, disturbed or otherwise, in a society that has often lost a capacity to value individual productivity, respect personal integrity and value human needs. That the. young survive and mature is a tribute to the resilience of humanity; the goal of this book in some small way is to try to enhance this process.

The manuscript was helped through many drafts by Mrs.

Cynthia Shuler to whom I am grateful. Roy and Francis Watts critically reviewed my comments on the problems of black youth. Alan Krohn was perceptive in his observations. Many medical students of the University of Michigan in their senior elective in adolescent psychiatry read various chapters and pointed out areas in which I had clouded issues with unnecessary jargon.

Reference

Miller, D. (1970), Parental responsibility for adolescent maturity. In *The Family and Its Future,* ed. K. Elliott, 23–38. London: Churchill.

ADOLESCENCE

PSYCHOLOGY,
PSYCHOPATHOLOGY,
AND
PSYCHOTHERAPY

1

Early Adolescence

Definition of Adolescence

Adolescent needs can be appreciated only if we know what we mean by adolescence. It is convenient to think of it in terms of an age range; there is a general assumption that it starts at about eleven or twelve and finishes at nineteen or twenty. Nevertheless, two rigid age limits are not a satisfactory way of delineating its span. What is adolescence varies from culture to culture and also from class to class in the same cultural setting. Adolescence can best be defined as "a process of adaptation to puberty" (Blos, 1962). An additional problem for parents, teachers, and society in general is that late developers whose puberty has not begun often behave as if they were adolescent and consider themselves as such. So, even to define adolescence in a general way as "adaptation to puberty" is not necessarily accurate. Adolescence can be understood if the world in which young people live, the way of life of their family, and the physical changes of growth are all considered. The personality of any adolescent boy or girl must also depend on their earlier life experiences; healthy adolescence depends to a large extent on a healthy infancy and childhood. Physical growth is an essential part of the creation of adolescence and the way young people behave. Without the changes of puberty, true adolescence is not really possible. Puberty and adolescence are the last great staging posts on the way to maturity.

Experience of Adolescence

The life experience of the individual adolescent depends on the way the world is seen and felt. Insofar as the social environment of an adolescent is concerned, where and how the family live, the job of the father and perhaps of the mother, and the school the youngster attends must matter. City, small town, or country living all make some difference, as does as pedestrian an issue as the size of a family's house and the number of available bedrooms. The way of life of the family obviously affects the behavior and experience of adolescents. Those parents who have brought up their children with a peaceful, loving authority may be reproached as being dull, old-fashioned, or "not with it," but their children will not noisily complain that they are uncaring. Highly permissive parents are often felt to be disinterested, even if their children see them as swinging. Children identify with the way families relate to each member; a turbulent, shouting family makes it more likely that the adolescent will express his anxieties in turbulence and noise; frozen families with little feeling produce children with a similar personality style.

Maturational or Chronological Age

Firm age subdivisions, if they could be attached to adolescence and its stages, would be very convenient. In many ways society attempts to do this, particularly in the school, where age tends to be used as a criterion of behavior, educational expectation, and school change. This preoccupation with age continues despite the fact that parents who have several children know perfectly well that the use of age as an assessment of expectations in adolescence is not reliable. One child may be quite mature at fifteen or sixteen; another may be physically and emotionally far behind this. From an emotional, educational, and social viewpoint, maturational age is more significant than chronological age, despite the socially induced preoccupation held by young people themselves over the latter.

Because they compare themselves to each other, adolescents tend to be preoccupied with the issue of fairness. In managing the lives of young people, concerned adults often get overpreoccupied with a similar issue: Will their actions appear fair to the individual youngster? Of course, what is truly fair depends on what is best for the adolescent's well-being, and all men are not equal, least of all because they are of similar age. So, apart from going along with the adolescent's concept of fairness, adults also tend to go along with the age sensitivity of individual adolescents. As part of their development to adult maturity, adolescents compare themselves one to the other on the basis of age, but society does not need to reinforce this. A thirteen-year-old boy, for example, makes many comparisons with others of the same age to see whose physique is more developed, who is socially more successful, physically able, or academic. Since in our society adolescents may compare their educational progress, which very much varies with maturational age, schools that expect performance based on rigid age norms may make it even more difficult for many adolescents to grow without unnecessary stress and strain. Even though there are variations in academic ability depending on the individual, a comparison made on the basis of age is certainly not a comparison of those of equal potential (Mussen and Jones, 1958).

Some of the confusion about typical adolescent behavior is resolved if the total developmental period is described in three stages. These stages often overlap to a certain extent, and some of what is described is present in childhood. The divisions can be seen more clearly in some social classes and cultures than others. Each stage covers about three full years, but there is obvious overlap between them. Furthermore, some qualities that are

typical aspects of both individual psychology and parent adolescent interaction in adolescence, are present in childhood, as well
as in some adult relationships. Similarly, some qualities high-
lighted in the early part of the age period are still present later.
Those young people who ultimately go on to some form of further
training after the age of sixteen show all these stages more clearly.
The stages are, however, less clearly defined in young people who
leave school at that age or earlier and who are then exposed to the
pressures of a complex society demanding more adult behavior.

Adolescent turmoil, about which there has been much argument (Offer, 1969) typically is seen in early adolescence, the
period of puberty, which lasts three years or more, from about
eleven or twelve until fourteen or fifteen. Midadolescence, the
period of identification, "This is what I am," and self-realization,
lasts from fourteen or fifteen to seventeen or eighteen; during
these periods oedipal conflicts should finally be resolved. Late
adolescence, the period of coping, lasts from seventeen or eighteen to nineteen or twenty. This last period is associated with
advanced training for specific roles in society. For young people
who leave school and attempt to earn a living at sixteen, late
adolescence is largely condensed into the midadolescent period.
Both middle and late adolescence may appear superficially as
periods of relative calm, especially in those who are conformists
(Lederer, 1964).

Early Adolescence—Physical Development

Puberty has been variously defined as the time of the first
ejaculation, when fertilization becomes possible, or as the second
stage of pubic hair development (Kestenberg, 1968), but if psychosocial change is significant, it is more helpful to regard it as a
period starting from the beginning growth of testicles in boys to
the time when there is active production of spermatazoa. In girls,
the era lasts from the onset of an increase in pubic hair, followed

by the budding of breasts, the beginning of vaginal secretion and the enlargement of breasts, to the time when menstruation begins.

These physical changes are associated with a rapid rise of seventeen ketosteroids in boys and girls, a greater production of estrogens in girls than boys, and a greater production of androgens in boys than girls (Nathanson et al., 1941).

Puberty usually begins at about the age of eleven plus in boys, ten plus in girls. Along with well-developed physical changes, it is associated with a rapid increase in the rate of growth. As pubertal changes occur, girls are suddenly likely to find themselves taller than boys of the same age. Because in childhood boys are bigger and heavier than girls, this change adds to the general feeling of confusion that both boys and girls experience. Between the ages of eleven and thirteen and for the subsequent two years the average girl is taller than the average boy of the same age for the only time in her life. After the age of fifteen to sixteen girls stop growing taller. Boys have their maximum growth spurt about two years later than girls, from age thirteen to fifteen, and they may continue to add a small amount to their height until the early twenties (Tanner, 1962).

Girls tend to gain weight; they have a period of puppy fat between the ages of ten and fifteen, and they tend to reach their adult weight after the age of eighteen. Boys put on weight fast in early adolescence and go on making small gains until nineteen or twenty. Most girls are well into the pubertal stage of development by the age of thirteen, most boys by fourteen, although a significant number of slow maturers—more often boys than girls —develop later than this. Late maturation is often hereditary. Often a girl's first periods are quite irregular and do not necessarily indicate that she is capable of bearing a child. First periods tend to be spaced further apart and last about a day longer, on the average, than would be expected in a fully mature woman. They are usually associated with premenstrual tension. The change in the shape of the larynx, which leads to boys' voices beginning to get lower in pitch and to break, occurs at the end

of the pubertal period in its last year. In boys, as in girls, there is
a gradual change in bodily shape: girls' hips get wider relative to
the rest of their bodies; in boys, the hips get slimmer. Boys become more heavily muscled, and hair appears on their face, initially in the moustache area and at the hairline at the side of
their face, then over the chin and neck.

In both boys and girls at puberty, sweat glands become more
active, as do the glands that supply oils to the skin and hair.
These sebaceous glands are sometimes apparently overactive during early adolescence, which may be one of the reasons for acne.
It is sometimes believed that this overactivity is related to diet—
sugar, acid, and candy, for example—but there is no clinical evidence of this. It may persist during middle and late adolescence.

Behavioral Changes at the Onset of Puberty

The first warnings of the onset of adolescence are usually
seen within families. At this time, parents may notice that children change in their behavior toward them. Boys of ten, for
example, often appear to become preoccupied with the sexuality
of their mothers. They may comment on how pretty they are;
they may contrive to touch their breasts as they pass them; they
may make comments that indicate that they wish to be in some
way their mothers' boyfriends. Similarly, girls become subtly
more feminine and more seductive with their fathers. These behavioral changes begin to be apparent, before there is very much
evidence of breast development in girls; there is, similarly, little
in the way of obvious physical change in boys. There are few
adequate studies of the relationship between physical change and
this type of behavior. All that can be said is quite general: Just
before the dramatic onset of puberty, children begin to try out
their ultimate roles as sexually aware men and women within the
safety of their family. These emotional signs of coming adolescence occur just prior to the beginning growth of testicles and

penis in boys, when there is low gonadotrophic and testicular androgen in the urine; in girls, the bony pelvis begins to grow and the nipples are beginning to bud, but estrogen excretion has not yet accelerated (Wilkins, 1965).

When children are besieged by the emotional impulses associated with the rapid changes of puberty, there is a further change in their attitude toward their parents. Clinical evidence indicates that early adolescents are as preoccupied with the sexuality of their parents as younger children, but this awareness is denied, and it is not evident from behavior. Early adolescents may strenuously deny their parents' ability to have sex, and, for this reason, it is often emotionally painful for them if their parents have more children. Their intense embarrassment may border on shame that their parents are not visible to the world as sexually "dead."

Early adolescence is associated with a beginning wish on the part of boys and girls to free themselves from those dependent feelings on their parents that they feel are childlike. Companions of their own age are used as support in what adolescents see as a struggle for freedom against parental domination and possessiveness. Allegations may be made, for example, when arguments about bedtime occur, about the lateness to which other children stay up. When going out with friends at night becomes an issue, parents are told about how late other children are allowed out. Similar problems occur with spending money, helping at home, doing homework, and having freedom to choose clothing. Pressure to obtain part-time work is similarly applied, and some children may be baby-sitting or running a paper route before they are sufficiently mature to handle the demands of such jobs.

Children use the comparison with friends of the same age to try and get more freedom and independence from their parents; then they assess themselves by the amount of freedom and independence they have managed to obtain compared to that of their friends. So it is inevitable that parents usually will not hear from their children of friends who have less freedom than they themselves. Parents are rarely told of the parties at which adults are present as chaperons. Instead, the adolescent may imply that all self-respecting fathers and mothers go out on such occasions and that their friends will see them as weak and inferior, if they have parents who stay around.

The adolescent concept of fairness is often used as an attempt, consciously or unconsciously, to manipulate parents. Everyone likes to feel that they are being fair and just; it is much easier to say "yes" than it is to say "no." Nevertheless, each family unit has its own standards, and there is no evidence that the way the neighbors bring up their children is a model for everyone. Parents want their children to get along with their friends, but significant adolescent relationships are not lost if clothes do not exactly match or if one youngster has to be home earlier than others. Often it may be a matter of some pride to boys and girls that their parents are insistent on certain standards, a paradox when they also use the amount of freedom they are given in the same way. When parents insist on standards, so do their children. In one school all formal clothing rules were dropped. The early adolescent girls then began to go to school in slacks. The boys were fiercely critical of this, and it became extremely rare for a girl to appear in other than a skirt and sweater.

Parents are used by their adolescent children as sounding boards against which to test feelings of independence. There is no expectation that every request will be granted. Adolescents, particularly in early years, tend to ask for more than they really expect to get; they are the model of the way government agencies behave when they ask the Treasury Department for money. Some fourteen-year-old boys will talk of asking their fathers for things just to see what they will do in reply.

For boys and girls early adolescence is a stage when the development of control over sexual and aggressive feelings begins to be particularly important. This is also the stage when the ability to feel like men and women and to see themselves as separate from their parents begins to be powerful. In childhood there is always some sense of separateness, which shows in such declarations as: "No, I don't want to come in to eat." In the teens this demand becomes more explicit: "Leave me alone."

Most early adolescents are still concrete thinkers, who limit themselves primarily to thinking about things (Piaget and Inhelder, 1958); as the years pass this type of thinking may change.

In understanding early adolescents there is an advantage in considering the needs, attitudes, and behavior of boys and girls separately.

A Comparison Between Masculine and Feminine Experience

Boys tend to be more physically uncomfortable about their bodily changes in size and shape than girls, although many girls experience a period of shy embarrassment.

The need to gain control over their own bodies and impulses, at the same time as they are developing feelings of separateness from their families, creates a particular problem for early adolescents. This is a time of rapid growth, often involving the experience of being out of control. With their dramatic growth in height, boys are no longer sure of their own bodies in space, and many become clumsy. Their voices change at just about the same time; although ultimately the voice will deepen, there is at first a startling variation in loudness and pitch, which can be increased by emotional stress. An additional problem for boys is that as their penis and testes grow larger, they become intensely aware of genital excitement, which is felt to be quite out of their control. Boys can gain active mastery over this state by masturbation: girls have no alternative but to passively accept the menarche. Boys can see what is happening to their bodies; girls do not know what goes on inside them. The passivity of girls and the available mastery techniques for boys are reinforced by traditional societal roles.

To cope with all this there is, in many adolescent boys, a period of apparent emotional withdrawal from the real world outside themselves. During this time both boys and girls may chatter, but they do not appear to be really interested in communicating their thoughts, feelings, or ideas to others, particularly adults. Nor do they appear very interested in hearing what adults have to say. "Are you deaf?" is a common cry from parents. Teachers who have contact with children over two to three years lament that youngsters who previously paid attention in class go through a period of six months or so in which they are restless, difficult daydreamers. In addition to this need to withdraw emotionally from others, early adolescents also develop a need to retreat physically from the adult world and their families. This carries implications for the design of homes and schools. Houses and apartments that give no space or physical privacy to adolescents may drive them on to the streets.

The Needs and Behavior of Boys

It is usual for boys to go through a period in which they are clumsy. They always seem to be falling over their hands and feet. Often in association with rapid growth they are quite lazy and disinterested in their appearance. It is at puberty that boys start to want to stay in bed in the morning for hours. Along with apparent laziness boys are also almost hyperactive from time to time. Particularly at bedtime they deny any feelings of fatigue in a way that may be reminiscent of a much younger child. Although pubertal boys may be generally disinclined to wash, they may suddenly appear looking devastatingly clean and well groomed. The early adolescent boy is highly vulnerable to fashion and copies the dress of older adolescents. Sleeping and bodily care are major battle grounds over which the dependence-independence struggle is fought. A boy insists he can make decisions but may forget to wash his hair, teeth, neck, and ears. The conflicts of early adolescent boys with parents may be more or less obvious. In those developing a healthy drive for autonomy, the conflicts are present, even when covered by a facade of apparent comfort.

When parents remind their sons of the necessity to look after themselves properly, these remarks are likely to be received with great offense. The pubertal boy may behave like an irresponsible child but feel as if he ought to be treated like a responsible adult. As a result, when parents react to his behavior and make the looking-after remarks and gestures that have been called for, the boy becomes angry, offended, or rebellious. Boys appear not to expect logical caring, parental responses, but they are not as angry if they get them, as they are if they do not. For example, if parents suggest to a boy who has difficulty getting up in the morning that he go to bed early, this may be felt to be a nonsensical and interfering suggestion. If such a boy is wakened in the morning, he may react as though his parents are sadistic monsters, demanding, lacking understanding, and so on. On the other hand, if parents fail to get their son out of bed, they are likely to be felt as uncaring and neglectful. It is as though the fatigue of early adolescence is used in the dependency struggle. If this behavior continues through later years in an aberrant way, is it a measure of psychosocial conflict alone and almost certainly has no physiological basis.

Male Striving for Independence

Early adolescent boys often are particularly intolerant of control exercised by women, in particular, their mothers. There is an unconscious attraction in being mothered, the strivings for independence of the male are never quite as clear and definite as they may appear on the surface. This is apparent when illness drives a boy to bed. Some cannot bear the dependence that is implied in being ill. As a result, early adolescents are often bad patients, disobey their doctor's orders, get up too soon, and do

not eat appropriately. Others appear to overwelcome the chance
to be babied; they may become difficult with their diet and constantly ask for attention of various sorts from either mothers, or
in hospitals, from nurses, aides, and doctors. Furthermore, early
adolescent boys are still unsure of their own manhood; to allow
themselves to be ordered about by women is intolerable. The less
secure a boy might be in his own manliness, the more rejecting
of mothering he becomes, but the more he is likely to provoke
his mother to tell him what to do; he feels ordered about by a
woman and then defiantly rejects this.

These two factors, the wish to be mothered and masculine
uncertainty, together may combine to make a pubertal boy as
resistant as a negativistic two-year-old. It often appears that a
pubertal boy prefers to have a blazing row with his mother over
minor trivialities—for example, failure to tidy his room—than to
simply pick up a few bits and pieces. Some mothers may feel personally hurt by their son's behavior, but it is really not a rejection
of a person, although it may appear to be so. It is a rejection of
mothering.

Providing that a man's role at home is valued, that wives
respect their husbands, it appears that boys take control and discipline from their fathers better than from their mothers, although they may also need to enter into competitive battles with
dad. Ultimately, the struggle with fathers is a struggle about
masculine assertiveness. Both parents in their relationship to
their sons, particularly when direct clashes are involved, should
be aware that if they win a point and their sons lose face and
pride in themselves, the victory is hollow.

Inevitably the young adolescent mixes up being independent
and being rebellious; in striving to be the one he almost necessarily becomes the other. Yet, in their rebellion the young imitate
what they see as the acceptable adult behavior of their parents.

Attempts to control a difficult, recalcitrant early adolescent
boy may require many changes in parental techniques from those
used in earlier childhood. Mothers may get help from their sons

by appealing to their masculine sense of chivalry; unfortunately, they may also get it by blackmailing them with tears. Fathers may get their son's cooperation by a genuine interest in their activities and by a preparedness to let them make appropriate decisions of their own. The father who emerges from behind a newspaper to bark out an order is likely to be less successful in helping his son or getting his assistance in household tasks. In early adolescence fathers can still expect from time to time that their sons will enjoy doing things with or for them. They are resistant when fathers are felt to be overprotective and over-demanding.

Pubertal boys have obvious problems over self-control. When frustrated, they may become so angry that they are near to tears; instead of talking, they may constantly shout. Often they are distressed about their own lack of control and, as mothers and fathers are seen as precipitating this, parents are angrily felt as responsible. It is not unusual for adolescent boys who feel under parental pressure to rush to their room with a dramatic slamming of the door.

Preoccupied with their own bodies, needing to gain control of their sexual urges and make them an emotionally meaningful part of themselves and their lives, and trying to reassure themselves that they are men and able to ejaculate, boys naturally masturbate (Winnicott, 1971). Those who never masturbate find it much more difficult to develop a feeling of genuine self-awareness. They do not easily come to terms with their own sexual feelings. They find it difficult to move beyond childhood toward the blending of sexual excitement and the expression of loving feelings that is the foundation of adult heterosexual relationships.

During early adolescence boys assess their masculinity primarily in relationship to other boys; girls are not a significant factor except in fantasy. Boys compare themselves to each other in ways that are acceptable to adults; for example, they compare their height, muscular development, ability at work, and competence in games. They also make comparisons that are less acceptable to the grown-up world. They compare their capacity to spit, to urinate, to ejaculate, and the size of their genitals. Similarly unacceptable to adults may be their spinning of prurient tales and loud-mouthed uncouthness.

At this stage boys may need to be emotionally involved with other boys in groups that may become gangs of a transient or more permanent nature. A group of boys gives its adolescent members the emotional support and sense of security that often prevent a return to the dependent feelings of childhood. Early adolescent boys who experience extreme psychological stress may depend on a gang to help them resolve their tensions. Dependence on their families is unacceptable to boys, both psychological and culturally, as a solution to anxiety. So if early adolescent boys are exposed to too much psychological stress, they have no alternative but to group together more formally and work out their anxieties on society. Unduly aggressive behavior on the part of an early adolescent boy is almost always a sign that he is under excessive psychological pressure.

Most of the time happy and comfortable young people who feel loved and valued are pleasant, alive, interested, creative, and generous. Healthy early adolescents are nevertheless difficult from time to time. Those who are always so well-behaved and conformist that they never give any trouble at all to their parents or teachers may be troubled. Such young people may not be able to allow themselves independent strivings ahead of their parents' and their society's wish to grant them freedom and responsibility. On the other hand, tolerant parents may let their children free themselves from their childish wishes so appropriately that there may be little external sign of conflict and turbulence. The complexity of society in large cities makes it improbable that this can always be a smooth process, but it is not impossible for the child of well-balanced, loving parents who have been able to take the stresses and strains of child rearing calmly and in their stride.

If parents are felt as too understanding, this may cause problems for their children, who never get the opportunity to feel that they win any significant struggle with parental authority. Good parents may thus experience a situation in which their sons relate to them as if they were harsh and tyrannical. Thus, a boy will get the satisfaction of feeling that he obtains something, despite the real absence of parental opposition; he may produce it in fantasy, if it is not there in fact.

Needs and Behavior of Girls

If, as is usual, the growth spurt of girls is less dramatic than than of boys, they do not go through a period of intense clumsiness. Depending on cultural pressures, girls may become intensely preoccupied with their physical appearance very early in puberty. Often, as with boys, their rooms are intensely untidy, the external chaos being a measure of internal confusion. Personal cleanliness is often not as much of an issue as with the early adolescent boy. Girls at this age may, however, still be cuddled by their mothers, so infantile needs for nurture can be directly met; the indirect babying sought by adolescent boys is less necessary.

Female Striving for Independence

Pubertal girls have different independent strivings from those of boys. They wish to free themselves from childishly dependent feelings, but they need to keep a different type of dependent relationship, if they can, with their parents, particularly with their mothers. Girls are always likely to find it tolerable to lean on their mothers for advice, even if they have set up homes of their own. The problem for girls is that they may retain a childlike dependence, instead of reaching a more mature level of autonomy in which an adult personality is able to turn to parents for a degree of emotional support.

The battleground for independence with boys is fought

largely outside the family. A boy proves his masculinity away from home, primarily with male friends, with girlfriends, and finally with economic self-sufficiency, the family getting the backwash of the struggle. Girls have their primary struggle for independence in the family group; ultimately, they partly resolve this by becoming dependent on lovers or husbands. A girl seeks economic self-sufficiency, but she is still likely to view this as transitional experience in her overall relationship to her world.

A girl's struggle is more dramatic in relationship to her mother than her father. Girls borrow their mother's clothes and actively criticize their mother's taste. At one time they feel their mothers are dowdy; at another they are felt to be too seductive with the family's male friends. Shopping for clothes with early adolescent daughters can be a hideous experience for their mothers. Either daughters spend hours cogitating over a dress, or, much less tolerably, they insist on buying clothes that their mothers feel demonstrate a lack of color sense or a lack of care for themselves.

Sometimes daughters willingly help their mother; at other times they are apparently reluctant to move and be helpful. Because they do not have as dramatic a growth spurt and use physical activity less as a tension release than boys, girls do not usually stay in bed as much as their adolescent brothers. However, both male and female narcissism are the constant preoccupations of adolescence; as with boys, girls too spend many hours involved with their appearance. Like their brothers, girls are easily angered and easily reduced to tears. They actively try out mothering roles and enjoy looking after small creatures, whether babies, puppies, mice, or hamsters. This mothering wish can also be seen in early adolescent boys who disguise their need to look after babies by being forced to baby-sit.

Very often girls just before and just into the pubertal period are chronic complainers, nothing is quite right. Whatever is done by parents appears not to satisfy them. Although filled with chronic complaints, particularly toward her mother, the early adolescent girl may often appear very seductive, particularly with her father. Just prior to the onset of puberty, the girl may want to sit on father's knee. In puberty she may wish to go to the films with him, and join in secrets with him, if possible, excluding her mother. Girls may appear to get along quite well with a slightly older brother; yet, with a group of girlfriends, they may join in hostile giggling and teasing that is calculated to enrage. Smaller brothers and sisters may be sometimes carefully looked after, at others casually disregarded; pseudomaternal care alternates with neglect. Sometimes early adolescent girls appear willing to help with household tasks, at other times apparently incomprehensibly, they may be as neglectful as they were previously helpful. All this is understandable as part of the girls' struggle to adopt a culturally acceptable feminine identity.

Some of the fluctuations in the mood of the early adolescent girl are related to the way the world is seen and to feelings that arise with minimal outside provocation. Boys in puberty, to some degree, try out their manly roles by being pushy and aggressive and testing the limits of external control. Girls may behave similarly, but they also try out being women by taking on mothering and homemaking tasks. However, just as from time to time boys collapse into an inertia in which they seem to give up the struggle, only to take it on again at a later date, so girls will attempt to be housewives and mothers for a while and then revert to childhood.

Many early adolescent girls are preoccupied with the feeling that they are insufficiently attractive. This is not related to any real relationship to boys but rather to their own opinion of themselves. They feel their legs are too fat, their hair too curly, their skin has a spot. This preoccupation with their own body and its attractiveness or otherwise may mean that girls are tempted to put themselves on diets. It may also make girls very reluctant to take part in physical activity in which they have to expose themselves to their peers. Many early adolescent girls refuse to swim or do physical exercise.

The early adolescent girl is often moody and tense; she daydreams and flings herself into activities. This is the age when visiting friends to stay overnight is just as important as when she was eight or nine; gossiping for hours is a common occurrence.

Like her brother, the early adolescent girl has a need for limits to be set, even though, in so many ways, the experience of girls in early adolescence is quite different from that of boys. Since their growth rate is not as rapid, they do not become as clumsy. Whereas a boy experiences more frequent erections and rapid growth at the same time, girls usually do not start their periods until after their growth spurt is over. Although early menstrual cycles are sometimes irregular, the premenstrual tension that is often evident in early adolescence can help girls by warning them that their periods are about to start. Regular periods are quite usual about a year after the process has begun (Montagu, 1946). Girls acquire quite quickly the feeling that menstruation is a natural and controllable event (Deutsch, 1944).

Girls in early adolescence can allow themselves to feel dependent on their parents when they feel anxious. Thus, they do not need their own age group for support as much as boys. Girls form one-to-one relationships, rather than larger groups. When adolescents are in a playground, both boys and girls may appear to be in large groups at first glance, but the girls' group is often a cluster of one-to-one relationships.

Development of a Sense of Femininity

Girls do compare themselves with one another, emphasizing breast size and the beginning of periods, but boys are always most important to them in the assessment, testing, and realization of their femininity. It is very difficult for a girl to be safely convinced of her femininity unless, as well as having a good father, she has in her life men who care about her, are not members of her immediate family, and who are not interested in using her sexually. Older men are often satisfactory in this respect: uncles, family friends, and young male teachers. Girls in early adolescence may use a fantasy hero with whom they can have an idealized love affair to reinforce their feminine feelings. Early adolescent girls, and those whose emotional growth is slow beyond this level, are often preoccupied with pop stars. Mass hysteria gives them the opportunity to release sexual tensions and anger towards male authorities. But pop singers are used by girls in a variety of ways, as is shown by the following clinical example:

> Ruth was a sixteen-year-old typist. As a child in England, she was evacuated with her mother because of the war. So through her early years until the age of five she had no man in her life, no father. After his return from the war, she was never able to get really close to him. Until early adolescence and the onset of puberty, Ruth was a tomboy. Soon after she fell for a well-known pop singer whom she had never met. By the time she was sixteen she was a leader of his fan club and had his pictures plastered over her bedroom walls, ceiling and bed. She tried almost weekly to get a job in his manager's office so she might be near enough to talk to him.

Often the overvalued member of the pop group is used by such girls to express contempt for the boys who are available and to protect themselves from real sex:

> Whenever Ruth went out with a boyfriend to a place where she might see or hear her singer, she would get wildly excited; by contrast she was at least cool to the boy she was with at the time. When the real boy attempted to kiss her, she would tell him that she did not think he could do it as well as her singer "friend."

Boys, sensing the sort of man that girls see as attractive, respond to this by copying the heroes in dress and appearance. It is not at all unusual in totally male societies, schools particularly, for the early adolescent boys to have male rather than female pin-ups. The boys appear to see the male pop hero as a model for themselves. These male pin-ups are one of the first signs of a boy's desire to make himself sexually attractive to girls; they are not usually any indication of overt homosexual interest.

Sometimes boys have responded to girls' worship of these heroes by attacking them. When in certain countries hysterical feminine screams were encouraged in theaters to boost the stars' reputations, boys who were in the theater with their girlfriends would sometimes wait at the stage door afterwards to attack the singers as they left. These assaults could have been the result of homosexual anxiety as well as heterosexual jealousy: At this stage boys' sexual interests have not yet taken their final direction; they can still be drawn to a glamorous male figure.

Adolescent Needs from Their World

Boys and girls in early adolescence, whether they are altruistic or selfish, ascetic or self-indulgent, have two principal needs from adults (Freud, 1958). They need, first, interest and emotional involvement and, second, external control of their behavior by the adult world founded on mutual respect rather than fear.

Early adolescents require from school a feeling that their environment is stable and secure. A school should be able to offer such adolescents external controls when they find difficulty in controlling themselves. Like all children, they are upset by constant changes of teacher, for the atmosphere in the classroom must differ from teacher to teacher: When new teachers arrive at a school the pupils must test the limits of their control.

Early adolescents need a school that allows them to try themselves out in a whole variety of intellectual, emotional, and physical activities. They should be able to experiment in different ways. If such opportunities are not given to them in early adolescence, it may be too late to do so afterwards.

Intellectual and Imaginative Growth
of Boys and Girls

Because of their preoccupation with their bodies, their internal world of fantasy, and their need to develop inner controls, early adolescents do not do as well with work that compels rote learning as they do earlier or later. If children are taught languages in the traditional way, and fail to make progress before puberty, a reasonable hypothesis is that they are unlikely to do much better during the turmoil of early adolescence. The price paid may be that of retarding the development of imaginative potential and perhaps more mature types of thinking. If such demands are made, young people are likely to feel that they have no capacity to cope with the frustrations involved. When they are again ready to learn in this way, by midadolescence, teachers have given up in despair and the adolescents feel they are failures.

Far too little is known about the development of thinking capacities in early adolescence. Adolescence is the time when the capacity for different types of formal thinking (Dulit, 1972) and abstract thought (Jersild, 1963) develops in most people, but at puberty bodily preoccupation consumes energy and attention; there is relatively little left over for academic work. This explains why adolescents at puberty go through a period in which they become less able to concentrate and work efficiently than is the case earlier or later.

The existence of different growth rates for boys and girls means that, until the end of adolescence, girls are always about two years ahead of the same age boy insofar as their imagination, capacity to abstract, ability to perceive the feelings of others, and the capacity to tolerate frustration is concerned (Symonds and Jensen, 1961). This means that if boys and girls are compared to each other in a school system, the boys may actively stop working, thus assuring themselves that they could have beaten the girls if only they had so wished.

Problems of Maturational Age Variation

There are particular difficulties in early adolescence around normal variations in physical development (Schoenfeld, 1964). Boys may experience the extreme embarrassment of having a transient enlargement of the breast area (Schoenfeld, 1962). Girls may develop a faint growth of hair across the upper lip. Both of these tend to fade as adolescence progresses. A developmental variation that causes particularly emotional difficulties is that of late maturation. Although this is sometimes associated with retarded growth, more usually, late developers are very tall. This is because they have continued growing at the average childhood rate of about two inches a year until puberty; they launch into their growth spurt from a taller level. Late development is more common in boys than girls, and, since it is never easy to be behind one's agemates, is always difficult. Both boys and girls in the development of a sense of self, make comparisons with other members of their own sex. Late maturation in boys is not ultimately harmful; such a boy may become a sensitive, perceptive adult more able to be in touch with his inner world than his normatively developing peer (Jones, 1957; Peskin, 1967). During adolescence boys may have problems when they feel they are weak physically compared to agemates of their own sex; when maturation occurs, they, nevertheless, do not feel inhibited and unattractive to girls. Their height may then make them feel that they have the edge over their competitors, apart from the fact that their longer period of maturational childhood makes it easier for them to cope with the physiological drives of puberty. Thus, ultimately, they have the emotional edge on other eighteen- to twenty-year-olds.

Girls who develop late may feel that they are unattractive and odd as people, because girls of their own age are interested in boys when they are not. They also feel, if they are tall, that it will be very difficult to find a boyfriend. Very tall women are often uncomfortable about their femininity if their height is a function of late maturation.

Although adolescents who mature late know that the physical changes will take place, they do not really believe it until they do. Boys, who experience this delay more often than girls, are liable to be teased for being "effeminate." They feel that since they do not rate in the comparisons their contemporaries make, they have to assert themselves in other ways. Sometimes they become very hard working, as if to prove themselves intellectually; sometimes they become assertive and rude. Late developers often make themselves gang leaders.

In a rigid academic system of education these young people are often wasted as they are slow to mature emotionally as well as physically. If they do not do as well academically as their contemporaries, they may be labeled as failures and act accordingly. Special efforts may have to be made to rescue them, though this is most difficult in an institution that mirrors society's obsession with the need for qualifications:

> Seventeen-year-old Alec failed to graduate from high school not because he was dull but through late development. He had to live with powerful resentment at losing all his friends. At a community college, he passed with excellent grades. In the meantime, maturation had occurred.

In most pupils the difficulties of puberty fade toward the age of fifteen. Then there can be a real flowering of talent. Those who are clumsily handled in their early adolescent years, however, or cannot cope with their problems, are likely to go on being restless, turbulent and insecure through all the stages of adolescence and perhaps into adulthood.

References

Blos, P. (1962), *On Adolescence*. Glencoe, Ill.: The Free Press.
Deutsch, H. (1944), *The Psychology of Women,* Vol. I. New York: Grune & Stratton.

Dulit, E. (1972), Adolescent thinking à la Piaget: The formal stage. *J. Youth Adolescence,* 1 (4): 281–301.

Freud, A. (1958), Adolescence. In *Psychoanalytic Study of the Child,* 13: 255–277. New York: International Universities Press.

Jersild, A. T. (1963), *The Psychology of Adolescence.* New York: Macmillan.

Jones, M. (1957), The later careers of boys who were early or late maturing. *Child Dev.,* 28: 113.

Kestenberg, J. S. (1968), Phases of adolescence. Part IV. Puberty growth, differentiation and consolidation, *Am. Acad. Child Psychiatry,* 7: 108–151.

Lederer, W. (1964), Dragons, delinquents and destiny. *Psychol. Issues,* 4:3.

Montagu, M. F. A. (1946), *Adolescent Sterility.* Springfield, Ill.: Charles C Thomas.

Mussen, P. H., and Jones, M. C. (1958), Self-conceptions, motivations and interpersonal attitudes of early and late maturing boys. *Child Dev.,* 29: 61–67.

Nathanson, I. T., *et al.* (1941), Normal excretion of sex hormones in childhood. *Endocrinology,* 28: 851–865.

Offer, D. (1969), *The Psychological World of the Teenager,* New York: Basic Books.

Peskin, H. (1967), Pubertal onset and ego functioning, *J. Abnorm. Psychol.,* 72: 1.

Piaget, J., and Inhelder, B. (1958), *The Growth of Logical Thinking from Childhood to Adolescence.* New York: Basic Books.

Schoenfeld, W. A. (1962), Gynaecomastia in adolescents: Effect on body image and personality adaption. *Psychosom. Med.* 24: 379–389.

———— (1964), Body image disturbances in adolescents with inappropriate sexual development. *Am. J. Orthopsychiatr.* 35: 493–502.

Symonds, P. M., and Jensen, A. R. (1961), *From Adolescence to Adult.* New York: Columbia University Press.

Tanner, J. M. (1962), *Growth at Adolescence,* Oxford: Blackwell.

Wilkins, L. (1965), *The Diagnosis and Treatment of Endocrine Disorders in Childhood and Adolescence.* Springfield, Ill.: Charles C. Thomas.

Winnicott, D. W. (1971), Adolescence, struggling through the doldrums. In *Adolescent Psychiatry,* Vol. 1, ed. S. C. Feinstein, A. Miller, and P. Giovacchini, 40–51. New York: Basic Books.

2

The Life Space of
Early Adolescents

Male and Female Roles

In most societies of mankind the male role is to master the environment (Gutman and Krohn, 1972), the female to carry the sensitive, imaginative maturity of the group. Since adolescence is also a period of preparation for adult roles, it is to be expected that these would be tried out during the age period. Thus, boys like to spend more of their time away from home with groups of their friends roaming around neighborhoods; girls spend time with one or two girlfriends around the house of one or another of them. Girls in early adolescence like visiting each other; boys tend to concentrate on and constantly visit the family of one of their friends, or they like to be away from any family at all in a local teenage hangout. Usually, there is one family, or even one yard, that is the gathering place of early adolescents; often this has been the favored place of the neighborhood young for a number of years.

Need for Privacy

Both boys and girls in early adolescence like listening to such loud music that all capacity to communicate in words appears to be blotted out. Similarly, both boys and girls have an intense, if intermittent, need for privacy from each other and their parents. Sometimes adolescents hang around their parents, saying very little yet appearing most interested in what parents and their friends may be saying. On other occasions early adolescents will spend hours by themselves. Adolescents want and need privacy (Winnicott, 1971) but are not always prepared to grant it to their parents.

In some families children are brought up with the assumption that physical privacy is unimportant. Parents may wander naked through the house. They may go into the toilet when their children are using it and the children may go into the bathroom when the parents are bathing. In childhood parental nakedness may be felt by children to be provocative and possibly worrying; in adolescence this may produce in children an inhibition of sexual feeling. If parents allow their adolescent children of the opposite sex to see them naked, there tends to be in this action an implicit disregard for the childrens' budding sexuality. Boys and girls may then get out of touch with important aspects of their emotional inner worlds. Just as the manliness of boys, when respected, makes parental control somewhat easier, the same is true for the femininity of daughters. Besides physical privacy, boys and girls in early adolescence need to keep secrets both from their parents and, to an extent, from other adults. Their fantasy and sexual lives are now kept secret from mothers and fathers, and insistence by parents that adolescents not be secretive can become a severe psychological assault.

Adolescents and the Expression of Anxiety

Early adolescent girls have quite different family relationships and personal problems than boys. Both socially and psychologically there is an expectation that they will be somewhat more tied to their home than their brothers. The essential difference in the psychology of boys and girls, insofar as family relationships are concerned, is that the adolescent girl can turn to her father or mother for help in times of crisis without feeling that she is experiencing an irrevocable loss of independence and face. In other words, when she feels anxious, she can turn back into her family for assistance. Furthermore, she is easily able to demonstrate her distress by obvious sadness and misery: The early adolescent girl can deal with her tension by bursting into tears. Thus, girls are more easily able to keep in touch with their own emotional lives. The early adolescent boy is still both culturally and psychologically encouraged to control the expression of unhappy feelings, although this varies among individuals from different ethnic groups. Second- and third-generation immigrants still show ethnic differences in the way they handle their feelings; some alcoholic Polish fathers in Hamtramck, Michigan, may still beat their fifteen-year-old daughters for disobedience. Since the children know that other girls may have the same experience, this potentially traumatic experience is less psychologically damaging than would be the case if an alcoholic WASP parent in Grosse Pointe behaved similarly to his daughter.

Although there is often pressure to control the exhibition of anxiety in what the subculture may see as an unmanly fashion, boys are as likely as girls to show their feelings in a dramatic way; door slamming and sulky silence are not unusual. However, boys are more likely than girls to show their distress by antisocial behavior at school or in the neighborhood. The girl in equivalent misery is likely to stay home. It is thus easier for girls to be offered understanding by parents than it is for boys; girls also often seem more appreciative and obviously aware that help is being given. If a girl shows her distress by weeping, parents are less likely to feel tempted to be controlling or punitive than they might be with a boy who is showing his anxiety by being aggressive. On the other hand, because they cause pain in the community boys are more likely to be offered some type of assistance. When girls do behave in an aggressive, antisocial way in school or in the community, however, they are less likely to be offered help; this unfeminine behavior is seen by adults and other children as too alienated to be tolerated. Since lower-socioeconomic-status black girls are allowed by their subculture to externalize aggression in both words and action, their behavior may be seen as incomprehensible by middle-class people from almost all ethnic groups. Socially acceptable outlets for aggression are more easily found by boys than girls, sports activities for example are more available to boys. It is when these techniques fail that the early adolescent boy is likely to demonstrate anxiety by involving himself in a series of misdemeanors at school or by failing to do his homework. Adults may then have to deal with the misbehavior, as well as the possible causes. It is easy to see how preoccupation with one may lead to neglect of the other. By the time girls act up in the community, if this is not socioculturally allowable, they are likely to be more disturbed than the equivalently misbehaving boy. Parents may find it acceptable when an overanxious girl stays too dependent upon them, although she may then be unable to make independent decisions as she grows toward adulthood; boys on the other hand, denied necessary emotional support from parents may build a pseudoindependence on shifting sands.

If they have been unable to ask for help with their conflicts by verbal requests, a usual situation, and their action requests have been misunderstood, both boys and girls may have to contain inside themselves too much insecurity to develop a satisfactory sense of their own autonomy.

Adolescent Vanity

Until the last decade the early adolescent girl was allowed by society to be more obviously preoccupied with her body than her brother. Boys may now show their interest in their own bodies by being openly concerned about their clothes, their hairstyle, and general appearance. This change in attitude toward male adornment does not apply just to adolescents. Society is now changing its attitude toward the adult male's narcissism: He may now wear hairpieces, and the use of male cosmetics by both adolescents and their fathers is growing.

An interest in their own feminine attractiveness has historically always been granted to girls. One problem for early adolescents may be that their parents or society may demand that they try to be attractive before they are emotionally ready for such an involvement. A girl may feel intensely feminine from childhood onwards. Apart from the promptings of overeager adults, this has little significance insofar as an actual relationship with boys is concerned. An early adolescent girl's interest in her appearance is associated with a more conscious awareness of herself as feminine; it does not mean she is ready to try out real sexual relationships.

Because girls are more directly modeling themselves on their mothers than are boys on either parent, the girls' task in developing a sense of autonomy is in some ways more complex than is that of their brothers. Although ultimately girls are not as intolerant of control from mothers as are early adolescent boys, in order to establish a separate sense of self, they may, for a time, be intensively and directly negative and defiant (Block, 1937). Mothers often get the feeling that nothing they do for their daughters is right, and life seems to be a grim battle. Maternal control, however, is not likely to be felt as a threat to a girl's growing sense of womanhood, unless she feels that her mother is really trying to make a baby out of her.

A particular difficulty for adolescent girls is likely to arise if they have beautiful and youthful-appearing mothers. Early adolescent girls may appear gawky and unattractive. Competition from a beautiful mother for the love and attention of men in generel, and father in particular, is a battle they feel they can never win. It is not uncommon for girls in such a situation to feel utterly despairing: They can never be beautiful; they will always be dumb and stupid; no one will ever want them. The daughter of a very beautiful woman may be in a position similar to the potentially academic or creative son of a very brilliant man. Children often need to feel they can be successful in areas of life in which their parents have not trodden. They do not want to do better than their parents of the same sex, while they are alive at any rate, and children do not compete when they know they cannot win. So a girl will find it hard to be successfully feminine if she sees her mother as too successfully attractive; similarly, a boy will rarely strive exactly in those areas in which his father is felt as very powerful.

Girls and Fathers

If controlling comments from a father are felt to be necessary, his daughter needs to feel that she is cared for and cared about. Overcritical fathers can be particularly wounding to their early adolescent daughters. Sometimes the comments are felt as persecutory, even though such was not the intention, because a girl is doubtful herself as to how attractive she might be. Makeup, a hairstyle, or a certain type of clothing may be tried with the basic idea of being more feminine and attractive; being told by father that something else was liked better is painful, but not as bad as being told to "take that muck off your eyes." An early adolescent girl's sensitivity may lead her to a distortion of the intention and meaning of remarks from adults; this sensitivity may create a situation in which the adults feel emotionally blackmailed. A pretense something is liked, when it is not, may then be made. Sometimes daughters may provoke their fathers to gain their attention in the struggle to feel appropriately loved, especially in competition with mother, brothers or sisters.

Male and Female Tasks

Just as is the case with more primitive societies, some tasks in Western culture are seen as masculine, others as feminine. In general, the former include those that require physical effort, the latter include homemaking and caring-for tasks. The distinction is crude, but it can be highly meaningful to the young who perceive some activities as appropriate to boys and others to girls. A pervasive concept among the intellectual middle classes, that men and women should occupy similar roles in all aspects is not likely to be held by early adolescent boys and girls. Insofar as household tasks are concerned, anxiety about roles may be reinforced when sons and daughters are expected to accept chores irrespective of the masculinity or femininity of the job. Early adolescents may be reluctant to help their parents, because this threatens their sense of autonomy, but it is often more acceptable to boys to engage in activities that they see as clearly masculine: obaining fuel, mowing the lawn, washing the car, taking out the garbage. Girls may more comfortably assist in making beds, washing dishes, and helping clean house.

Boys are more likely to be sensitive about the masculinity or femininity of jobs than girls, because at an equivalent age they are probably less sure of themselves than their sisters. What is felt as manly varies from family to family, but to some extent the masculinity or femininity of any piece of work is associated with class attitudes. Washing dishes is not felt by an English middle-class adolescent boy to make him effeminate; some working-class young people do feel this. In such situations, perceptive parents tend not to ask their sons to perform such household jobs.

Adults may, however, be confused about the sexuality of certain tasks and become overanxious lest they be seen as inappropriate. It may not be recognized that in secure masculinity there is the capacity to be feminine and motherly; in femininity a capacity to take charge and master the external world. So boys commonly enjoy cooking, and it may take time for some adults to accept that this does not necessarily lead to sexual confusion.

A group of staff running a psychiatric adolescent service became very concerned when it was suggested that cooking be a vocational activity for boys as well as girls. They thought that an implicit message about role confusion might be given. One year after this project started, they recognized that the boys would not feel less masculine because they enjoyed this activity. Similarly, in high schools, cooking as an activity may be very popular with many boys, particularly those whose aggressive behavior implies an overprotestation about manhood.

A major worry for parents is often to get their early adolescent children to take their fair share of household tasks. It often appears that young people prefer to mow the neighbor's lawn rather than their own. Similarly, they will commit themselves to baby-sit for others rather than for members of their own family. The reluctance to help parents may be partly because of the possible financial gain in working for others, partly because it helps young people to feel more independent if they are doing jobs for relative strangers.

Adolescents and Money

Sometimes parents attempt to resolve their adolescent's wish to be independent, while still having to help in the family, by paying their children for jobs they do around the house. This may create in children an expectation that they will never have to do something for nothing. A balance needs to be struck. The expenditure of early adolescents may partially be provided for by the amount they are able to earn, partially by a possible allowance from parents. Situations exist in which early adolescents can earn substantial sums—golf caddying, lawn mowing, and baby-sitting—yet they may have no real sense of the value of money; since it is earned, it can be squandered. Thus, many parents feel the need to control the spending of their children, yet substantial earnings may make it hard to justify this. In those societies in which it is more difficult for adolescents to earn money, by the time they are able to work they may know better how to spend

their salary. Over the age of fifteen or sixteen an allowance may
no longer be necessary, because sufficient money can be earned;
younger adolescents may thus be given a larger allowance than
their older brothers and sisters; this is sometimes a cause of sibling
conflict.

Adolescent Conformity

The less sure a boy or girl feels about his or her sense of
autonomy, the harder it is to be helpful to their parents. Similarly,
the less support is obtained from a network of involved peers and
extraparental adults, the more difficult are intrafamilial relationships.

If an early adolescent is over anxious about a sense of self, it
is as though such independence as is felt will be given away if
parental wishes are accepted. On the other hand, those children
with no sense of independence may be highly conformist. An early
adolescent who never complains and is never felt to be a problem
by adults is probably in emotional difficulties. All adolescents
are highly conformist to familiar stereotypes (Taba, 1953), but
depending on the weight of family pressure and the passivity of
the adolescent, some are more obedient than others. Boys may
clean house for domineering mothers; girls regularly may wash
cars for seductive fathers. When adolescents feel unfairly used,
however, the task may be performed but ways of showing resentment may emerge. The job may be badly done; parents may need
to nag; opportunities for success may appear to be almost deliberately spoiled. Adolescents are experts at crucifying themselves to show the world of adults its inadequacy.

The untidiness of early adolescent boys and girls, the
reluctance to wash, to brush teeth, to keep clothes clean, may
mean that adults who care about the appearance, surroundings,
and hygiene of their children are in for a two- to three-year
struggle. The external chaos with which early adolescents are

often surrounded is a measure of their preoccupation with themselves and an inability to be bothered with the world of reality. Sometimes external disorganization is a measure of only this, sometimes of the adolescent's internal emotional confusion. Untidiness may also be one more manifestation of the struggle to be independent against the unconscious wish to be dependent. The implicit request is to be looked after, but the caring actions may be resented. Thus a struggle over mothering is successfully fought (Levy and Monroe, 1938).

Adolescents and Community Organizations— The Function of Gangs

The community relationships of boys and girls help or hinder their developing sense of manliness and femininity, which is strengthened or weakened not only in the family group. Extraparental adults are important for the natural development of personality, but in early adolescence boys and girls of the same age group are particularly significant. Peer-group relationships are consciously felt to be more essential to security than those with nonparental grown-ups (Fainberg, 1953). With either missing, smooth personality growth through adolescence is immensely difficult. For the early adolescent the role of a grown-up is to provide a social structure of acceptable and unacceptable behavior, to surround the individual with a world that cares, and to offer ideas and feelings with the recognition that only part of what is said will be immediately absorbed into the personality. If adolescents work in a social system that obviously fails to meet their growing needs, the adults who run the system are often felt to be inhuman. Early adolescents doubt the strength of the controls inside themselves. Consciously aware of restlessness and tension, early adolescents unconsciously look for control, support, and understanding, not only from parents and other adults whom they know and like but also from their agemates. As a general rule, boys will seek groups of friends of about the same age as themselves, with up to six months to a year difference. They will tend to form "in" and "out" groups in which people whom they know and like are felt to be superior to others. Although early adolescents tend to have a packlike relationship with each other, usually playing and chasing about in groups of six to eight, gangs in a formally structured sense, with leaders and followers, are likely to occur only in two situations. First, they may meet a temporary need related to the reality in which the youngsters find themselves and their state of psychological development. Gangs may be formed over real or imagined slights by an out-group, and in such a case the gang normally has a very short life. Second, a gang may develop from the possession of a club room, either in the home of one of the boys or if they can find it, in a disused shack or something similar. These gangs are not usually highly organized except sometimes for a specific task. Although daredevil defiance of the rules of society with mildly sporadic antisocial behavior, such as petty theft, is common at the beginning of puberty, only if the emotional climate is difficult for the boys do they behave antisocially. This again is likely to be transient. However, if adolescent boys grow up in neighborhoods or communities that lack facilities to meet their needs, more structured gangs with a longer life are common (Miller, 1958).

Most gangs are found in emotionally and physically underprivileged neighborhoods, schools, or penal settings. They may sometimes be found temporarily in more affluent districts in which there is little or no relationship between adults and children and there are few local outlets for adolescent creativity, imaginativeness, or aggression. Affluent neighborhoods, however, usually tend to be spared persistent gang activity as they are less physically constricting than ghetto areas. Since there is more space to move about, tension can be relieved by diffuse physical activity. It is also easier for more affluent adolescents to relieve inner boredom and emptiness by change. The mobility of such young people in early adolescence may be helpful; this is less true later in the age period except for certain specific situations, travel, for example.

In many parts of the United States the gang tradition is strong. In the black ghettos and among other immigrant or deprived communities gangs are common, and they map out their own neighborhood areas—their turf—over which they jealously guard their rights. In neighborhoods in which there is little or no social stability because too many people have moved too often or, if, in other ways, developmental needs are not met—for example, the absence of asexual male love from fathers and others—early adolescent girls may also form themselves into gangs (Crane, 1958). Often the appearance of these has a particular plaguelike quality. They may be constructed for a particular task: blackmailing and robbing weaker members of the junior high school, swamping a department store area with children, making it easier for theft to take place. This type of gang usually does not have a long life.

The quality of neighborhood social life may be such that formal gangs are created. In these circumstances, after a preliminary probationary period that may date from childhood, adolescents may stay in them for a number of years. Membership may stretch well into the middle or late period of adolescence (Block and Neiderhoffer, 1958). Usually by the time puberty is over the need for gang activity has gone, although men are always interested in friendships of a fairly superficial kind with groups of their own sex.

It is fairly clear that one function of a gang with boys is to give them external support to help make emotional maturation possible. Often gang controls are very strict. Boys who will defy any limits that their parents may try to put upon them will accept highly formal rules in their gangs. They may disobey their parents but be most obedient to the strictures of their gang. Early adolescents may similarly be highly reluctant to wear clothes or adopt hairstyles about which parents insist, but such young people may be eager and willing to obey the varying fashion demands of their own age group. School dress codes may be disapproved; gang emblems are cheerfully worn.

Even when adolescents do not form gangs and are not playing in groups, they often like to wander about in groups together. These groups tend to hang about in the same neighborhoods, the same street corner, or the same back alley. The groups may move restlessly to and fro, but they do not generally move very far from their home area, except from time to time when a whole group of boys will suddenly move for a night to a new neighborhood. This may become a group tradition, and there is a regular foray to a club, cafe, or discotheque at the other side of town. This phenomenon is more usual in the middle years of adolescence, when adolescents can drive cars, although it may be present with the younger age group. It is sometimes associated with older boys looking for girls whom they fantasy will be easily available sexually—rather like the fantasy late adolescents might have when they travel to a foreign country.

Early adolescent boys and girls have a need for space. They need the opportunity to play competitive games that are organized by adults and also to take part in activities they organize themselves. Boys, in particular, need the opportunity for unstructured play that allows them to have physical contact with each other. Early adolescence is particularly the age in which boys engage in play fights with each other and friendly punches are traded. If the environment fails them, or if they are in poor control of themselves, these can spill over into a more real aggression (Opie and Opie, 1969).

Apart from the need for physical contact sports and games, boys as well as girls, need outlets for their imagination and sense of creativity. If these are present in a neighborhood or a school, along with the opportunity to be safely adventurous and to withdraw from adults, it is unlikely that any formally structured gangs will be created. If all these possibilities are missing, then gangs will almost certainly be produced that begin to have a life of their own.

Relationships with Adults

Although adult company may be willingly accepted by early adolescent boys and girls, they tend to be wary in their relationships with grown-ups. Because they distrust themselves, they tend to distrust others. This wariness means adults are tested to see what they are like: Do they lose their tempers? Are they kind, firm, weak, or over-permissive? Do they show any capacity to convey to a boy or girl that feelings are respected and understood? Young adolescents are ready and prepared to accept direction from people they respect and admire. This admiration usually has to be earned. Involved adults have to show that they have qualities that early adolescents can understand.

Desirably, those adults whose relationships to early adolescents are involved in helping them gain control of themselves should be able to be a part of the adolescent's life through the middle stage of the age period. This means that adults who have been tested and found worthwhile can then be used as individuals upon whom, to an extent, young people can model themselves (Miller, 1969).

Young adult males are necessary to a boy to help him develop and reinforce feelings of manhood, to a girl to reinforce feelings of femininity. If adolescents are lucky, they will find a teacher, a relative, or friend whom they can respect, admire, and like. If they are less lucky, none of these will be available. They then become more involved emotionally than would otherwise be the case with the folk heroes of the present generation: a pop star, a blues or soul singer. Sometimes a revolutionary hero, usually a foreigner about whom less is known, and therefore, fantasy is easier, can be worshipped. For both boys and girls older women may symbolize safe mothering.

Music

Along with, and sometimes without, the preoccupation with singers and musicians, early adolescents are nowadays preoccupied with music itself. This has been brought about partly by the communications industry, which has sold music in order to sell records, partly to meet personal adolescent needs. Passive entertainment is only one aspect; music is particularly enjoyed because of the exciting quality of its sound and the rhythm it gives to the movement that is necessary in early adolescence to relieve tension. Early adolescents do not play music loudly because their hearing is less sensitive than that of adults (damage to the hearing apparatus due to excessive noise is not rare in the young). Loud music is partly a cultural habit, partly it is played with an awareness that loudness is an irritant to adults, partly it is a way to blot out thoughts and fantasies that the young may wish to avoid.

Sexual Relationships

Early adolescent boys are not genuinely or actively interested in girls, who tend to be seen as worthless and are criticized for being weak and soft. The attitudes about girls present in the eight-year-old boy are still present, because feelings of being inadequate are always just on the border of consciousness. Young adolescents always fear they will be unable to control themselves, for boys in early adolescence are interested in sex mostly as it affects their own bodies. Clinical examples demonstrate this problem. Sometimes older sisters of fifteen or sixteen may tease and provoke their younger pubertal brothers. It is as though the girl needs to see just how far she can go in provoking an outburst from a rivalrous male. On occasion this may lead to tragedy. One seventeen-year-old girl, in a family where verbal communication was minimal and parental interest distant, was knifed by her brother in the following circumstances:

> Kenny was a fourteen-and-a-half-year-old boy who was about two years into early adolescence. He and his friends were preoccupied with magazines such as "Playboy" and "Penthouse" and

often his sister would get these for him. She would also ask him if he yet had a real girlfriend. Furthermore, she would engage in wrestling matches with him. Many boys, threatened by such behavior might have lost their tempers; Kenny never did. One night as he was watching television, his sister began to shave her legs in the adjoining room. The boy went and got a kitchen knife, wrapped the handle in a towel, and entering her room began to attack his sister with it. As they struggled, the telephone rang, the boy stopped the fight and answered it.

He was horrified to discover how badly he had wounded his sister and was almost completely unaware of what had happened.

Kenny's dissociative murderous episode had obviously been precipitated by his sister's consistently provocative behavior. In this pubertal boy there was an intense mixture of aggressive and sexual impulses; usually these were isolated from consciousness and not translated into behavior. When the provocation became too great, the violence ensued. The clinical problem was to decide how dangerous Kenny might be, but as is so often the case, the behavior of a disturbed adolescent demonstrates some of the problems of normal growth.

It is obvious from the behavior of early adolescent boys and girls that they use a variety of techniques to get control over their sexual feelings. In their groups early adolescents tend to tell each other dirty stories and toward the end of early adolescence, they may circulate dirty pictures to each other. Pornography is particularly the preoccupation of the pubertal boy just before the middle stage of adolescence is reached.

Adolescent jokes are designed to shock adults and preferably must be about subjects of which adults would disapprove (Freud, 1905). In those parts of society where ordinary sexual matters are no longer a subject for adult shock, jokes told by early adolescents now begin to have a mildly perverse tinge, including such topics as lesbianism and homosexuality. Adolescents with parents who are still puritanical tell jokes about straight sex and snicker about normal intercourse.

Sexual jokes told by boys are also associated with behavior that demonstrates their preoccupation with their genitals and those of other boys. It is common for boys to attempt to debag each other in scuffles. Where boy's clothes still have fly buttons, they commonly play games with each other to tear open the fly; this is a preoccupation with exposure and nonexposure.

Masturbation

Jokes, physical play, and masturbation are all used by early adolescent boys as part of the process of gaining control over their own bodies, particularly control over feelings of sexual excitement. Toward the end of early adolescence boys very easily experience genital tension. They go through a stage in which they experience an erection with little or nothing in the way of external stimulation. When sexual feelings were thought to be properly hidden, many boys found this a shameful and embarassing occurrence. The shame and embarrassment, however, are now more related to feelings of lack of control rather than of the shamefulness of sexuality.

It is a psychological task of early adolescence in boys to begin to tie together a feeling of sexual excitement with the physical changes that take place when an erection occurs. Boys who tell dirty stories to each other are trying out their own control of their feelings. They stimulate their sexual fantasies, but, when these occur in a group, they control their bodily expression. Pornography allows sexual excitement partly because it is stimulated from outside the self, thus fantasies are other people's responsibility, are socially acceptable and need not be felt as incestuous. The relationship between social acceptability and incestuous anxiety is demonstrated by the following clinical example.

A fourteen-year-old Irish immigrant boy had his first emission when he was thirteen. At that time he was living in a primitive part of Ireland and shared a bed with his two sisters, one older, one younger. Both his parents were in bed in the same room. This lifestyle continued in the new urban environment and six months after the move Don began to have "seizures." These were investigated for physical causes and only when all investigations had proved negative was referral made to a psychiatrist. No one in the neurological investigation had checked the boy's sleeping arrangements.

The move to the city had meant that the boy moved to a school in which sexuality was freely discussed, a situation that did not exist in Ireland. Don now had social permission to be sexual and here was confronted with his incestuous situation. Unable to masturbate as did others, he had "seizures" instead. A change of sleeping arrangements and brief therapy focused on the "normality" of his conflict led to rapid resolution.

It becomes important to boys toward the end of early adolescence to know that they can ejaculate. They discover this either by masturbating, a natural activity of this age period, or by nocturnal emissions. Masturbation is associated with the discovery that ejaculation can take place. Its importance to boys is obvious in the slang words they give it. *Spunk,* one English swear word used to describe ejaculatory fluid, used to mean bravery. *To come,* another way of describing the act of ejaculation, also means to arrive.

Masturbation itself is described by words that also say a good deal about attitudes in terms of budding manhood. A middle-class British private school description is to *flog off,* which has meaning in terms of aggression. *Beating* is used as a slang word for the act in the United States. In America *jerk off* is a typical adolescent slang expression for masturbation, and it can be no accident that *jerk* is a slang term describing someone who is inadequate. An English working-class descriptive word is *wanking,* a word that appears to have a variety of derogatory connotations. In the First World War a wonk or wank was a useless seaman or an inexperienced naval cadet. The pun on the word *seaman* (ejaculatory fluid=semen) is striking. In East Anglican dialect *wanky* means feeble, and at Felstead School in 1892 *wanker* was the school word for a stinker. Since working-class boys tend to be more contempuous of masturbation than middle-class youths, as is obvious from the derivation of the slang word, so working-class adolescents tend to abandon masturbation before their middle-class agemates. Working-class boys, however, tend to have earlier sexual relationships with girls, though these are often loveless and thus masturbatory in quality.

Adults and older adolescents sometimes contemptuously recognize the childish quality of the masturbatory act as something associated with growing up; they talk of boys playing with themselves.

Masturbation is an act that is clearly self-centered. It is a way in which boys appease feelings of loneliness and isolation and a technique by which boys gain control by physical means over their own state of sexual excitement. It also attempts to tie together psychological feelings and physical experience, sexual fantasies with the experience of tumescence and detumescence. Finally, it is used to relieve conscious feelings of sexual frustration. There is a quality of aggressiveness in the act in older boys, as it implies that the purpose of women is only to satisfy men.

It is not uncommon in some societies for early adolescent boys to engage in mutually masturbatory acts with each other. Sometimes this is a part of a group activity; sometimes two boys may masturbate each other. This type of activity does not necessarily indicate the ultimate development of a homosexual involvement. When boys masturbate themselves in front of other boys, the exhibitionism is a way to confirm to each other that sexual feelings can be held in common; it is a primitive way of confirming manhood. This is reinforced because such an activity is disapproved of socially; it becomes a way of defying the standards of the adult world.

Mutual masturbation between two boys in early adolescence is rarely associated with feelings of love and affection. Often when the boys in question like each other before such an act, they are unlikely to do so afterwards. This is because such an activity, although often a transient part of development, is felt by the boys who take part in it, as meaning that they are going to be exclusively homosexual. Boys whose primary orientation is heterosexual do not want to put together in the world of their feelings, love, affection, and sexual excitement in relationship to a member of their own sex. Either group masturbatory activity or mutual masturbation more usually occurs when boys are under stress; it is particularly likely if their environment fails to meet their needs. This is a common situation in neighborhoods that have few outlets for constructive activity for adolescents and in schools or penal settings that are too rigid or too permissive. In neither situation, one of which offers too little, the other too much freedom, do adolescents get the amount of responsibility they can handle, a prerequisite for satisfactory emotional growth.

Despite the wide dissemination of knowledge about the normality of the act in the last twenty-five years, masturbation is still a subject of concern and anxiety both to some boys and their parents. It is often believed to weaken boys and lead eventually to their being unsatisfactory lovers and husbands. Some boys who do not easily make friends and do not get the opportunity to compare personal experiences with other boys, think that they are odd if they masturbate. Others believe that it is harmless, providing it is not done excessively. The definition of excessive varies from individual to individual; some feel it is excessive to masturbate daily, others once a week.

It is inconceivable that any boy can physically harm himself in normal masturbation, and it is impossible to define excessive frequency from a physical standpoint. But the anxiety that can be produced because of the fantasies associated with masturbation can be intense. A boy wrote the following letter:

Frankly speaking, because I got into the habit of masturbating so often (usually two or three times a day even at home), it is

obviously less easy to "come off" each time. To counteract this
I find I have to think along more and more perverse (for want
of a better word) lines. . . . By the way, sucking and kissing of
boy's pricks and balls also enters my thoughts, which is what is
most distressing, after I have "come off."

The loneliness and isolation of this boy was intense. He had
few friends and was facing the painful experience of having a
father who was ill of cancer. He could not tell his parents anything of the anxiety he suffered; they did not even know of his
loneliness. To have told them even this would have been to
abandon the tenuous sense of autonomy he experienced.

Just as the male of the species can have intercourse with a
frequency that varies with his sexual drive, the willingness of his
partner, and his general state of fatigue or tension, so the frequency of masturbation relates to the first and last of these. The
physically active young male cannot become weak and debili-
tated by masturbating, nor is it possible to deduce that a boy
masturbates because in some way he shows socially inadequate
behavior.

Psychologically withdrawn, isolated, lonely boys who spend
too much time alone may be masturbating during these periods.
This means that for them masturbation becomes a poor substitute
for genuine human relationships; it is no accident that often adolescents who take LSD continue to masturbate during the drug
experience. With a failure to make meaningful emotional relationships, the act of masturbation becomes the equivalent of the
thumb sucking of the lonely infant.

A common sight in classrooms is for some of the early adolescent boys to be manipulating their genitals at the back of the
room. This is a measure both of general physical tension and
boredom. Sometimes young adolescents tend to sit with their
hands covering their penis; these are anxious boys who are
unconsciously ready to ward off an attack.

Masturbation in early adolescent girls is less common than
with boys. Girls do not generally experience the same feelings of

focused sexual tension as boys (Kinsey *et al.*, 1953). Their need for sexual bodily contact is first experienced as a need to be hugged and cuddled. Sexual arousal in a girl is a slower process than with a boy. Although fantasies give some satisfaction, women have to learn from experience that genital manipulation followed by vaginal penetration is emotionally gratifying. Some girls never have this experience and have intercourse only as a payment for being held and cuddled. Other women can enjoy external manipulation of their genitals but get no satisfaction either from penetration by the male penis or from the awareness that they have given their sexual partners a significant emotional experience.

Tense, overanxious pubertal girls often experience a diffuse physical discomfort that they discover can be relieved by genital play. Sometimes this extends to the use of an artificial penislike object; a tampon may be used, but this is relatively rare. Girls who masturbate have much more shame about this act than boys, who now mostly accept it as normal, at any rate consciously. Girls often feel that they are behaving in an unsatisfactory, perhaps emotionally sick, way. In girls masturbation is often a response to stressful situations; it is not a necessary act on the road to mature sexual development.

References

Block, H., and Neiderhoffer, A. (1958), *The Gang*. New York: Philosophical Library.

Block, V. L. (1937), Conflicts of adolescents with their mothers. *J. Abnorm. Soc. Psychol.*, 32: 193–206.

Crane, R. A. (1958), The development of moral values in children. *Br. J. Educ. Psychol.*, 28: 201–208.

Fainberg, M. R. (1953), Relationships of background experience to social acceptance. *J. Abnorm. Soc. Psychol.*, 48: 206–214.

Freud, S. (1905), Jokes and their relation to unconscious. In *Standard Edition*, Vol. 8. London: Hogarth Press, 1960.

Gutmann, D., and Krohn, A. (1972), Changes in mastery style with age: A study of Navajo dreams. *Psychiatry*, 34 (3): 289–301.

Kinsey, A. C., *et al.* (1953), *Sexual Behavior in the Human Female.* Philadelphia: W. B. Saunders.

Levy, J., and Monroe, R. (1938), *The Happy Family.* New York: Knopf.

Miller, D. (1969), *The Age Between.* London: Hutchinson.

Miller, W. (1958), Lower class culture as a generating milieu of gang delinquency. *J. Soc. Issues,* 14: 5–19.

Opie, I., and Opie, P. (1969), *Children's Games in Street and Playground.* New York : Oxford University Press.

Taba, H. (1953), The moral beliefs of sixteen-year-olds. In *The Adolescent: A Book of Readings,* ed. J. Seidman, 592–596. New York: Dryden Press.

Winnicott, D. W. (1971), *Therapeutic Consultations in Child Psychiatry.* New York: Basic Books.

3

The Middle Years

Physical Changes

In the middle stage of adolescence physiological and anatomical changes in connection with growth are still taking place. Boys show a marked rise in testosterone levels, mature spermatozoa are found, and facial and bodily hair continue to increase (Talbot, *et al.*, 1952). The hairline of boys begins to develop a slight peak. Acne is common. In boys, the years fifteen, sixteen, and seventeen are most commonly associated with this period; in girls, the time covered usually includes the years fourteen, fifteen, and sixteen. Pregnancy at this time is possible; there is a great increase in estrogen excretion and an increase in seventeen ketosteroids. A girl's voice changes its timbre, the change not being as dramatic as with boys, and she too may develop acne. The body takes on its final feminine shape, the ovulatory cycle becomes stable, and growth stops.

Confirmation of Identity

In their relationship to the world-at-large, middle-stage adolescents often show the beginning of this age period by demanding to know the reason for the rules set by society. There can be a short space of time, lasting six months or so, when authority appears to be almost totally rejected. The end of early adolescence is thus marked by extreme psychic turbulence that points to the onset of the development of a firm feeling of identity: "This is what I am." Identity can be defined as a conscious sense of individual uniqueness (Erikson, 1963). When they are sure of their own identity, adolescents can finally free themselves from childish dependence on parents and begin to establish a new relationship with them as grown-up sons and daughters. They remain open to new experiences and a changing self-concept from then onwards, even as adults. Identity foreclosure, the development of a rigid sense of self, to an extent, represents a failure to develop an adequate sense of inner freedom. This can be a suitable adaptation to everyday life; the price in terms of personal rigidity may be high.

From infancy, children model themselves on their parents and to some extent on other adults; during midadolescence this need for other adults as potential models reaches a peak. The midadolescent boy has a particular need for an adult male with whom to identify, although he may also incorporate into his personality the tender caring qualities seen in more mature women. Identification is the process by which the individual takes into his personality the qualities of people as he sees them and the way they seem to get along with each other. To make this possible, it is necessary for adults other than parents to show boys that they are interested in them over a period of years. It is also important that these adults be seen as valuable to the boy and to society-at-large. There is, for example, some evidence (Gold, 1963) that delinquents are more successfully helped by adults whom society obviously regards highly than they are by people whom society does not apparently value. Girls identify with their mothers more directly than boys with either parent. They not only identify with extraparental adults, the nonsexual affection of adult males reinforces their sense of worth as women.

Types of Identification

Identification may be either a conscious or an unconscious process (Erikson, 1968). Since the first models with which children identify are their parents, it is not surprising that other people used as models by adolescents often have qualities remarkably like the parents, though the adolescents may not be aware of this. The new adult becomes a "mediator" for identification with parents, allowing adolescents to be like their parents but to feel independent of them. For example:

> Kenneth, a sixteen-year-old boy, had a father whom he perceived as rather outgoing, active, and sexually very successful. He said he despised his dad and did not wish to be like him. Kenneth was extremely shy and inhibited. After six months the French instructor at his school changed, and the boy perceived the new teacher as an outgoing, charming, uninhibited person. He came to the conscious decision that he would very much like to have a personality similar to that of the French teacher.

Kenneth imagined that his teacher was, like all Frenchmen, extremely successful with women. He was unaware, when he felt this, that the qualities that he saw in the teacher's personality were remarkably similar to those that he thought his father had. He could not identify with his father directly, because to do so would have meant that he could not see himself as separate from him: He could have no feeling of independence. So he needed the teacher to make identification possible.

Adolescents may consciously decide that there are qualities in other people that they would wish to have and that differ from those of their parents. One boy found himself attached to certain mannerisms of his geography teacher. He decided that this way of relating to people would be a comfortable and agreeable one for him. He consciously copied these mannerisms; at a later stage in his development they became so much a part of his personality that he was no longer aware of his original copying process.

An American boy of sixteen met another boy whom he saw relating to people with a "European" ease. He himself was rather shy, and he decided that this way of relating was a highly appropriate one. Therefore, he set out to copy it. By the time he was nineteen, other people noticed how "European" he was.

Very often boys and girls who are emotionally involved with adults may unconsciously behave like them without being at all aware of it.

In a hospital in the United States, one physician was responsible for looking after a boy of sixteen and a girl of thirteen. The girl, while on the hospital campus, saw the boy walking at some distance from her. His walk was so much like the walk of his physician that she ran after him calling out the doctor's name. It was only when she reached him that she realized her error.

The boy had begun to copy the doctor's walk without conscious recognition that this was happening.

When the identification model is unlike the parents, the process of identification may enrich the personality, but it can also cause many problems. This is particularly likely if the people available as models come from a cultural background that is different from that of the adolescent, a probable experience for children living with their parents in foreign states who may go to schools in the countries where the family is temporarily residing. When there is a common language, the problem can be quite subtle. American children in London during their midadolescent years often attend English schools, as their parents may not wish them to live a ghettolike existence with other Americans. After three or four years they tend to develop the identity of English boys and girls:

One American boy who was unsure whether he wanted to go to

college in the United States or Great Britain unconsciously had a British accent while talking of England, and an American one while discussing his home. It was as if he attempted to retain a partial identification with his parents through his American accent.

Not all identifications are positive; if the most significant aspects of the environment are felt as brutal and aggressive, then these are the qualities that are taken into the personality. Those adolescents who were concentration camp victims during the war may, as adults, have many of the aggressive qualities of their guards. The adolescent victims of brutality are rarely able to adopt a more tender attitude towards humanity. If girls are so exposed, they are often unable to be loving wives and mothers. Boys are more likely to be in some type of penal setting than girls during midadolescence, exposed to the depersonalized degradation of such a setting, they are likely to become adults who are cold, distant, and harsh, who degrade both their own humanity and that of others.

The attitudes and feelings adolescents sense in others and adopt for themselves vary among ethnic groups. In children of Finnish descent in the Upper Penninsula of Michigan, commonly the adult male still does not express open tenderness. Traditionally, the man is silent in his home, is not very communicative, and does not display warmth. Many of his conflicts and impulses are released by an open-air life of hunting and fishing, some by an intense preoccupation with high school sports, others by the excessive use of alcohol. One of the major problems in that society is that alcohol tends to be used by the young in the same way as it is used by their elders, although more recently other drugs have been added.

The responsibility of adults is that adolescents identify not with what adults want to be but with what they are; the sad feeling of some parents that their children pick up their worst qualities may be justified.

Sexuality

Most high school students probably do not engage in full sexual relationships, and most academic adolescents still inhibit genital seuxality (Deutsch, 1967). At the same time as he needs the adult male as a model, the midadolescent boy becomes gradually ready to try out his manhood. Initially, boys daydream about girls they do not know, often older women (Offer, 1969); and as they move through the age period, they begin to experiment sexually with girls, thus assessing sexual prowess. At the end of the early adolescence, the girl feels ready to try out her own femininity; to try herself in the role of an adult woman. The midadolescent girl is looking for a boy to love. Even to the boy of seventeen, however, the sixteen-year-old girl who loves him is all too often a medal that he will proudly display to his contemporaries. During the middle stage of adolescence, other boys are still more important for the assessment of individual masculinity than relationships with girls.

> Tom, a sixteen-year-old, in grade eleven was referred to a psychiatrist by his somewhat puritanical, middle-class father because, during a furious row with him he had admitted to having intercourse with his girlfriend of fourteen. The boy said, "He doesn't understand that everyone in my group has fucked a girl—he is trying to make me soft or something."

Apart from those who are responding to sociocultural pressures, and even among that group, girls need to try out loveless sexuality activity *only* if they are *so* psychologically under stress so that they are unable to tolerate feeling frustrated and unloved. This state may be produced by serious conflict and deprivation during adolescence or the absence of supportive adults, particularly men. Fathers may have been the only men in a girl's life, or developmental immaturity may have been produced by an unhappy childhood. Girls brought up in one-parent families without father substitutes, those with fathers who have abandoned all semblance of an understandably masculine role differing from that of mother, or those who are members of an isolated family group are particularly at risk. They are likely to be tempted to try out and reassure themselves of their femininity by becoming sexually involved with a boy in much the same way as a boy normally does with girls. It is also likely that they will need to discuss this competitively with other girls—a discussion that has a different flavor from talking of a love affair to an intimate girl friend.

Boys confined to all-male environments, providing that their integrity is respected in other ways, are much less psychologically threatened than girls in an equivalent situation. Masculinity during midadolescence can still be assessed if girls are not present, whereas girls cannot perceive themselves as becoming acceptably feminine in the absence of boys or interested adult males about whom fantasy is possible.

During midadolesence social-class differences in attitudes to sex become startingly apparent. Working-class boys, both black and white, often appear to be relatively uninvolved emotionally with their girls, although they may have intercourse with them. For such youth the double standard is still common. Such boys may say that if one is in love with a girl, she should not be spoiled by premarital intercourse—if she is prepared to allow this, she becomes worthless. It is as if she ceases to be good when the boy has sex with her, a striking comment on his own sexuality. Open aggression toward girls is often acceptable in such groups. Many a working-class boy sees nothing wrong in slapping a girl's face if he dislikes her behavior. He feels that if he does not do this, the girl will not think him man enough.

Middle-class boys on the other hand, despite the fact that sexual freedom is said to be increasing, still cannot allow themselves much early heterosexual experimentation and tend to have intercourse two years later than working-class boys (Schofield, 1965). Clinical observation indicates that many regard

masturbation as acceptable for a longer period of time than
would working-class youths; this is still true into young adulthood. A twenty-two-year-old white, middle-class, medical student
will freely admit to masturbation at times when he has no
sexual partner; this admission appears intolerable to either
a black socially mobile student or to a young white worker in an
automobile factory. Middle-class boys often assess their masculinity, when they finally have intercourse, by their ability to give
their girlfriends an orgasm, and they like to feel that they are
emotionally involved with their partners. Working-class boys,
however, regard the sexual possession of a girl as satisfactory
proof of masculinity.

More and more, middle-class boys no longer appear to feel
that their wives should necessarily be virgins. Both they and
working-class boys seem convinced that a virgin who has intercourse with a boy will inevitably need another lover when the
affair breaks up. This idea has been going around for decades,
and from a great many case histories it appears to hold true.

Middle-class adolescents appear to be more likely to use
contraceptives than those of the working class. Many insecure
boys, however, find it intolerable to have their girlfriends use
either a contraceptive pill or an intrauterine device. Secure men
find it inconceivable that intercourse might be preferable with
anxiety over possible pregnancy. In the male psyche, however,
fertility is equated with potency; boys like to know how much
seminal fluid they can produce and how forcefully it can be
ejaculated. Boys who are unsure of themselves may prefer to
have sex with no contraceptive at all and may insist that
intercourse feels better when their girlfriend does not use the
pill.

> Jim, age seventeen, saw a psychiatrist, complaining of impotence.
> He said that sex with his girlfriend was fine until she began to
> use the pill. Then, he complained, she wouldn't leave him alone
> sexually, and he insisted that intercourse felt better when no
> contraceptive was used.

Anxiety about homosexuality, despite the Gay Liberation Movement, is common among all social classes. The need to conform to the way of life of contemporaries is intense, and the homosexual boy is painfully aware of his different orientation.

Vocational Choice

Young people in their midadolescent years begin to develop their first real sense of the future. They now begin to ask: "What sort of person am I?" During midadolescence there begins to be a definite idea of career choice, although this may not be more than preliminary sifting (Porter, 1954). For the first time the midadolescent is capable of saying with a degree of certainty: "This is what I like." The choice is less likely to change during midadolescence than in the early adolescent years. A career choice made before the age of fourteen or fifteen is almost always unrealistic. Only those early adolescents with special talents— artists, musicians, and mathematicians, for example—appear capable of making an early choice with any certainty that this will be their vocation, although they often face intense boredom in the usual high school situation. Furthermore, they risk rejection by their peers because they are considered odd and unusual (Hollingsworth, 1926).

Need for Stable Relationships

All developing human beings need a stable environment, but the midadolescent often appears to have less stability than any other age group. This may be because society has been fooled by the superficial appearance of physical maturity in many adolescents and assumes that they are as mature as they look. Society does not seem to understand that midadolescents need to have a three to four-year period of stable relationships with adults. If helpful adults are not available anywhere in their lives they then find it very difficult to make secure identifications. Statistics kept by juvenile courts often show that a peak of delinquent behavior occurs at the change point from junior high school to high school in those school districts that isolate all early adolescents from the rest of the school system. Anxiety about leaving a known environment is one possible reason for this, but anti-social behavior may also occur because the junior high schools, except for those children engaging in athletics, drama, or the school orchestra, commonly do not provide children with stable extra-parental adult relationships. With great difficulty, because of the structure of the school, a stable peer group may be found, but a change of school now threatens this stability. Delinquent behavior may become a protest against the loss of developmental security.

The response of girls to the loss of significant anchor points in society was clearly described by a young schoolteacher in Britain. Talking of the behavior of girls in their last year at school at fourteen-and-a-half, she said that for the first six months of their last year they seemed extremely interested in what they were doing in the classroom and highly involved with each other and with her. In the last six months it was as if they changed completely. They were concerned only with acquiring material possessions and boyfriends; they saw obtaining a boy at any cost as quite crucial. The teacher wondered whether this change in behavior was due to a failure on her part.

The evidence from clinical work is that this overpreoccupation with materialism and boyfriends comes from despair. If an adult is felt by adolescents to be a worthwhile person and then seems to reject them, the good attitudes that the youngster feels the adult possesses may also have to be discarded. The girls in this teacher's class saw the possession of things as an answer to the anxiety aroused by losing someone they respected and admired. In the United States equivalent situations occur when young adults develop an apparent interest in the young via "rap

sessions" in a school, stay for one semester, and then casually go
on to other things.

The pain caused to midadolescents by having to lose significant adults too early appears in many ways. Often drug-taking
begins, as the midadolescent realizes that the outside world is on
him long before he is ready to face it, in typical high schools
adolescents who have usually experienced repeated changes of
teacher often seem by this age period to despair of adults as having anything worthwhile to offer. On the other hand, the resilience
of youth can be striking, and they never seem to give up hope.
In one high school riddled with apparent racial tensions the
adolescents wrote on the hall walls: "Will no teacher ever talk
to us." In another school, apparently the victim of racial confrontation, both black and white students made the same demands
for interest and involvement from the staff.

The stages of adolescence overlap, and the delineation is not
as definite as these paragraphs suggest. Adolescents who stay at
school show a marked stage of early adolescence. In those who
are still pupils from fourteen to eighteen, perhaps bound for college later, the midstage is also marked. In those who go to work
after sixteen and are not given further education, the last two
stages do begin to overlap; they have an exceedingly short
period of midadolescence. Nowadays the speeding up of identification processes brings many problems and produces little
satisfaction for the individual or for society. This is especially
troublesome, if the networks of society have broken down. Young
people then have no pride in their own productivity. Society be-
wails the loss of pride in vocation; the loss is of pride in oneself.

References

Deutsch, H. (1967), *Selected Problems of Adolescence*. New York:
    International Universities Press.
Erikson, E. H. (1963), *Childhood and Society*. New York: Norton.
_____ (1968), *The Young Man Luther*. New York: Norton.

Gold, M. (1963), *Status Forces in Delinquent Boys.* Ann Arbor: Institute for Social Research, University of Michigan.

Hollingworth, L. S. (1926), *Gifted Children, Their Nature and Nurture.* New York: Macmillan.

Offer, D. (1969), *The Psychological World of the Teenager.* New York: Basic Books.

Porter, J. R. (1954), Predicting vocational plans of high school senior boys. *Pers. Guid.* 33: 215–218.

Schofield, M. (1965), *The Sexual Behavior of Young People.* London: Longmans.

Talbot, N. B., *et al.* (1952), *Fundamental Endocrinology from Birth through Adolescence.* Cambridge: Harvard University Press.

4

The Life Space of
Middle-Stage Adolescents

By the time early adolescence is over, boys and girls are beginning to feel themselves, in an emotionally meaningful way, to be autonomous individuals. They are obviously involved with friendship networks of their own and begin to demand freedom from parental interference. Parents tend to become concerned as to whether or not they are giving their children too much freedom and responsibility; fathers of daughters of fifteen or so may become anxiously aware of the real or fantasied sexually predatory nature of young males. In the conflict areas of society—drugs, sexual permissiveness, styles of dress, language—adolescents enjoy shocking their parents. In mid-adolescence increasing self-control is acquired; actions are performed because boys or girls feel them to be appropriate. Often the newly acquired values of youth are unconsciously similar to those parents have been trying to instill (Bath and Lewis, 1962). Nevertheless, both boys and girls feel that the concepts and ideas they have are original. A sense of self, along with a growing awareness of the needs of others, are perceived by adolescents as coming from the wellsprings of their own personality.

Midadolescence is the period when the young should develop a final sense of their own identity. In the middle years of

adolescence many begin to know what they would like to do
with their lives although firm decisions may not be made before
young adulthood. A delay in decision making is more likely with
the academic adolescent, although the sixteen-year-old school
drop-out may try several jobs before finally settling on a career
and faces a higher statistical chance of unemployment than the
high school graduate.

Initial Turmoil

If adolescent turbulence is present, the first months of midadolescence are commonly a time when it is most obvious, particularly in boys. It is almost as if some boys wished to check,
as they gain more freedom and responsibility, that external controls will prove that dependent needs can be met. At the same
time, as part of the struggle toward independence authority
figures are provoked: A boy of sixteen may agree that he will
be home at eleven o'clock; he may arrive home at two in the
morning refusing to say where he has been. Apart from the failure
to keep the time commitment, the boy's behavior may have been
responsible; lack of a comment may be understood as uncaring,
and more irresponsible behavior may occur. A verbal protest
may be seen as fairly meaningless; a withdrawal of privilege, although perhaps appropriate, is likely to leave the boy feeling
misjudged and mistreated. It is as if these adolescents need to
test the quality of people in their environment before they can
use them as models. Adults are put under a good deal of stress;
boys may be intensely negativistic, difficult, argumentative, destructive, sometimes antisocial, and, at times deceitful. Particularly with first-born children, this behavior may make parents
anxious because of the lack of prior experience as to what the
young are like.

This phase of negativism is often the period of the omission
lie: The truth, but not the whole truth, is told; information is not

freely volunteered. The impression is often gained that defiance has become an end in itself. This defiance may be crucial for development; it is a further attempt to assert autonomy.

Adolescents brought up by overpermissive parents may now lack all controls; overrepressive parents may produce over-passive and compliant young people. Because of the adolescent's overt hostility, some families abandon all attempts at control; they apparently feel unable to cope with openly expressed anger from their children. Given the complexities of modern society, however, few can function without parental support. As with younger adolescents, this is more tolerable when it comes from fathers. Mothers and their mothering still represent a great threat to autonomy because dependent needs are still great. Sometimes boys may cope with changed feelings by being with-drawn from adults and highly uncommunicative: Sometimes they may plunge into activities. Youth clubs or political organi-zations on the extreme left or right may be joined. Some may find themselves in ways society considers social: They may in-volve themselves in sports for the first time or may begin to work very hard at school to get emotional support from their teachers. Some adolescents now involve themselves with drugs, delinquen-cies, or perversions, often in order to see themselves as mem-bers of a special group, rather than for satisfaction from the activity itself.

Girls may not appear as negative as boys; the transition to the middle stage of adolescence may not produce a crisis with adults. It is much more likely for a girl of fifteen to feel anxious that she is unacceptable to boys. All her friends are considered to be more successful in having and keeping boyfriends. A girl's problems are more likely to be personally felt, less likely to be played out in the community. Sometimes a girl has to prove ac-ceptability as a woman by throwing herself at the head of the nearest available boy.

In early adolescence a boy's bodily preoccupation tends to be secretive or mentioned only to a best friend or other boys.

Boys are aware of the significance of the growth of pubic hair, the increase in the size of genitals, and the general growth of muscles. Unless pressured by society, boys do not become interested in outward appearance to attract girls, although they are susceptible to the demands of fashion, until midadolescence. Girls are concerned with being attractive before they really want a boyfriend and may be more involved with securing parental approval about their appearance than boys; a long struggle over clothing style and hair length tends to be a male prerogative. The struggle with girls is usually of short duration and occurs particularly as part of a conflict with mother. The issue is often one of taste—the length of a skirt, the amount of cosmetics, whether or not jeans should be worn—although beneath this there may be, unconsciously, a struggle about sexual exhibitionism. An alliance between mother and daughter is a particular aspect of the middle period of adolescence. When this occurs, mothers may expect their daughters to be helpful in the home, and girls are more likely to respond to an implicit family expectation than boys. Obvious grumbling and discontent is now less likely with a girl than with a boy.

Emotional Attachments of Girls

Not only do the family relationships of midadolescent girls differ from those of boys, their external relationships are quite different. Boys, as men, are always comfortable in large groups. They like being in teams, they are comfortable with many diffuse friendships, and they are happy if they have one or two very close friends. When no stable peer group is available, male personality development is hindered. If boys do not have special friends, this is not a major stumbling block on the way to adult maturity. A particular buddy is a desirable bonus that is given to a boy by life (Jersild, 1963, pp. 254–255). Girls need one-to-one relationships more than boys. Without these, the capacity to form heterosexual relationships is impaired. Large groups do not provide an acceptable substitute.

Insofar as clothing, superficial behavior, and appearance is concerned, girls are conformists, but they do not become emotionally involved with a large group in the same way as boys.

Whether or not a girl is at ease with herself depends not only on her life experience as an infant and child within her family but also on experiences during puberty. Girls need their fathers as asexual lovers. At first early adolescent girls are competitive with mother, seductive and charming with father. By middle adolescence girls need to have known men and boys who are not members of the immediate family, who will not be involved in a sexual relationship, but who will care about them.

In early adolescence many girls who are given the opportunity are interested in riding horses; they not only ride, they also groom and feed them and clean out stables. Girls in puberty are intensely interested in the mother-offspring relationships of small creatures—mice, hamsters, rabbits, dogs, and cats. In midadolescence they become much more interested in small babies.

Girls at the beginning of midadolescence may also develop "crushes" on slightly older girls or women (Cole and Hall, 1964, pp. 256–259). If these are grossly exaggerated, the indication is that a girl is under educational or social pressure or that she has received insufficient mothering; her needs to be loved are not being met. The crushes of the beginning of the middle stage occur partly because girls are not yet ready for emotional involvement with boys; partly they indicate a fear or anxiety about being unattractive to the opposite sex. Sometimes crushes are directed toward obviously different people, almost as if the other girl has desirable qualities that emotional contact will help the individual acquire. An older girl often tries out mothering roles in such siuations, which, for those with confused feelings about sexual roles, may become lesbian.

Midadolescent girls become involved with the necessity to formalize their own emotional experiences. They are great keepers of diaries, in which they may pour out, for their eyes only, their intense hopes, fears, loves, and hates (Jersild, 1963, pp. 28–29). Both the crush and the diary are only the background music to a girl's assessment of her femininity. In fantasy in early adolescence, in reality by the middle stage, the assessment of desirable womanhood is played out in relationship to men and boys.

Parents and Children

Fathers now need to convey to their daughters that their feelings and ideas as young women matter. Boys can hold forth in their groups and to an extent, compensate for what they see as adult and paternal disinterest. For girls this compensation is not so readily available. If they complain outside the family group about fatherly neglect, they are to an extent, implying their own lack of attractiveness. This is somewhat similar to the later situation with boyfriends; if boys reject girls in an unkind way, many girls see this as a function of their own unattractiveness rather than of male discourtesy.

Parents have conflicting needs about the growth of their children into adulthood. Mothers and fathers may both be reluctant, unconsciously, to see their children grow up and leave home. Fathers often get job satisfaction, mothers who are full-time homemakers may try to hang on to their children, since to allow them to grow up creates a situation of relative unemployment. Because girls are more obviously dependent than boys, the reluctance to have adolescents leave childhood behind is more likely to be a problem between mothers and daughters than between mothers and sons.

In a serious and meaningful way parents may find their children questioning attitudes, beliefs, and behavior. Some parents perceive themselves as growing with their children, others find it almost intolerable to have their ideas contradicted and may dismiss both their children and their ideas as rude and inconsiderate. Children may then retire into themselves in a sullen fury and despair. The sexuality of their children may be felt as an emotional threat by parents who may feel their own sexual potency to be declining. Parents who have themselves had an unsatisfactory sexual adjustment may unconsciously provoke sexual activity in their children (Johnson, 1953). The frigid mother may live vicariously through the sexual activity of her promiscuous daughter (Miller, 1958).

As young people move away from the ties of the nuclear family, some parents begin to see that they are unable to change the personality characteristics of their children; at this time marriages that are fragile may begin to disintegrate.

Overpermissive parents may create great anxiety in their children, who may continue to behave antisocially or self-destructively until external controls are offered. Overly rigid parents are likely to produce in their children either a dishonest negativism or a desperate compliance. Adolescents need the amount of responsibility they can handle. There are no rules for this, but the growing adolescent shows his parents that they must let growth occur. Adolescents who are overcompliant do not give their parents signals that indicate that they are ready for more responsibility.

Most girls are ready to try out their role as women by the middle stage of adolescence, but some girls are well into late adolescence before they feel ready to involve themselves in a meaningful way in the complexity of a human relationship with a boyfriend. Social pressures make a difference in this respect. In some parts of the United States there is social pressure on early adolescent girls, originally parentally precipitated, but now peer-induced to "date" boys. This behavior may be thought by some adults to be cute, a measure of its shallowness. It represents a false sexuality in girls who are not yet ready for a meaningful emotional relationship.

Dating practices vary depending on social class, economic

status, and religious affiliation (Crist, 1953). Immigrant groups often differ from the host society for two to three generations depending on their isolation, educational techniques, and the closeness of kinship ties. Girls from financially or emotionally underprivileged families are likely to have intercourse earlier than those from more secure groups; although girls from the upper-upper social groups tend to behave in a similar way to those from lower-lower socioeconomic strata. This is because both experience essentially similar types of upbringing; neither are looked after by their mothers, and they have a similar contempt for external objects—the very rich because they are so easily obtained, the very poor because they rarely have any of significance. Early school leavers and delinquent girls who may be educated in residential, single-sex schools may have intercourse before equivalent girls who are going to graduate from high schools (Schofield, 1965). Girls from those rare schools with an environment that respects the growing needs of adolescents appreciate that boys and men can like them for themselves; girls from environments that do not do this are more likely to seek sex in order to feel valued.

Girls who put a high value on academic achievement do not seem able to involve themselves at any serious emotional level with boys until toward the end of late adolescence. Clinical evidence indicates that academic overinvolvement tends to create emotional immaturity. The parents of girls who are seeking university entrance may try to discourage boyfriends because this will spoil academic chances. Such a girl may acquire a boyfriend as a symbol of successful parental defiance or may be a relatively isolated member of an academic community.

> Karen, a beautiful nineteen-year-old student, was referred to the student mental health clinic because, despite excellent high school grades and SAT scores over 1300, she was failing academically. Her usual work load was to go to the undergraduate library for approximately six hours nightly after classes. She had one girlfriend, no other social relationships. In high school she had a

grade point average of four and had been told by her parents that friendships with boys would mean inevitable academic failure.

She was unable to accept that her life was inadequate during an initial psychiatric assessment. She went to a psychotherapist as obediently as when her parents told her to avoid boyfriends.

The Academic Girl

Many academic girls are overcompetitive compared to the equivalent type of boy. Girls often may overconcentrate on studies because of internal conflicts or in order to deny important feminine qualities. Sexuality is not all that matters about a girl, but without such an expression of her femininity, life is often felt as empty. Middle-stage adolescent girls are not at ease in being competitive with each other or boys. Competitiveness is much more the prerogative of male psychology. Girls who are forced into competitive situations may have to suspend important aspects of feminine psychology: tenderness, creativity, and the particular capacity to care for others. Under stress girls may find it increasingly difficult to make meaningful and important emotional relationships (May, 1950). Further, excessive academic pressure, to which adolescents in the middle stage may be exposed, may make it difficult for them to mature independently from their parents. The demand to produce academic work when natural needs are to be in touch with a physical or emotional self may mean that young people cannot really envisage standing on their own feet independently of their parents. Passing of requisite examinations or making appropriate grades in school is taken as a sign of satisfactory maturity; this may be false. The adolescent who is not growing emotionally and learning to be autonomous of parents may appear to do well at school, perform satisfactorily in the first two years of a university course, and then, in the last year, do less well. Adult status, instead of being a delight, is a threat, emotional upset is a last attempt to cling to the benefits of childhood.

Stressful overcompetitive situations may seem only to delay some aspects of emotional maturation. However, as with unsatisfactory jobs, some adolescents become emotionally isolated and depressed; by overconcentrating on academic work, their level efficiency declines. Such individuals spend more hours at books than their level of academic achievement or the standard of the subject demands. This overanxious behavior is more likely in those who come from small, isolated nuclear families in which academic achievement is overvalued. Many girls fail to reach their academic potential because the competitiveness of the academic world primarily meets the needs of boys. Nowadays many attempt to solve their identity conflict by becoming aggressively involved in feminist movements.

Falling in Love

Girls mature faster than boys (Wilkins, 1965), so they are likely to be interested in boys two or three years older than themselves. The more uncertain girls are of themselves, the more likely they are to plunge into prematurely intense relationships with boys or, sometimes, with very much older men. Girls who fall intensely in love at fifteen, who feel they cannot live without their boyfriends, may be unconsciously trying to repair an emotional deficiency of early years.

Even without an excessive need for affection, a first love affair in the middle years of adolescence, unless it ends by mutual agreement, almost always ends with pain and sorrow for a girl. When girls fall in love and enter into a sexual, loving relationship, they rapidly want it to be permanent. Although boys may say that they will love the girl forever, they cannot mean it before they are well into adulthood, as their primary psychological task is environmental mastery. In sexual relationships they do not accept long-term responsibility until they feel secure in their vocational responsibility.

Even the well-adjusted girl reinforces her sense of feminine worth in a love affair, the end of this may make her feel unlovable as well as unloved. A satisfactory feeling of womanhood is associated with a capacity to feel creative and imaginative, to be productive in academic or vocational achievement and in homemaking activities. But girls and women do not feel complete as people until they have felt loved by a man. When they feel this love, they ultimately want the relationship to be permanent, and they want to bear their loved one's child. When a girl falls in love, these womanly needs come to the fore. In the relationship between the sexes, there is a need for both physical and emotional ties. The possible intensity and completeness of the one is not balanced by the other during middle-adolescent years.

Significance of Sexual Relationships

In the young the wish to experiment and test out capacities is often of greater significance than in later adult years. Adolescents need to find out about themselves in relationship to another person; this includes the need to discover their own sexual capabilities. Until a boy has actually had intercourse, he cannot know for sure that this is something he can do; until a girl has experienced an orgasm, she does not know whether she has this capacity.

In those cultures that allow this, adolescents in their middle years are likely to have sexual intercourse, but the intensity of exploratory needs as against tender loving needs may create a conflict. A boy may not necessarily boast about his sexual activity, but unless he is unconsciously seeking a maternal substitute, the need for a tender, loving relationship with a girlfriend is likely to be secondary to his drive to obtain genital pleasure. In girls, these needs are reversed; their primary need is for a tender, lov-

ing relationship; only secondarily, at any rate before they had
had sex, have they a need for sexual exploration and excitement.

Girls find dependent needs tolerable and emotionally acceptable; intense sexual excitement occurs only at the culmination
of the act of intercourse. A girl first must allow herself to feel
and to be dependent on a boy for feelings of sexual readiness to
receive him to come to the fore. At this point, girls have glandu-
lar and vaginal discharge; most girls do not experience this as a
frequent sensation without an actual sexual relationship.

By the time a boy engages in a heterosexual relationship, he
will have ejaculated many times, having experienced a solitary
orgasm either in masturbation, nocturnal ejaculation, or both. In
a heterosexual experience, boys seek an enhancement of an experience that to an extent they have already had. Only secondarily are they likely to seek a loving tender relationship. Along with
a possible wish to feel in love with a girl, the exploratory wish for
sexual experience is more conscious with a boy than with a girl.
Loveless sexual intercourse indicates that a girl insufficiently
values herself; this is less likely to be true with a boy.

Problems of Sexual Permissiveness

Sexual permissiveness poses a dilemma in present-day society. There is still parental and societal pressure against premarital
intercourse, but there is also a pressure to early active heterosexuality. A girl who remains a virgin, even in midadolescence,
may feel that she is missing out on special experiences that she
suspects that her girlfriends are having. The pressure that exists
among midadolescents to ignore parental interdictions is reinforced by some parts of the communications industry, although
adolescents who are able to conform to family standards are
protected from this.

The acceptable moral attitude is appropriately protective
of the emotional needs of girls. A compromise in parental atti-

tudes because of a fear of rejection by their daughters is unhelpful. Acceptable moral codes may or may not be listened to or even apparently heard, but a potential way of life is offered young people that even those who ignore it may ultimately adopt. If adults understand the needs of boys and girls and if this is reinforced by a girl seeing her own loving parents, then they can be heard. When an obviously happily married mother talks about human needs to her daughter, the girl will find it hard to believe that her mother sees all men as predatory when she is urged to restrain her sexuality until she is older. When a parental marriage is unhappy, a daughter may feel that her mother is trying to prevent, in an envious way, a relationship that she herself has never had. An unloving parental home is likely to harm a girl's capacity to make loving relationships but may drive her to seek them. Silence about sexual relationships may be a function of parental embarrassment but may be seen as an unconscious encouragement to become overinvolved.

A type of Victorian conservatism, liberally applied by loving parents, is the attitude that is likely to be most helpful to their midadolescents. It is reasonable for parents to expect to meet their daughter's boyfriends. Similarly, to allow daughters (or sons) to visit strange homes where the parents are going to be out, is not felt by children to indicate that they have loving parents, whatever might be said. It is helpful to adolescents in this age period for parents to be fairly restrictive, to insist, for example, that their children be home at night by a certain time. In some neighborhoods, this may arouse a feeling that parents are being overprotective; young people will angrily complain that their parents are old-fashioned and that restrictive behavior prevents friends of the opposite sex from being interested. When their children are angry with them, parents face the problem of feeling unloved; there is no doubt that it is easier to say "yes" than to say "no." But an angry daughter is less likely to be emotionally hurt than a daughter whose parents cannot tolerate her anger when immediate gratification is denied. Those young people who have been surrounded all their lives by loving and caring adults can weather many storms; those adolescents who have been brought up only by one parent or with a father who is disinterested or often away from home are more vulnerable. A rejection that to one individual is only hurtful, to another is a painful blow that may temporarily hinder further emotional development.

Social Aspects of Feminine Identity

The attitude that achievement is less important for girls than for their brothers ("they can always marry") is now less usual than previously. However, the awareness that a girl is likely to marry, and thus perhaps have her economic needs met, may save her from externally applied academic competitiveness.

The imaginative and creative potential of both boys and girls is neglected by the educational system (Vernon, 1968). Girls who are particularly involved in academic studies need a special recognition that nonacademic school subjects matter. These few schools that value the artistic endeavors or unusual imaginative potentiality of pupils suffer in two ways: either grade-point averages are seen as an indication of worth by universities or, alternately, the refusal of local communities to support school taxation has meant the cutting back of vocational or nonacademic studies.

In the middle years of adolescence girls need outlets for their interest in mothering:

> At a youth center in the slums of London, three girls brought their babies to show their friends. So intense was the interest in mothering that the youth council began classes in child care for the sixteen-year-olds.

When girls are given the opportunity to look after little ones, they usually enjoy this; it becomes important for them to be able to baby-sit for their own small brothers and sisters, as well as for other people's children. This need to care for others could be met if schools gave opportunities for responsibility to look after younger children. If young people are part of a social network, a typical example is traditional small-town life, the opportunities to be helpful to others are more easily arranged; in urban society this has to be sought.

Career choice begins to be an issue in midadolescence. The prospect of unimaginative and unskilled jobs faces those who drop out of school. If schools provide an interesting, exciting experience—a rare event in twentieth-century America—a dull job is even more difficult to tolerate. Activities that teachers find desirable are unlikely to be of concern to employers. If tasks are repetitive, unimaginative, and not needing responsibility, only partial involvement takes place. With such employment, other outlets to prove self-worth are necessary; education can prepare people for this.

Jobs that do not reinforce a sense of value are likely to lead to an overpreoccupation with an immediate need for a boyfriend. This preoccupation may become very obvious in the last months of school. Lovers are needed to fight off potential feelings of being unloved and unlovable. When boys are used in this way, they tend to experience the girl as clinging and demanding; the girl may then be devalued and rejected.

An alternative attempt at a solution is that girls may act towards all boys as they imagine boys behave toward them, moving promiscuously from person to person. Other girls may be isolated, depressed, and withdrawn.

External Controls for Midadolescents

If parents are respected by adolescents, the latter behave in a psychosocially appropriate way because of what is said rather than because of fear of what might be done. The physical control of adolescents at fifteen or sixteen and over is impossible, and physical struggles with boys and girls of this age are an unhappy way of trying to assert parental dominance.

As one of the anchor points against which the middle adolescent matures, parents are still needed in many ways. Mothers still provide a model of femininity to their daughters as well as other imprints of how the parents of adolescent children should behave.

Parents, however loving, cannot protect their adolescent daughters when reality stress becomes excessive. Parents are not omnipotent, but under stress adolescents appear to retain this childlike concept. When adolescents find themselves hurt by life, they may irrationally blame their parents for not having protected them. An equally difficult problem for the parents of adolescents is that they can no longer protect their children. When young people are hurt by reality, parents tend to blame themselves (Jersild, 1963, pp. 246–247).

In the middle years of adolescence daughters may still take their parents' advice about many things: boyfriends, jobs, and girlfriends. Thus, parents can still protect children from ill-chosen friendships. However, some relationships appear to be picked provocatively to provoke a parental response and prove that they still care. At the same time, an attempt may be made to prove autonomy. This midadolescent behavior may appear in chronological late adolescence.

> Janet sought help at the age of twenty-one because she was afraid that she was becoming promiscuous. The daughter of a controlling Jewish mother and a distant father, she began her first love affair at age seventeen with a nineteen-year-old college student. She lived with him for three years and was happy with him. Although he was Jewish, her parents disapproved of him because he was too "hippie." She ended the relationship and then had an intense affair with a gentile boy that lasted three months. She was

so afraid of what her mother would say about this relationship that she never told her parents about it. This boy abandoned her. She then fell in love with a twenty-three-year-old medical student who was also Jewish, and her parents approved. After three months, despite a happy sexual relationship with him, she felt herself attracted to a gentile law student.

It is clear that Janet sought autonomy from parental domination by picking boys of whom they disapproved; at the same time she provoked their intense anxiety about her.

At midadolescence some young people may be beyond parental control, refusing to take advice or direction. Such adolescents may repeat in their friendships the disappointment that they already feel with their parents. The adolescent who is beyond parental control is a young person at risk; inner controls are not usually strong enough to offer self-protection in present-day society.

Sexual Relationships of Middle-Stage Boys

The boy in his middle adolescent years is still assessing his manhood in relationship to his own age group; such boys are not yet ready to begin mature relationships with girls. Their main interest is in taking rather than giving, in a semipublic rather than a private heterosexual relationship. For example, boys of sixteen or seventeen, may not object to rather exhibitionistic public necking at parties. They commonly adopt a take-it-or-leave-it attitude to girlfriends. They will rarely admit to their male friends that any girl has the capacity to hurt or influence them. Boys sometimes discuss the details of highly intimate sexual experiences with male friends, and the opinion of a friend of the same sex matters more than that of a girl.

A boy of fifteen or sixteen, actively interested in possible girlfriends, may find it difficult to find a girl of a similar age. An exception to this is that boys who were in the active growth phase of puberty at the age of eleven or twelve may be physically very mature males at fifteen; older girls of sixteen or seventeen may find them interesting. It was once a prevalent idea that older girls might involve themselves with younger boys because these were less sexually threatening. This is untrue. Some older girls may choose physically mature fifteen-year-old boys who may still have a strong need to be mothered. Because of the strength of their physical needs, as against their relatively weak emotional controls, these boys are more likely to seek impulsive gratification in a full sexual experience than are older boys at the same stage of physical maturity. Physical maturation is not a measure of emotional maturity, but expectations are often based on the former. Too little may be expected from those who develop late, too much from those who mature early. Usually fifteen-year-old boys are not sexually interesting to girls of the same age, who are looking for older boys. Thirteen-year-old girls who might find sixteen-year-old boys interesting may not interest them. A boy of fifteen to seventeen thus tends to go through a developmental stage in which there are few girls available; this period of sexual frustration allows many boys to sublimate sexual drives into other important areas of masculine mastery and development.

Not all adolescents have celibacy thrust upon them. For some, sexual exploration is allowable at the beginning of the midadolescent years. A working class boy of fifteen or so, physically mature, may have exploratory intercourse with a girl of fourteen or fifteen. In general, those who have regular early sexual intercourse are less likely to be members of those groups of society who will be academically trained members of the community.

Midadolescent boys, although still struggling against dependent wishes, begin to feel more meaningful autonomous by the end of the age period. Parents begin to notice an increased capacity on the part of their children to care for themselves. Appropriateness in dress and hairstyle may not be that of parents, but it is acceptable to their own age group.

There is much discussion about adolescent rebellion, less about adolescent conformity. Adolescents are highly obedient to what they sense as implicit rather than explicit group demands, whether their group is mixed in age or contains only peers (Reames and Sadler, 1957).

Extraparental Adults in Midadolescence

All through adolescence adults known, liked, and respected primarily by young people themselves and their parents, secondarily by society-at-large, are important in emotional development. These necessary grown-ups may be the parents of childhood friends (usually these are made before the age of ten), or they may be adults who occupy a significant role in an adolescent's life. In the school system athletic coaches and drama, art and music teachers keep an interpersonal relationship long enough to be of developmental value to adolescents. Other teachers rarely relate significantly to their charges at a meaningful emotional level. Often neighborhood adults may provide the emotionally meaningful extraparental figures in the lives of middle-stage adolescents. One set of local parents will provide a home away from home for a whole group of young people. Sometimes they hold open-house even when their children are away. These are people who have a particular quality of warmth and tolerance that appeals to the adolescent. They may be older than most parents. They often offer an emotional, safe, culturally more stereotyped picture of mothering; plump, not-too-well-groomed mother figures are the ideal image for adolescent boys, particularly if they are not their own mother. These adults may provide a friendship network that is used by boys and girls in two ways. First, they are a refuge in times of crisis; their home can provide a haven when an adolescent feels at odds with his own parents; it is somewhere to go to be accepted. Second, as young people strive to move away from the dependent feelings of childhood, since they no longer have to struggle with the turmoil of puberty, they can emotionally involve themselves with other people. To prove that they are no longer children they may move away from home and literally put distance between themselves and their families. In any case, they enter in some degree of emotional withdrawal. Some adolescents may stop communicating with their families; adult friends then become important both to provide an anchor point against which growth away from the family can take place and to become identification models.

Nonparental adults are used differently by both boys and girls. Girls need to feel valued by extraparental adults in early adolescence; boys have this special need two or three years later, especially in the middle stage. At the time when adults are most significant to boys, girls are beginning to seek heterosexual relationships with older boys. Boys in midadolescence make relationships primarily with other boys, secondarily with other adults, and only when more maturation has taken place with girls.

Adults who are liked and respected may be seen by boys as people whom they would like to be like. How such adults are seen does not depend only on what they actually are but more on the way the individual adolescent looks at them. Parents are the initial significant models for their children, implicitly showing them what is is like to be adult. Adolescents, particularly boys, cannot agree that they wish to be similar to their parents. A five-year-old boy may say that he wants to be just like dad, this is inappropriate for a fifteen-year-old, who is more likely to announce that he has no wish to be like his parents because they are at best old-fashioned, at worst stupid. The qualities a boy admires, however, as he sees them in others, are very similar to those of his parents; of this he is unaware.

Relationships with adults outside the family obviously widen the horizons of young people, not only because they provide ideas but also because they offer themselves as models of human beings different from the adolescent's parents. Thus, contact with grown-ups help enlarge both an adolescent's way of looking at the world and the breadth of his own personality. Although adolescents do not usually learn better just because they like the teacher, this quality of child–teacher relationships is still present in the teenage period. A good relationship with an adult enhances the value of formal academic and vocational education.

As young people grow through the middle years of adolescence, they begin to take on more adult responsibilities. There are many ways in which this is done. By the time this age is reached, money and its spending begins to be seen quite differently by parents and their children. Boys may begin to earn part of their allowance, in some countries all of it, and resent having to ask their parents for a weekly sum. The development of future orientation of young people now allows money to be saved; parents who give their children allowances may now begin to give them a checking account.

Problems of Academic Education

It is questionable whether adolescents who do not enjoy academic work should attempt to go on in higher education. If they do, they are likely to find the years through adolescence burdensome. Many who feel forced to go on to an academic education, when they have no real wish to do this, do not last in a university course. They either drop out of a university or fail to make the grades that would be expected according to their intellectual potential (Wise, 1958). Early specialization or an early commitment to a specialty that does not change is likely to make the problem worse. This is a particular problem with the children of doctors, where the wish to study medicine represents a childlike early identification with a parent and has never become part of an adult self. When maturation does occur, such young people may abruptly leave medical school. In some medical schools this is known as the "doctor father" syndrome. Often, however, the offspring of doctors who study medicine consciously identify more with other physicians than with their fathers.

During midadolescence formal, propositional or abstract thinking develops (Piaget and Inhelder, 1958), although the process of change from concrete thinking has been going on through puberty. Formal stage thinking means that possibilities can be considered. It is common for formal thinking not to develop fully even in academic adolescents, although in most it does. Some can match standard problems with standard solutions, others work on inspiration although often they have no idea why they think as they do (Dulit, 1972). There are divergent thinkers who can often freely develop a variety of answers; standard method users are convergent thinkers who focus down in a concrete fashion on the right answer (Hudson, 1966). The modern school system generally seems to prefer the latter type of thought, which may explain why convergent thinking is common, even among those who potentially could be more divergent.

If all goes well during the middle adolescent years, the move towards independence will go quite smoothly. Parents will be able to offer their children increasing responsibility, which they will be able to handle. During these years parents may expect to meet their son's male friends, but they should not necessarily expect to meet their girlfriends. Neither should they expect to hear detail's of their son's intimate relationships with members of the opposite sex. Boys and girls who need to tell their parents intimate details of their sex lives are failing to develop a satisfactory feeling of self.

Adolescents and Work

Now that the days of craft apprenticeships are over, adolescents who become fully employed usually do not make their first job their final one. It is a rare adolescent who finds work that will meet vocational and emotional needs. Adolescents do better in those firms that are interested in them as a total personality. Alienating tasks that do not involve the whole personality tend to be badly performed. Adolescents are able to be actively and vigorously involved in jobs they are offered, provided that personnel of firms are prepared to care about the sort of work life the young people might be having. If the relationship between the management and adult employees is unsatisfactory, the same is likely between all adult workers and the younger staff. If adults take long breaks and are interested in maximum return for a minimum involvement, young employees gather that this is a desirable behavior. Apprentices may be criticized by senior employees for failing to perform tasks they are asked to do; but young people may only be copying the world of immediate self-interest and greed that they see around them.

Idleness is particularly demoralizing for young people. Most jobs probably do not expect enough from adolescents in terms of time or energy. A shorter working week may be appropriate for the middle-aged; if the task is interesting, it does not meet the needs of the young. Young people are likely to stay in jobs where adult workers are interested in them as people. The routine nature of some industrial work makes interest and concern from their superiors, as well as adequate opportunities for further education and recreation, essential if tasks are to be well performed.

Boys in the middle years of adolescence still use older adolescents and young adults to obtain emotional support. They need the continuing opportunity to mix with them in social and recreational settings. Middle-stage boys vary their relationships to their peers as well as to adults depending on their emotional needs, a function of internal experience as well as external reality. Sometimes isolation with peers is sought, sometimes constructive activities with adults. At times it may be preferable to laze time

86   ADOLESCENCE

away; sometimes the opportunity for constructive activities in
the community is essential.

The middle years of adolescence are a time full of the
excitement of discovery. The world feels new and fresh, and the
young feel that it can be changed. They are critical of adults and
themselves, and they are intolerant of failure. Only with adulthood do the young first begin to discover that they are little more
than a leaf in the wind insofar as life is concerned; only in late
adolescence can they begin to develop a real tolerance for the
weakness of others.

References

Bath, J. A., and Lewis, E. C. (1962), Attitudes of young female
    adults towards some areas of parent–adolescent conflict. *J. Genet.
    Psychol.*, 100: 241–253.
Cole, L., and Hall, N. I. (1964), *Psychology of Adolescence.* New
    York: Holt, Rinehart and Winston.
Crist, J. R. (1953), High school dating as a behavior symptom.
    Marriage Fam. Living, 15: 23–28.
Dulit, E. (1972), Adolescent thinking à la Piaget: The formal stage.
    J. Youth Adolescence. 1:4: 281–301.
Hudson, L. (1966), *Contrary Imaginations.* New York: Schocken
    Books.
Jersild, A. T. (1963), *The Psychology of Adolescence.* New York:
    Macmillan.
Johnson, A. M. (1953), Factors in the psychology of fixations and
    symptom choice. *Psychoanal. Q.,* 22: 475–496.
May, R. (1950), *The Meaning of Anxiety.* New York: Ronald Press.
Miller, D. (1958), Family interaction in the therapy of hospitalized
    adolescent patients. *Psychiatry,* 21: 277–284.
Piaget, J., and Inhelder, B. (1958), *The Growth of Logical Thinking
    from Childhood to Adolescence.* New York: Basic Books.
Reames, H. H., and Sadler, D. H. (1959), *The American Teenager.*
    Indianapolis: Bobbs-Merrill.

Schofield, M. (1965), *The Sexual Behavior of Young People*. London: Longmans Green.

Vernon, M. D. (1968), The development of reality construction in children. *Br. J. Psychol.,* 39: 102–111.

Wilkins, L. (1965), *The Diagnosis and Treatment of Endocrine Disorders in Childhood*. Springfield, Ill.: Charles C Thomas.

Wise, D. M. (1958), *They Came for the Best of Reasons: College Students Today*. Washington, D.C.: American Council on Education.

5

The Later Years of Adolescence

Physical Changes

The late stage of adolescence, though essentially a psycho-social event, is still a period of physical growth in the male. As male genitals reach maximum size, usually between the ages of sixteen and eighteen, there are changes in the hairline, and a well-formed "widow's peak" appears. The larynx reaches its maximum size at about the same time, and more body hair may appear, usually at least a typical male distribution of pubic hair with a hairline stretching to the navel. Arrest of skeletal growth does not occur in men until twenty to twenty-one, and it is not until then that adult levels of seventeen ketosteroids and testosterone finally are reached (Hamburger, 1948). In girls, adult physical status is reached at sixteen to seventeen, but late adolescence may stretch beyond that age as part of the moratorium available to many young people. Unlike the first two stages, late adolescence is not a period of very obvious physical change.

The Coping Period of Life: Its Age Limits

The late adolescent is basically concerned with trying out the personality structure that has been built over the years since childhood and with learning to cope with the complexities of adult society and adapt to the usual stresses of everyday life. This is to some extent still, like the middle adolescent years, an era of personal consolidation, but environmental mastery is now possible. With a firm sense of self, the adolescent finally learns to cope with the complications of adulthood. Since the concept of late adolescence is not based on physical development, it can be given fairly definite age limits. These depend on social class, economic status, nationality, and ethnic group. Furthermore, the ambivalence of society means that, on the one hand, the adolescent may be considered an adult; on the other, such young people are also treated as if they were quite irresponsible.

For those who go to universities, late adolescence covers the years between seventeen and the early twenties. For young people in jobs, late adolescence lasts a much shorter period of time; it may be over by eighteen or nineteen. This variation depends on society's expectations. Effectively, the student is given the right to further education, is allowed a certain amount of irresponsibility in the social sense, and, in exchange for this, is expected to abandon certain adult privileges, the right to earn a living wage, for example. In the United States it is not unusual for a student to work his way through college; such an individual really holds two jobs — one, unpaid as a student, another, paid, often in a relatively menial occupation.

Those young people who go out to work, except in certain trainee posts, are expected by the age of eighteen or so to have undertaken adult responsibilities. Students are given grants or loans; therefore, they should be appropriately responsible and not make a nuisance of themselves. On the other hand, young workers are encouraged to spend their not inconsiderable earnings with a high degree of irresponsibility; if they marry, however, they find their incomes will barely support adult sexual maturity. The establishment apparently has less concern about the aggressive "antisocial" behavior of young workers than about the behavior of university students, perhaps because the former are thought to be essentially conservative, although for many of the latter this is also true.

Society attempts to resolve its confusions about young people by making them legally adult at the age of eighteen. Mixed feelings about this are demonstrated by the fact that in England late adolescents are to be allowed to stay in the residential care of children's authorities until they are nineteen. Some states are struggling not to allow eighteen-year-olds free entry to bars. On the other hand, adolescents of seventeen are tried in adult courts and sent to adult prisons. The confusion of society is understandable in that inner maturity is reached in late adolescents at quite different ages for different groups.

Maturity of Late Adolescents

The late adolescent boy should be able to forgive both his mother and father for their failures and omissions. In doing this, he will be able to establish a true loving relationship with his girlfriend. He will forgive her "maternal" nagging, which he himself may provoke; he will be seduced by her feminine being; and will accept her sense of loss and anxiety without anger. He will understand the depths and variations of his girlfriend's moods and understand the variations in her trust in him, both sexual and otherwise. A girl always needs a loved individual to bolster her self-esteem and feeling of worth. While retaining attachments to her mother (Lample de Groot, 1928), she is able to vary between intense involvement with herself and profound involvement with her mate and their children. She is the mainstay of the family structure, and men are almost totally dependent on her for their sense of masculine worth. Yet, in the modern world, she may compete equally with a man for jobs and economic status. She needs her mate to tolerate the illogical and dependent behavior that may occur as a part of a response to her menstrual cycle; he must know that she is vulnerable to psychic pain just before menstruation begins. The love affairs of late adolescents as they plan a future are the grown-up version of "house" played by children. To reach full sexual maturity, the late adolescent girl needs conditioning and training of her sexual organs in coitus with a man she loves. Sometimes a girl thinks she is unable to have an orgasm because she has had occasional intercourse with a boy she does not love. There is no evidence that this is truly so until she fails to reach complete sexual satisfaction in a loving, long-term relationship. Orgasmic insufficiency, then, is often due to a failure to accept physical femininity, a need to have pain inflicted, a desire to thwart masculinity, all of which are due to a failure to resolve these infantile dependent and sexual conflicts aroused by relationships in the nuclear family (Bonaparte, 1953).

In fields other than sexuality, by the time late adolescence is reached, signs of mature behavior should be very apparent. Maturity can be measured by a capacity to be loving, to wait for emotional satisfaction, an ability to consider the future and the control of aggressive and hostile impulses. The future will be influenced by actions in the present; an adult can tolerate anxiety without an immediate need to act to alter the situation irrespective of consequences. The issue of maturational age is still important during late adolescence. Variations in physical maturity, emotional growth, and, hence, academic achievement still persist as a result of late maturation to puberty. Such a late developer is likely to continue to experience those earlier feelings of insecurity that have not yet been resolved by time. However, during late adolescence when, paradoxically, there is generally less disparity between maturational and chronological age than was the situation earlier, society is less rigid about age as an indication of potential, particularly in the academic field. Performance expectations are no longer attached to age by society, but immature adolescents may experience difficulty because of their expectations of themselves. This is particularly an issue in sexual and social relationships. Hard data is typically difficult to acquire, but it appears in clinical practice that a significant number of nineteen- to twenty-year-old students with anxieties about their sexual attractiveness reached physical maturity later than their peers.

The Academic Adolescent

Provided that the foundations of personality integration have been satisfactorily laid during childhood, early, and mid-adolescence, the late adolescent can try himself out as an individual. Late adolescence can also allow for further emotional growth. This may be especially necessary for those whose lives have been unduly complex, many academically able adolescents fall into this group (Kinsey *et al.*, 1953). This means that many reach higher education still highly vulnerable to reality stress, which adds to the task of schools and colleges with late adolescents. More is involved than preparing them for a vocational existence; universities have a responsibility to help their late adolescent students to be young adults who have to learn, along with the enrichment of intellectual sensibility, to cope with a general responsibility to society, to develop a sense of personal worth, and to ensure a sense of continuity with their society and cultural and human heritage. Quite apart from the problem of late maturation to puberty, an educational system that values an early forcing of academic achievement inevitably produces a large number of late adolescents who are still emotionally immature. Yet most institutions involved with education during the late teens behave as if the psychological foundations of the personality have been quite firmly laid in each of their charges. Even when educational authorities recognize the need for peer groups and teacher stability in junior high schools, most high schools do not provide any consistent peer-group and teacher relationships for adolescents of seventeen to eighteen. Universities appear to have abandoned all responsibilities other than in the provision of student mental health services for the emotional care of their charges. Adolescents in large universities live in dormitories with no emotionally supportive social structure, no rules, and no adults with inter-personal relationship skills in charge. That the legal age of major-ity is now eighteen does not mean that this age group can tolerate academic and emotional stress without feeling cared for by older adults. In factory assembly lines the same holds true and industry generally appears to accept no responsibility for the emotional well-being of its young charges. Interestingly, only the armed services provides a structure of emotional support for the young. The young who feel worthless need to be given significant oppor-tunities to feel useful; in the navy, army, and air force, such individuals normally do get this opportunity. Unpopular wars tend to spoil a system in which dependent needs can be met in a socially acceptable way, thus allowing support for a sense of masculinity.

Autonomy Struggles of Late Adolescents

All adolescents should have as much freedom as they can capably handle and as much responsibility as they can tolerate. They should have "caring for" duties and an opportunity to be useful to the community-at-large. Late adolescent girls, in particu-lar, suffer because it is hard for them to feel valued as women except in sexual relationships. The separation of late adolescents from the caring roles in society is likely to be much more painful for the girl than the boy because her mothering needs are greater. If late adolescents are given too much or too little responsibility, they retain the capacity to behave in highly self-destructive ways: quitting jobs, dropping out of school, or being almost pointlessly aggressive.

The wish to leave school does not always stem from the failure of the immediate environment to meet needs. Sometimes it may be an attempt on the part of the young people to free themselves from what they feel is a childishly dependent relation-ship with their parents. The more a university or high school meets the needs of late adolescents, the less likely it is that youth will see dropping out as a way of asserting independence. In some societies there is a natural time gap between leaving high school and entering college. Entry into the latter is gained two semesters before actual admission begins, which gives late adolescents time to explore their world and themselves by wandering freely throughout their own and foreign countries. This is normally true in England. In the United States, however, entry in the fall semester immediately after the completion of high school is almost always obligatory. This provides a continuous process, but does not give adolescents a necessary period of exploratory freedom.

Education of Women and Minority Groups

One major stress at this period comes with social mobility. The adolescent from a nonacademic family who has become academic has learned to express his views in a way that is strange to his parents. A change in the techniques of communication is also a problem for immigrant children who are educated in their new country but whose parents retain their original language and culture.

The child of the black ghetto who obtains an academic education is likely to feel in a similar conflict with his nuclear family. The black American may find that education threatens his tenuous sense of cultural identity; education for a poor black, as for a poor white, may begin to move the individual into a different social-class group with different communication techniques. This may partially help to explain the apparent failure of integration of minority students in universities. Faced with a realistic hostility, minority students often have a fantasy of extreme hostility from the world-at-large where it does not exist. Clinging together in the face of real and imagined hostility also tends to reinforce group identity. Socially mobile black students, however, are also fighting their own wish to move away from their own ethnic background into the ranks of the affluent host society. Thus, minority students often sit together in classes and social mix with other ethnic groups is rare (*The Michigan Daily*, 1972). The well-documented studies on the effect of education on communication techniques (Bernstein, 1961), when applied to black Americans, may help explain the apparent hostility and anxiety felt by many. The hostility is perhaps a manifestation of identification with the aggressor, the white host society. It may also represent anxiety about being pulled away from tenuous ethnic roots. The ethnic identification of Africans depends on their tribal roots; the Hausa are not the same as the Yoruba, although they share a common skin color. Blackness is no more a measure of ethnocentricity than "whiteness." So black Americans, when they seek an identification with an African Hausa may be in the same position as the descendant of a Scotsman who seeks a common identity with a European Serbo-Croat. Given the nature of the black American identity, which is a newly budding plant, those who are acquiring the upwardly mobile skills of the larger society may find it difficult to know what they really are. The anxiety created by this also creates intragroup hostility, which leads to tensions among black students being high. As one individual said, "We are putting each other down." The black student is in a somewhat similar emotional situation to the British working-class university student who gains entry on the basis of scholarship; he, too, feels the loss of his cultural base. The latter student, however, is not admitted on the basis of ideology, as is often the case with the student who may help fill the affirmative action program of a university, its minority quota. If such a student feels pulled away from his own group by education and consequent social mobility, his conflict is that much greater. Hence, the black student must cling to his peers to reinforce a sense of ethnic value about which he is at least unconsciously ambivalent.

A mixed feeling about education is also present in minority-group parents and in those lower socioeconomic groups whose children achieve academically. On the one hand, parents are immensely proud of the academic success of their children; less consciously, the response of nonacademic parents to their children's academic progress is often resentment. Such parents may fear the "loss" of their children. The adolescent from a nonacademic family may reciprocate this feeling. Whichever attitude is conscious and dominant may make for academic success or failure (Taba, 1953). In some ways, the minority student is better off than the socially mobile white student. Although there is intragroup hostility, the former gets peer support at the very least, as well as larger group reinforcement both from the majority and minority. The white student who is conflict-ridden as a result of social mobility is offered no support by peers or adults in his college. In many large universities students have no effective contact with faculty members. Even where universities have a tutorial system, in which there should be a close relationship between staff and student, tutors are often unaware of the psychological stresses to which their students are exposed. The tutorial system is, in any case, no substitute for confidential guidance on intimate problems. Students are unlikely to tell their tutors about their worries, partly because they fear that these confidences may prejudice the references they need for future employment.

Girls often cope with anxiety by allowing themselves to feel dependent on their parents. When girls move up in the world and go to college, they do not lose their particular need to turn to their mothers. It is not uncommon for anxious girls to feel that if they continue their academic education their life will be intolerable; they are afraid of finally losing their mothers. Such girls often give up further education because of physical health, because they do not want to go on, or, sometimes, because of a more obvious emotional breakdown. Another solution is to try to seduce a young man, who the girl hopes, will want to make this affair permanent. She begins to feel that if the young man really loved her he would want to marry her. This is like the problem that exists with some girls earlier in adolescence. The nineteen-year-old man may not be willing to commit himself to an indefinite relationship. Such a young man is often assessing his manhood by trying out the role of a "husband"; he is not yet ready to make this a formal step. The girl is anxious to stabilize the relationship because she feels that she has lost emotional contact with her own parents. She becomes depressed when the relationship ends, particularly because the "loss" of her own family leaves her with no one upon whom she can rely.

Parental Roles in Late Adolescence

Although by late adolescence, parents can have remarkably little overt influence on changing their children's personalities, they can, however, still help to create emotional comfort or discomfort for their young. The role of parents in late adolescence is really to help confirm their children's steps to final adult roles in society. If they fail to do this, the split between generations is likely to be reinforced; those late adolescents who reject the standards of official authority to an extent are rejecting the standards of their parents. This is desirable, for otherwise society would remain static; the problem for parents is to accept the idea that their concepts may be rejected by their children. This does not mean that parents are necessarily rejected as people. If parents have been successful in that role, their children, as free, independent adults, will inevitably disagree with them on some issues, although they ultimately tend to agree on fundamentals.

Late adolescents often reject parental beliefs and attitudes if they feel these have been imposed for hypocritical reasons. Parental oversensitivity as to what the neighbors might think creates a social face that may be one reason given by adolescents for rejecting parental standards. Adolescents who are themselves intensely conformist may reject their parents' norms as too conformist, although to different standards. For example, parents who go to church on Sunday because of what the neighbors might think may have children who reject organized religion but join different religions or political organizations with a fervent religious zeal.

Late adolescents often identify with the attitudes they claim to deplore in their parents' generation. A group of young people prepared to bully and hound those they consider dissident will criticize the older generation for allowing fascism to develop and for bullying minorities; only the victims change.

In this last step before formal adulthood it is almost inevitable that some young people will have conflicts both with society and with their parents. Problems with authority at home may still be present. Late adolescents should see themselves as adults in relationships to their parents. However, at the end of childhood, holdovers from earlier parent–child relationships are almost inevitable. In the modern world, young people have difficulty mastering the environment and facing impotence in many areas of life. The anxieties of the final step to adulthood arouse a temptation to draw back to childish dependence. The presence of parents can be a provocation to behave in a childlike manner. Angry defiance may be a way to struggle with dependent needs aroused by the imbalance between social stress and the ability of the individual to cope with this. Family quarrels may be a result of a projection of conflicts about dependence. In late adolescence some degree of intergenerational clash is almost inevitable if the adulthood of their children is accepted with difficulty by parents. Some have problems because they recall consciously and unconsciously the small children they reared as they relate to grown-up sons and daughters; others spoil relationships as they may want to lean on their children as the latter grow up. The strength of childlike feelings in the late adolescent may be matched by a parental need both to infantilize and unconsciously to be an infant. This may lead to adolescent withdrawal from any family contact. The possibility of an extended family in the next generation is hampered; the overconcentration on the nuclear family, which causes so much stress to individuals within it, is thus perpetuated.

All human beings occupy a number of different roles and the "self" that is apparent in one may not be the same as in the other. Sometimes an adult role in the community is not a measure of independence within the family. The highly successful businessman may not be autonomous in other ways. Children may settle for being only sons or daughters. Overdependence on the original family is a common cause of marital breakdown.

John, a twenty–two-year-old student, who was highly dependent on his parents, married a twenty-year-old nursing student. His marriage to a potential nurse seemed to represent a wish on his part to continue to be looked after. The girl, however, a product of a broken home and was herself seeking to be fathered. The more dependent she became on John, the more he withdrew alleging a need to study. Sexual relationships between them almost ceased and finally she made a suicidal gesture.

In a joint interview with a psychiatrist, a condition of relative safety, John announced that he wanted to leave his wife—"she can have the apartment and I will go home to live with my folks." He had been unable to be frank with his wife, previously suggesting only that if she went home to her mother she could be well-looked after "for a week or two."

If parent–child dependence remains intense during late adolescent years, the precursors of the forty-year-old adult clinging to a seventy-year-old parent may be present.

Intense rivalry between siblings with much aggressive competitiveness is almost always a measure of difficulty between parent and child, and, not surprisingly, unresolved dependency conflicts may be played out in quarrels between siblings even in late adolescence.

Kenneth had an intense struggle over dependence on his mother. An eighteen-year-old student, he would go home on the weekend and tell her all the details of his university life. He would also call her on the telephone each week. However, whenever he went home, he would quarrel violently with his about-to-be-married twenty-two-year-old brother. Father, a withdrawn accountant, was a distant shadow in the house. Kenneth had sought therapy because of his anxiety over sexual conflicts, which were related to his inability to allow himself to be close to anyone. The patient perceived his brother as being controlling, bossy and demanding; all qualities possessed by his mother but not consciously perceived by him.

When sibling quarrels continue into late adolescence, they still may be a projection of tension. It is not unusual for one sibling to criticize or dislike in the other qualities that are unconsciously disliked either in a parent or the self. Kenneth, in the above clinical example, thus showed a typical response: He was unable to feel close to his brother because of unresolved rage with his mother. As he matured in therapy, he became more distant from his mother and aware of warm feelings toward his brother.

Tasks of Late Adolescence

The late adolescent is learning to cope with life with minimum support from parents. In a very remarkable way this reproduces some of the same emotional situations of earlier childhood. Children learn new skills attempting to cope with a variety of testing situations: climbing trees, playing at some distance from their mothers, fighting and tumbling about with other boys and girls. They cope with these activities successfully, providing their mothers are available. If they should hurt themselves and if their mothers are not accessible, as, for example, in the tower blocks of low-cost urban housing, children either lose trust in parents, become overdependent on peers and child-minders, or they withdraw from meaningful emotional contacts with others. Children use newfound physical powers to conquer physical obstacles and assess their own skills; late adolescents do the same in relationship to life in general with their newfound personality strengths.

They test themselves against the real world and its demands to prove their own competence as adults in work, school, play, and social and personal relationships. If the relationship with parents is good, turning to them for help and advice does not imply a loss of personal integrity. If parents are not available, because of earlier personal or social difficulties, the late adolescent, who feels unable to cope with sexual or aggressive impulses, turns either to another adult, his peer group or he gives up a serious attempt at autonomy. Alternately, he abandons further attempts at personality growth, foreclosing his identity. The perpetual student falls into this category:

> Frank was a twenty-seven-year-old medical student who began to have academic difficulties in his junior year. He repeatedly failed examinations and was referred to the medical school's psychiatrist for an opinion about his academic underachievement. He was the son of rigid, overcontrolling, Roman Catholic parents. He was brought up with an overwhelming sense of how sinful it was to give in to one's own impulses—this denied his own capacity to be loving and sexual. He was polite but distant with his parents. After completing his undergraduate degree he sought a postgraduate qualification in physics. Two years before his doctorate he became dissatisfied and one year later applied and was accepted for medical school, providing he undertook certain postgraduate courses.
>
> His answer to his own dilemma of on the one hand failing as a medical student and feeling happy with it as a chosen career was to apply to go back to physics. His plan was to complete that and then return to medical school. He could not envisage the possibility of psychiatric help, nor was he prepared to accept "advice" from his counselor, his parents, or his peers.

Late adolescence, which seals the individual's sense of continuity with his family and his ethnic and national group, is also the period of separation from childhood (Terman *et al.*, 1947). As with all transitional stages of development, new roles are tried out before they are consolidated. These involve separation from a previous way of life. Late adolescence may, in a sense, be a series of transitional experiences designed to help in the final consolidation of identity. Temporary separation from home is one way of doing this. The three-year-old who first plays away from home casts an eye to make sure home is still there; late adolescents may make a significant physical separation from their home by going on vacation without their parents. This has a different emotional meaning from going away to school in that a vacation away from the nuclear family is much more a free-choice decision. The identification with parents is often clear, and the type of vacation taken by an adolescent is often similar to that of his family. Relatively affluent adolescents may choose to hitchhike even though they could afford the fare. The type of vacation taken by parents, however, is unconsciously copied; Blackpool, England, becomes Rimini, Italy; Miami Beach becomes Cannes, France. Children who have always been sent to camp in later adolescence may vacation with parents; parents who have always motored on the European continent have late adolescents who take a jeep to Turkey, Afghanistan, or India.

Vacations are not just a way of identifying with and separating from parents. Late adolescents wish to see the world through their own eyes. A vacation may be a wish to be adventurous, to meet new people and new situations. Experiences that in the past could be obtained in day-to-day living are now sought by young city dwellers in their travels. An unplanned vacation is commonly used to find a sexual partner who will provide new forms of sexual experience without the risk of incurring the responsibility inevitable in long-term relationships.

> Judy, an eighteen-year-old girl, was allowed by her parents to travel in Europe over a long summer vacation. At home she had a steady boyfriend but had never had an orgasm while having intercourse with him. Apparently, to have done so would not just mean her total acceptance of his masculinity, it also implied

an emotional dependence. While in Greece, France, and England, she had short-term sexual relationships with three boys; in each of these she had orgasm. A brief relationship in her home town was as unsatisfying as the longer term one had been. She understood in her psychotherapy that, among other things, the short-term relationships abroad represented a freedom from the risk of being vulnerably overdependent.

Vacations offer the opportunity for the equivalent of shipboard or clubcar relationships; intense intimacy is possible with none of the problems involved in long-term situations. Frankness is safe because it comes with no strings.

Late adolescents have other techniques of enhancing the weaning process from childhood. Even when they live in the same city as parents many prefer to share an apartment with friends, often returning home on weekends only to do their laundry. Very often, particularly in the first year or so at school, children who live some distance away return home two to three times a semester and then may quarrel with their parents, as if to reassure themselves that parents are still there and to prove to themselves that parents are not needed. Sometimes individuals leave home before being ready to do this:

Faye, a nineteen-year-old girl, was angrily dependent on her parents, so much so that they still applied curfews when she went out at night. She decided to become independent. Her parents suggested that she move into a dormitory, but she refused to consider this, being unable to find a roommate. She moved into an apartment by herself. She did succeed in finding a loveless sexual relationship for a time. Nevertheless, the whole experience was one of intense isolation. The failure of this attempt to reach emotional autonomy and independence led to her return home. She then sought psychiatric help for a fairly severe depression.

Faye's overdependence on her parents led to a futile attempt at rebellion rather than a transitional move to autonomy. A move leading to social isolation is an unsatisfactory attempt to resolve dependent feelings and does not indicate the likelihood of creating an autonomous way of life.

Apparently, socially acceptable situations may be used as a way of defying family standards. Superficially conformist but really defiant, domineered young people may choose a partner of whom their parents disapprove; often their choice is as domineering as the original nuclear family. Unwittingly, individuals may repeat the emotional experiences that they seemingly wish to escape most.

Often marriage is used as an attempt to gain freedom from overdependence on the nuclear family. The overdependent partner is likely to seek an inappropriate level of emotional support from a spouse. Marriage is not a solution to late adolescent maladjustment; "if only he would marry," should be "if only he were able to marry."

Sexuality may be used as part of an attempt to assert autonomy in ways other than matrimony. This is true in the genesis of some types of homosexuality, the choice of sexual partners of whom parents will disapprove, and exhibitionistic sexual activity of which parents are aware. Pubertal boys overdependent on mothers may leave masturbatory traces on their night clothes or sheets, a seductive and provocative gesture. Late adolescents may similarly take sexual partners to their bedrooms in the parental home. Whether this represents a provocative piece of self-assertion depends on the family codes. Some families accept extramarital sex; others regard it as anathema. Some girls may tell their mothers about a first sexual experience, but healthy adolescents do not discuss details of their sexual affairs with their parents. Young people who believe in premarital celibacy may, after an episode of impulsive lovemaking, marry or promise to do so as an attempt to expiate guilt. The sexually more experienced individual may use the sexual relationships to fight their partner's parents. A relatively passive, dependent young person may then have the unconscious satisfaction of watching the struggle of powerful people, the spouse and parents.

> John, a rather gentle nineteen-year-old boy, was brought up by Southern Baptist parents. He met a twenty-one-year-old girl on campus who eventually seduced him. At this point, he asked her to move into his apartment and to marry him. He took her to his home for a frozen vacation experience in which his parents complained to him about his girlfriend, and his girlfriend complained about his parents. After his return to school, he began to suffer from premature ejaculations as well as a reluctance to have intercourse with his girlfriend. He sought counseling help for this.
>
> It was apparent that he was now as angrily dependent on his girlfriend as he previously had been on his parents.

Parents who are permissive in their attitudes towards sexuality may have children who have to find other techniques of self-assertion; drugs that differ from those used by the family are typically an attempt to show autonomy. Marijuana is the current drug of choice, as it has been from time to time throughout history.

Educational underachievement in the children of ambitious parents is a passive–aggressive technique of self-assertion (Goldberg, 1962); the rebellious thwarting of parental wishes is mistakenly believed to create emotional independence. Late adolescents' failure to equip themselves for the world may ensure continuing dependence, if not on parents, then on society or one of its subgroups. The academic drop-out may be as highly dependent and rebellious a person as the lower-socioeconomic-class juvenile delinquent.

Late adolescents may not ask their parents' opinions about ethical, racial, political, and religious beliefs. All through their developing years, however, children have been picking up parental attitudes about these. This is demonstrated when a parent of a late adolescent dies. A surviving child may handle mourning by identifying most obviously with the dead parent and seemingly become exactly like him or her. This is only possible when all these attitudes are already internalized, even if they were not previously obvious.

Most late adolescents have a fairly smooth passage to adult life, but all the way through adolescence and childhood there are things children do to justify anxiety and concern. Most of these are the equivalent of minor roadblocks on the road to maturity, but overanxious misunderstanding may give some of them more weight than they deserve. More usually the difficult behavior of adolescents may carry implicit requests for assistance. If these are ignored, early maladjustment can become more serious.

The success of the late adolescent in accepting and enjoying adult responsibilities depends on how responsive his family environment, society, and school have been in meeting his needs. Their responsiveness can make all the difference between collapse in a crisis or the determination to profit and learn from the upset.

Adolescence is the last of a series of stations on the way to adulthood, which is demonstrated by a capacity to love and by the attainment of full mental and physical potential. Adults do not envy the opposite sex. The adult woman may have a career, but she is quite willing to acknowledge her wish to bear children; she is able to give and receive sexually in a love relationship. The adult male likes work, enjoys sex, and is capable of a tender loving sexual relationship with a woman.

By the end of adolescence, individuals have a belief in a personal affiliation with certain symbols such as the flag, national songs and dances, and the nation as a whole; they have an individual identity as well as a collective one. Individuals believe in the importance of their national and ethnic groups and should be able to participate in their own culture. Collective identity also depends upon communication through language, the sharing of moral values, and a political organization to share group policy. This depends, partially at any rate, on society's setting up social organizations by which identity systems can be maintained. In other words, the social organizations of society are required to provide the mechanisms for maintaing human motivations in large-scale organizations as well as to provide a sense of personal identity. In adolescence there are particular social organizations that are significant in the reinforcement of individual and social mental health. These are necessary for personal and cultural identity and give a sense of personal and social continuity. They are the family and its extended networks and the educational and religious systems of society. The failure or success of the latter, given the disintegration of extended family networks, are crucial and justify separate consideration.

References

Bernstein, B. (1961), Social structure, language and learning. *Educ. Res.*, 33: 163–176.

Bonaparte, M. (1953), *Female Sexuality*. New York: International Universities Press.

Goldberg, M. (1962), *Research on the Gifted*. New York: Teachers' College, Columbia University (Mimeo).

Hamburger, C. (1948), Normal urinary excretion of neutral 17-ketosteroids with special reference to age and sex variations. *Acta Endocrinol.*, 1: 19–37.

Kinsey, A. C., *et al.* (1953), *Sexual Behavior in the Human Female*. Philadelphia: W. B. Saunders.

Lample-de-Groot, J. (1928), The evolution of the Oedipus complex in women. *Br. J. Psycho-Anal.*, 9: 332–365.

Taba, H. (1953), The moral beliefs of sixteen-year olds. In *The Adolescent: A Book of Readings*, ed. J. Seidman, 592–596. New York: Dryden Press.

Terman, L. M., *et al.* (1947), *The Gifted Child Grows Up*, Vol. 6. Stanford: Stanford University Press.

The Michigan Daily (1972), Editorial. March 18.

6

Youth, Society, and the Family

Social Networks and Personality Growth

It is apparent from the consideration of personality and physical development that for successful emotional, intellectual, and physical maturation, adolescents need both to be able to face pressures in the immediate environment and to be cushioned against them if they become excessive. For all people, maximum emotional support is gained from caring human relationships.

Except for those who experienced primary poverty, until the Depression in the United States and the outbreak of the Second World War in Europe most children were brought up as members of a fairly stable network of grandparents, aunts, uncles, and family friends. In Africa and Asia children are still members of a "tribal" society that offers support to individuals and makes them less vulnerable to stress from outside. There is always someone who matters, who can be turned to for help and emotional support (Bott, 1957). Child rearing is shared among many individuals, chosen by blood ties, cultural and religious custom, and friendship networks. In Western Europe and North America this child-rearing group is now much smaller (Riesman, 1950): An isolated unit of parents, brothers, and sisters cannot fully meet the needs of the adolescent, however well intentioned its aims. Religious figures usually fill only formal societal roles, and the culture no longer provides other supportive figures. Teachers no longer impinge significantly on the personal lives of children, and there is a dearth of emotionally involved youth workers.

Adolescents find it very difficult to bear the dependence they feel when their immediate family offers its direct emotional support. But if they cannot accept this from their fathers and mothers, they often have no one else to whom they feel they can go (Kandel *et al.*, 1968). Yet, anthropologists have argued that the nuclear family is not even the basic and elementary social unit of mankind, although a mother–child bond and a father figure are necessary in a child's life (Fox, 1967). In the past a large social group encompassing many ages provided a haven when an individual's conflict with his parents got to be too much for him. The youngsters were involved with people and a way of life they could admire and adopt. From this viewpoint, it was not harmful if adolescents attended schools that failed to consider emotional needs: Teachers were not necessarily the only significant adult models for their pupils, and the social organization of the school did not necessarily have an implicit way of life with which young people might need to identify. As the networks of family friends and relatives disappear, particularly in large cities, and as society becomes more fragmented, a greater responsibility is put on the only extraparental adults with whom the adolescent has contact—teachers and other professional workers with young people. Schools often have to provide the environment in which young people learn a way of life, and teachers must become the adults on whom adolescents can model themselves. The episode described by one middle-age man is too rare today, and the supports he got in his youth are less easy to find:

All my family attended the same school, and everyone in the town knew everyone else. We had a history teacher who was eccentric, and everyone teased him, particularly my cousins. I well remember being punished for something they had said about him. Looking back, I don't think I minded very much.

Social Stress and Adolescent Turmoil

Adolescents very often respond to a lack of social support by disturbed behavior. Maximum delinquency rates are found in the conurbations, particularly in the unneighborhoods of big cities, among the towering apartment blocks and sprawling houses, as well as in obviously derelict slum areas. In Chicago the gangs of Woodlawn have developed a system in which children of eight or nine become junior members. As in many black ghettoes of the United States and in slum districts in Europe they define their own areas, map out their turf (Block and Neiderhoffer, 1958). Rehousing, which has often ignored social interaction, has not changed this pattern and in some cases has reinforced it.

Rapid change in a community can create adolescent turmoil when previously it was not apparent:

In the space of five years, a Scandinavian industrial town increased in population from 50,000 to 80,000. In place of the old tribal environment there were now large numbers of small families in the town. Individual adolescents became isolated from sources of social support. They were aware of changes in teen-age life in other parts of the world and they became very discontented. There had been for many years in the town a religious sect that insisted on puritanical conformity from its adolescents. Compared to the larger adolescent group these young people behaved in an unusual way. But until the change in population there had been no community problem and good relationships had existed between the small religious group and the larger adolescent group. As the population grew dramatically, this small sect was assailed as a "minority group." Large groups of adolescents from the town jeered them as they left their church, and these taunts led to fighting. The town authorities responded superficially and punitively by increasing police patrols and tensions ran very high.

Young people would find life difficult enough if their only problem was a loss of the "tribe," but they tend to be exposed to increasing social stress without a corresponding increase in social support. Some of these stresses are imposed by inconsistent demands from adult society: It is important to work and earn, but money is apparently "easily" acquired, and our economy depends on some of it being wasted. Sex is healthy and natural, but it is not supposed to happen before marriage (alternately, whatever moral code an adolescent might have, there is a tendency, because of social pressure, to feel that one does not rate as a virgin). Marriage is a sacrament, but it is treated more and more casually. Parents go to church, but children must not have religious education in school. Education is important, but lack of money forces schools to function on a part-time basis. Frustration must be borne, but every effort is made to prevent children feeling it. Magical solutions are purveyed to the population nightly on television, but when young people seek their own magic with drugs, society violently disapproves. The effect of all this is that self-destruction is often felt by some adolescents to have dignity. This is understandable because of the unforgivable way society ignores their need for a secure life. The presence of the atom bomb as a possible coda to their civilization, as well as the constant pollution of the earth by industry, shows adolescents that it is perfectly possible for them all to be obliterated by the action of their elders. This situation is similar to that in the thirteenth century at the time of the Black Death, when bubonic plague swept through Europe. Then the responsibility was projected onto a minority group, the Jews. Nowadays, children hold their parents responsible for the balance of terror. I have never met a thoughtful, academically able boy in his early teens who did not remind me of this.

Adolescent Techniques of Communication

Society-at-large exposes youth to increasing stress. But even
in small social organizations, there are many ways in which it
fails to provide the necessary supports. One of these is by not
recognizing the implicit message in disturbed and difficult adolescent behavior:

> June had good parents who provided her with a stable home.
> But they were an isolated family, and the girl had no links with
> grandparents, aunts and uncles, or family friends. The family
> occupied an apartment in an affluent suburb. Her school was one
> of the best in the neighborhood, being very well equipped, but
> most staff did not appear to understand that many children in
> their care needed them as significant adults in their lives. They
> were also apparently unaware that the sheer size of the school
> was quite overwhelming to some children. As is usual, June and
> her friends were not able to look on the school as a place they
> could use after school hours.
>
> At thirteen, June began to smoke marijuana. She and her
> friends frequented a cafe near the school that was known to be
> a center for drug pushers. When this was discovered, June's
> parents and teachers, believing that the drug was not addictive,
> responded just as if she had been caught smoking tobacco. For
> the following year she smoked marijuana regularly either after
> school or after breaking out of her bedroom at night. At four-
> teen, she began to have sex with a musician whom she thought was
> twenty-two—he was actually some ten years older. One day she
> told her mother that she thought she was pregnant, and she was
> at last referred for possible help.

June was behaving as a troubled child for a year before
anything was done. Neither her parents nor the school social
worker had understood the importance of the request for help
implicit in the marijuana smoking. Sometimes it appears that the
drug intoxication of an early adolescent has come to be as acceptable as alcohol in adults. There was no evidence that other school

staff had any training in the techniques of talking with children in individual interviews. June felt the school social worker, who was responsible for the emotional care of some 1,800 children, was hopelessly inept: "All she does is lecture at you." No particular effort had been made to close the cafe. Although some parents and teachers were worried about it, nobody had called the attention of the police to its presence. June's father ultimately did this and a number of drug dealers were arrested; the cafe continued to be a source of drugs for local teenagers.

Importance of School—Family Communication

If there is no regular contact between the school staff and parents, teachers are likely to be unaware of a pupil's family difficulties; they will not realize that upset behavior at school may be caused by these troubles. Sometimes teaching staff are not well trained in understanding adolescent psychology. Furthermore, teachers usually do not have contact with young people for more than one class period a day for more than two semesters, so they are often unaware either that there has been a change in the way a youngster behaves (for example, from being withdrawn to becoming restless) or that such a change in behavior may be a request for help:

> John, fifteen-and-a-half, went to a technical high school in the inner city that was largely for young people who did not have sufficient ability to be successfully academic. Administration was interested in the school's extracurricular groups, in particular, its band. The principal was interested in proving how academic some of his intake could be in spite of earlier failure. He therefore tried to ensure that as many high grades as possible were obtained at grade twelve.
>
> John, whose father was a crane driver and whose mother worked in the school canteen, was thought to have academic

potential. John went to see a family practitioner complaining of
several months of recurring headaches; the doctor thought he
was too difficult to talk to and sent him to a psychiatrist.
Although he had been frequently absent from school, the school
administration was satisfied to assume that he was medically ill.
When the psychiatrist asked about his progress, the reports from
his counselor were that the staff did not think that the boy had
reached his academic potential. He said that the boy's home was
without problems and that the staff could not understand why
John had become a little restless recently. This restless boredom
had been criticized by his teachers, but it had not made them feel
that there was anything particularly wrong. His change in
behavior was not thought to be particularly significant.

In his first interview with the psychiatrist John was shy and
withdrawn for about thirty minutes, then his story emerged. For
the last two years his father had been very depressed; for weeks
he had spent hours kneeling on the floor weeping, watched by
John, his mother, and his brothers. Because of this depression he
had lost his job, the family had been short of money, and his
mother had been forced to go out to work.

The boy also made a complaint more typical of his age
group. The eldest of three children, he felt that he got no special
privileges; for example, he and his younger brother were sent to
bed at the same time.

In a second interview John spoke of his sexual anxiety; in
particular, he was worried about masturbation. He thought he
did this too often and as a result he would be "weakened" and
would be less successful with girls when he was older. He also
complained bitterly about the quality of the teaching at his
school. He said that the teacher read from a book and expected
the boys to spend most of the period just taking notes.

In reply to a question John, said that he never spoke in a
relaxed way to teachers in his school. He couldn't remember
spending any time with an adult other than his father; more
recently the family practitioner had tried to talk to him for the
first time.

The boy had no idea what career he wanted. He did not see
himself as an unskilled worker, but neither did he wish to work

in an office. He said that, since he had to leave school soon, he thought he might as well give the whole thing up now and look for any job that came along. Nobody had ever discussed with him what he thought about himself, what he might do when he left school, what books he might read, what were the possibilities of further education. He seemed to feel that only one teacher cared at all but "he is busy." Father mostly watched television, or "he tells me what to do." Psychological tests showed that John was bright enough to obtain good grades. When he knew this and realized that if he worked hard enough his chances of passing were reasonably good, he relaxed.

In a third interview, thinking about his wish to work outdoors and meet people, he began to wonder about the Post Office as a possible career. By this time his headaches had ceased, and he was no longer intermittently absent from school.

If John had not had a perceptive family practitioner, which is a matter of considerable luck, it is highly probable that no help would have been available to him.

Why Adolescent Disturbance Is Not Helped

To be more effective with young people adults need to understand the nonverbal signals of early adolescents, whose words are often not as meaningful as their actions. It is evident that John's acute withdrawal, shown by shyness and headaches, was not "heard" by most adults around him as shouting distress to the world.

A lack of interviewing skills can also lead to adult failure to help young people even though intense efforts at help are made:

Peter, fifteen, went to a boarding school at the age of nine. At ten he and two other boys were seduced by one of the teachers.

This came to light because his mother noticed that he was more and more withdrawn when she and her husband went to see him. Finally when the story came out the principal urged her to seek advice from a psychiatrist to try to discover whether or not the boy had been in any way emotionally damaged by the episode. The mother became extremely angry at this. She said later that she felt that the principal was telling her that she was a failure as a mother if she could not handle the situation herself. She withdrew her son from the school. Through the ensuing years the family noticed that the boy seemed to be unreasonably bad-tempered: he was unusually difficult with his younger brother whom he would hit in an apparently impulsive and meaningless way. From time to time he stole from his parents.

Evidence of psychological damage was also apparent from his failure to develop many of the "normal" interests of boys of his age. Although he was physically well into puberty, he had no awareness of, or interest in, sexual feeling. Nevertheless, the family went along assuming that the boy would "grow out of it." At the age of fifteen-and-a-half he was involved in stealing at school. He was then referred to a psychiatrist for an opinion.

Why was Peter not helped at ten? One major factor was surely the school principal's unawareness of how frightening his suggestion of possible psychological assistance could be, with its possible implication of madness. He may well have tried to use his authority in a way that turned out not to be helpful. The parents partly felt that he was really responsible for what had happened to their son. His mother was, in any case, anxious that she was not a sufficiently good parent. This typical failure of communication shows how important are the techniques of interviewing, both with young people and their parents.

A further reason for the failure to help emotionally disturbed adolescents is that too many people still see these difficulties as frightening. Often adults overlook anxieties and tensions in young people and are quite happy, provided that the youngsters look normal and do not offend them. Sometimes disturbance is recognized but there is a reluctance to seek specialized help. For example, teachers are often afraid to tell parents that they think a child needs psychological help. They may often worry if one boy or girl sees a psychiatrist; they think the expert will make unreasonable demands on the school, or other children will react with hostility. Although an adolescent may be ashamed of his first visit to a psychiatrist and may tell his friends that he is going to the dentist, he almost always tells them the truth afterwards, and it is very rare for him to be teased unless he is in a generally unhappy school. Initially a fear of madness may deter adolescents. When they see a psychiatrist this usually ceases to be a continuing concern.

Antipsychiatry is more common among adults than adolescents. There are still some grown-ups who think that psychiatry is nonsense and other who think that a psychiatrist is involved only in the treatment of the disturbed and is unfit to express an opinion on "normal" youth.

Meaning of Emotional Disturbance

The idea that the needs of the disturbed are fundamentally different from those of others is quite naive, as is the idea that there is an absolutely healthy and an absolutely ill personality (Menninger, 1963). Most people swing between mental "health" and "illness." An episode of bad temper, for example, when young people become overwhelmed with rage and incapable of adequately appraising reality in a sense is "sick," but this is something that many human beings experience on many occasions. Likewise, withdrawal from the real world and a preoccupation with what is going on inside oneself—being "lost in daydreams"—is evidence of "illness," but it is also something that most human beings, particularly the young, experience from time to time.

Need for Social Stability

There are other ways in which the needs of adolescents for social stability are ignored, in particular, school changes occur too often at times that are maturationally inappropriate. Many people do not know what the emotional needs of the young are; perhaps because of their own emotional conflicts they find it difficult to understand significant aspects of adolescent psychology. The junior high school system, which covers grades seven through nine creates a school change usually at age twelve. This means that children lose the external support provided by known teachers and contemporaries just when the physiological tension of puberty is at its height for most of them and they are besieged by internal turmoil.

The particular need for external stability at this time can be understood from a brief glance at development from childhood. Children at the age of five, even in those societies where school does not begin compulsorily until seven, have already some emotional involvements outside their own families: They are obviously interested in learning and playing with other children in the neighborhood, and they should be comfortable in being away from their homes with other children for a few hours at a time. Nevertheless, these children are still highly dependent on their families in a way that is acceptable to them and society.

At puberty, at the same time as they experience increased emotional turbulence, the young begin to seek those significant emotional involvements outside their own family that are part of the final steps to adulthood, and they are less willing to accept dependence. Because of this they have a particular need for the support of known adults and stability from their social environment outside the family. By just over thirteen-and-a-half it would appear that in the United States, most boys are well into puberty, as measured by the beginning growth of pubic hair and testicular enlargement and most girls have nearly completed this developmental stage in that menstruation has begun (Group for the Advancement of Psychiatry, 1963); therefore, the logical school changing age is thirteen-and-a-half.

Problems of Neighborhood Integration

Most family practitioners, youth workers, and teachers will agree that they have not been well trained to deal with the crises of youth. Nevertheless, the concern about the effects of inflicting unnecessary stress on young people, which inevitably produces more intense disturbance and more frequent adolescent crises has not led to effective social action. Underprivileged adolescents especially are often under greater stress than the more secure.

There is a certain social and psychological blindness shown in some educated majority and minority attitudes toward the black population and other ethnic minority groups in the United States in the search for integration. Similar attitudes also exist towards immigrant communities from India, Africa, and the West Indies in Britain. It is generally held that the concentration of an ethnic group in certain areas is bad, and it is argued that these groups should integrate as quickly as possible into the host society. The wish for rapid integration is put forward by those anxious to destroy racial prejudice; it ignores the fact that both the majority and minority groups have to change.

In all societies throughout history immigrant groups have clung together in certain localities. Even in relatively tolerant societies, it has usually taken several generations for immigrant groups to melt into the population. This was true of the Huguenot refugees in Britain in the seventeenth century and of the Jewish immigrant wave from the Russian territories around the Baltic at the beginning of the twentieth. By keeping together and retaining their cultural identity, present-day immigrant communities in Britain provide a healthier social environment for the rearing of their children and adolescents than the native population. The immigrants maintain the extended kinship and social networks the natives have lost. It is not surprising that their adolescent population has a considerably lower delinquency rate than the white, British-born citizen.

The black American, on the one hand, seeks a reinforcement of an attenuated ethnic identity but, on the other, seeks a mutual tolerance that history shows only an integrated society can produce. The resources necessary to provide a decent environment and adequate vocational and social opportunities to ensure that blacks and others have the economic and social possibilities enjoyed by sections of the white population are, nevertheless, not made available. Islands of low-cost housing in more affluent neighborhoods and poorly conceived tower blocks are not a substitution for adequate employment opportunities and neighborhood enrichment.

Educational Stresses Affecting Youth

If there is conflict among adolescents in most school systems, such disturbed behavior is almost automatically blamed on the pupil's skin color; sometimes parents are blamed; sometimes the innate badness and sickness of individual children. There is little tendency to look at the social organization of the school and at pupil–staff relationships for possible causes. As a result, there is little discussion of the failure of the general social organization of the American junior high and high schools to meet adolescent needs, although much is written about classroom teaching (Miller, 1973). A preoccupation with the open classroom and permissive education cannot hide the fact that, in most schools, there is no recess period, often only twenty minutes may be allowed for lunch, and the classroom period may be fifty-five minutes long with five-minute breaks (Miller, 1970) for children to move across the school. One thirteen-year-old boy may be part of six to eight groups a day with an equivalent number of differ-

ent teachers. As a result, despite the heroic efforts of some individuals, it becomes difficult to know individual young people,
particularly those who do not call attention to themselves. A
further difficulty is caused by the fact that in any one school
either academic or nonacademic education is likely to be im-
plicity highly valued, whatever is explicitly stated. On the whole,
nonacademic adolescents are more likely to leave school at sixteen. Career choice, in the nonacademic parts of the school system, is thus likely to be forced on young people during early
adolescence when they may just be emerging from a time of
turbulence. Nontracked classes are often taught in a way that
suits the academic pupil but not his less-able contemporary,
which disillusions nonacademic pupils and makes them all too
likely to drop out of high school. The school drop-out is ill prepared to make a vocational choice for social, academic, and
psychological reasons. In those school systems that move to
a three-year high school at grade ten, adolescents change
from junior to senior high school at the psychologically inappropriate age of fifteen; they lose the adults upon whom they
begin to model themselves before this process has been completed.

In many societies academic adolescents face equivalent difficulties to the nonacademic. In Britain, in order to obtain the
requisite examination standards, adolescents are forced to choose
a series of subjects that they may come to dislike. They can then
find no way of getting out of their choice without expense to
themselves psychologically—and to the state and their parents
in hard cash. Also, ever-changing standards of university entrance make it difficult for adolescents to know the level of
academic achievement expected of them. Academic adolescents
in the United States are forced to chase grade-point averages in
order to enter prestigious universities, which often exploit under-
graduates with huge classes taught by teaching fellows in order
to finance and maintain the standards of graduate education upon
which their reputation stands.

Social Stresses Affecting Youth

All these uncertainties and rigidities make it hard for boys and girls to develop a satisfactory feeling of self. Those who reach adolescence with great personal and family security can cope with this; the vulnerability of others is reinforced. In many towns and cities throughout the world on any fine evening, scattered throughout the major squares or streets, there are dozens of young people sitting, watching the world go by; they have really nothing to do and nowhere to go. This is a clear demonstration that they feel there is nothing valuable and worthwhile for them. This is true in New York and London, of Ann Arbor and New Haven. In Greenwich Village, the King's Road, and Carnaby Street, the restless moving to and fro proclaims young people's inability to find significance in their lives. Adolescents who feel valued by their world are more able to develop a secure personality. Not all young people who hang around are lost, but too many of them for comfort suffer in this way.

Stress is also inflicted upon the young because present-day society seems to have lost the technique of assessing how much responsibility adolescents can handle. Sometimes they are given too much. Parents may go out and leave their fifteen-year-old children to have parties with no adult present. Sometimes too little responsibility is offered. Society does not appear to value what adolescents are able to produce; the money they earn is often not needed by their families, and academic young people can all too easily fail to get the higher education they seek through no fault of their own. Natural devices to relieve this tension and help coping mechanisms to assist in handling aggressive and sexual impulses are hard to find.

Those who have suffered childhood disturbances can find in adolescence a second chance for mature development if they are lucky enough to be exposed to people who understand and can meet their emotional needs. As his personality changes, a young person can reorganize his way of seeing the world: The failures of infancy and childhood can be rectified in adolescence. Although not all authors agree (Masterson, 1967), some children who have felt persecuted by life can in adolescence almost automatically correct this emotional distortion. In addition, there are some parents who cannot get on with small children but can help those who are more grown up. Some young people, unlucky enough to have had a disturbed childhood, are thus more fortunate in adolescence; their age presents them automatically with surroundings more appropriate to their needs.

The Spartans exposed their young to physical stress in order to toughen their society. This was a conscious decision, but, eventually, so much was demanded that by killing its young the society destroyed itself. Social stress applied to youth may produce similar effects in the Western world. Because of this it is very difficult for parents and other adults to know how much an adolescent's behavior is a function of family interaction and how much depends on stress in society-at-large. The conflicts of the present generation of young people are blamed variously on parents and on the environment. Blame is always sterile, particularly because of the nature of the adolescent age period, which is concerned with the interaction between physical growth, emotional development, and society's pressures. There is an additional dissonance between the expectations young people have of themselves and those held by society.

This has been called a permissive society. It is true that the range of stimulant and sedative drugs available to young people has increased; the decline of sexual prurience has led to doubt for many about acceptable sexual behavior. Nevertheless, society might more appropriately be considered confused and anxiety-ridden. As a result, the world of adults often appears neglectful, uncaring, and alienating in the eyes of the young. Many people are apparently preoccupied with surface behavior and appearance, but few are able to show that they consider the feeling and sensitivity of others. For example, the neatly dressed delinquent boys who call themselves "greasers" may arouse little public concern; long-haired, untidy-looking "freaks," who turn their aggression in on themselves by taking drugs and who perceive themselves as "heads," are thought to be a particular menace, although they are less dangerous to others.

Techniques of Reducing Social Stress

Young people need to find both physical outlets to release the inevitable tension produced by growth and social pressures, and they need opportunities for goal-directed constructive behavior. Changing society as a whole is an unreal wish but smaller social systems who are sufficiently motivated can more easily change in a planned way.

The available organizations that could be more responsive to the needs of youth are schools and youth clubs. Schools should not merely be centers of learning; they should also provide anchor points from which adolescents could develop their personalities and reach out into the community-at-large. Among all the adults who work with the young, teachers thus become the most significant. Schools could become places in which the potential of their pupils is enhanced. Schools can be centers of learning with the opportunity for creative activity and the goal of teaching pupils how to live (James, 1968). If adolescents enjoy education, as they should, school should improve experiences in the real-life situation of the community. The school should be a center for the life of young people from which they can become productive adults. The better the school and neighborhood, the easier this becomes; in underprivileged areas, particularly, good schools are most needed. The Israelis, for example, put the best schools with the best teachers, who are specially paid, in the most underprivileged neighborhoods.

Rich and poor schools both need to provide social systems able to meet developmental needs. Youth activities provided by churches and other voluntary bodies should not just offer guided vocational and recreational activities; the opportunity to be helpful to the aged and underprivileged is particularly needed by young and old (Miller, 1973). A youth center to help bridge the generation gap with trained volunteers and minimal planned activities is needed in any one community along with centers that provide a variety of other activities. The youth organizations in any one community could work together to ensure that they did not reduplicate facilities; thus, they would give young people the opportunity to move spontaneously to the type of activity that would meet a current emotional need.

There are schools and youth organizations that are sensitive to adolescent needs in the total community. However, these are exceptional; most youth facilities, of whatever type, are not aware that changes in society have thrust upon them a new role—one for which they have not as yet equipped themselves.

The idea of the generation gap has led adults to believe that they have no say over the way adolescents think and behave and there is a tendency for both groups and individuals to give up. Communication between the generations does not necessarily have to break down. Many parents still retain great influence over their children (Offer, 1969, p. 186), even if an apparently despairingly oppositional response is present because of mutual, if transient, misunderstandings.

Parental Uncertainty and Adolescent Stress— The Role of Experts

Some adults have become uncertain as to how they should behave as parents. This is probably a special problem of the twentieth century. Parental uncertainty has been present since the end of World War II; an insecurity applies also to the difficulties parents may have in deciding how best to bring up their adolescent sons or daughters.

Advice given by experts, which is designed to be helpful,

can paradoxically cause greater parental confusion. This is partly because experts tend to tell parents how they should behave (Ginott, 1965)—sometimes even telling them the words they should use in certain typical situations—partly because different experts tend to give contradictory advice. Even if all the experts agreed, a highly improbable situation, if parents behave as they are told, rather than in a way that is spontaneous and natural to themselves, they appear to their children as false.

Individuals who are unsure of themselves may seek security in the written word, but the security they receive tends to have shaky foundations. There are many reasons for this. No author can assess the capacity for understanding of his readers. If more is expected of children than they can produce, they are made anxious and uncomfortable; the same is true of their parents. If people are offered advice about how to behave and then are unable to follow through with the actions required, they are likely to be very uncomfortable. It is rarely helpful, for example, to tell a mother who cannot stand up to her son's angry feeling that she should do this. If she had been able, the chances are that she would already have done so; the advice will only make her more guilty.

Today many parents appear, unfortunately, to have little capacity to feel themselves valuable. It does not help to tell such people how to behave with their own children. The temporary feeling of security that may be obtained by being told what to do may have two effects. It may increase parental uncertainty, so that dependence on advice given becomes greater and greater, leading to the economic success of the advice purveyor. On the other hand, if the ideas offered are felt to be strange, they may imply to people the uselessness of their own opinions; good advice may then be rejected or, worse, slavishly accepted. In any case, if adults are doubtful about their own capacity to be good parents, telling them how to behave may make them feel transiently better, in that it may relieve their immediate worries, but it will not make them feel worthwhile. People can be comfortable about being told what to do only if their own ideas and wishes, which for some reason were felt as unacceptable, are confirmed. Forcefully presented alien ideas may make people temporarily submerge their own feelings; they lead to no permanent solutions. Apart from this, many attitudes are based on social class and ethnic group; experts are often middle class in their behavior and judgmental orientation. Such experts may be unaware of this, and unwittingly may try to inflict on their eager listeners a foreign way of life. If parents act their roles as fathers and mothers with a newspaper column, a paperback book, a social worker, or a family practitioner as the stage director, this will create within them and their children a feeling of inner confusion. Children are not fooled when parents do not behave naturally and spontaneously, and they sense that something is wrong in their relationships. This feeling may not be articulated, but it is present.

Parental uncertainty is a reality and adds once more to adolescent turmoil and stress. That direction is rarely helpful does not make help impossible. One principle of adult psychotherapy is that the individual patient should not be told how he or she should behave. Good therapy respects the ability of adults to make their own decisions. Using the same principles, advice on how to behave is generally not useful to parents, although it may offer a deceptively simple solution to difficulties. Knowledge about the reasons for human behavior may be of real assistance. Understanding offered without strings respects the ability of people to make their own decisions and reinforces their sense of worth.

Parental Confusion

There are a number of reasons why parents should be confused about the behavior of their adolescent children and doubtful about how to respond. Many of today's parents of adolescents were children just before the war and were adolescents while it lasted. Since their fathers may have been in the armed forces, many adults often have no experience of being fathered themselves from 1941 until 1945. This can mean that neither the fathers nor the mothers of today's young people may know how a father should behave towards an adolescent boy or girl. As a result, children may see no real difference in the behavior of their parents towards them, a situation that causes particular problems in early adolescence when boys and girls have to struggle with their mothers to fight their own internal wish to be mothered and to thus develop a sense of autonomy. If both parents are felt to be equally "motherly" then the child can find no support within the nuclear family at this time. This confusion about parental roles, which is currently being elevated to a philosophy, reinforces the anxieties among parents that have been created by changes in child-rearing techniques. Those who insist on equal roles for both parents lay foundations for generations of disturbed adolescents with internal confusion about their own identity.

The Depression and Second World War led to an intense dissatisfaction with the nature of man. It was thought, rightly, that if man were less anxious, he would be less aggressive. Changes in child-rearing techniques were proposed and the fashion since the last years of the 1940s has been for parents to consider the emotional needs of their children as they show them in day-to-day relationships. This is another reason for parental and, thus, adolescent anxiety. In infancy attempts at need fulfillment include demand feeding (children are fed when they show behavioral evidence of hunger) and toilet training (children are demonstrably ready to be clean) (Spock, 1945). The recognition of stages of human development (Gesell and Ilg, 1943) meant that many people knew of probable behavior at certain ages and had expectations on the basis of this. The independent striving of two-year-olds gave rise to the phrase "the terrible two's." Parents who were aware of this tended to handle situations with "Let us do this together," rather than "Do it," and "Let us clear up your toys," instead of "Put your toys away." The easy relationships of the three-year-old to his world gave rise to the phrase "the trusting threes"; the competitiveness of four-year-olds to the "ferocious fours"; the equableness of five-year-olds to the "fabulous fives." However, these catch phrases based on chronological age aroused as much confusion as age norm expectations in adolescence when the child matured more rapidly or more slowly.

In spite of confusion, significant changes in child rearing have taken place, with a very real effort made on the part of parents and health educators to meet children's needs. Nevertheless, some who do not physically suffer may still be neglected and emotionally deprived, an almost inevitable state among the realistically underprivileged. Confusion between needs and wants, when people do not recognize that "I want," is not the same as "I need," may lead to similar emotional deprivation among the more affluent.

The concept of the generation gap is not new. Parents who were not themselves brought up to have their needs met are unsure how to do this with their own children. Fathers and mothers of today's youth were commonly brought up by parents who were reasonably firmly convinced that they knew what they were doing was right and that they, as parents, knew best. Starting from infancy, the parents of today's adolescents were told as children how to behave: Toilet training was early, often at two to four months, rather than as nowadays from around eighteen months to two years. Feeding was by the clock at stated intervals from the time of delivery; there was no attempt to wait until the child cried, see this as a demand to be fed, and meet this need. There was at that time a consistency between the upbringing of the two generations. Mothers brought up their children as they themselves had been reared. Apart from being more comfortable themselves because of self-assurance, fathers and mothers were not likely to be in conflict with their own parents about child-rearing techniques.

A different situation probably existed when today's adolescents were infants. Interested grandparents were likely to feel that the then-modern child-rearing techniques were strange and unusual. Although such grandparents may have tried not to interfere, they almost inevitably demonstrated any disapproval they felt. Based on their lack of understanding, grandparents questioned whether it was justified to change the fairly rigid manner with which they had reared their children. That children's needs as they express them should be met, instead of basing expectations on a preconceived notion of what children ought to be doing, was difficult to justify. The state of current youth was used as a criticism to justify child-rearing conservatism. Without an imprint of the experience of having their needs met when they were children, and lacking support from their own parents, the insecurity of today's parents of adolescents was reinforced. The problem was compounded because often husbands who returned from a wartime deprivation of having felt unloved sought undue mothering, at any rate initially, from their own wives. Thus, the fathers of children born just after a return from a wartime experience are likely to feel intensely competitive with them.

Children need the security of parents who are genuinely sure of themselves or, at least, who are honest with themselves. A child is likely to be in difficulties if he has a parent who, while uncertain about what to do or how to behave, pretends certainty. If there is an absolutely right way to bring up a child, which is doubtful, it is better for a parent to be wrong with conviction than right with uncertainty. An adolescent is more likely to be mentally healthy and develop into a secure adult if parents comfortably do the theoretically wrong thing than uncomfortably try to do what is thought to be right. Parental uncertainty causes distress to both chidren and adolescents.

Today's parents also experienced a youth that was quite

different from that of their children. The behavior of the present generation of adolescents may, in many ways, resemble behavior in the twenties more than in the thirties (the years of Depression) or the forties (the years of the war). The meaning of adolescent behavior now confuses parents. Long hair used to mean effeminacy; bright clothes for the male were unknown. Sloppiness meant confusion. Those who were affluent were usually considered well adjusted. There was no difficulty in the adolescent finding a reason for his existence. His parents were in economic need, his society needed his warlike efforts to defend itself against enemies that were acceptable to all the population, or there were politically just causes. Anxiety about sexuality allowed the Puritan morality to be acceptable, and efficient communication experts did not surround each antisocial action with a halo of interest, thus reinforcing its desirability. Parents consciously try to give their children a better youth than they had themselves; often they then envy children for enjoying something not previously available.

In adolescence parents may unconsciously create more confusion by trying to change the way of life of their children, sometimes by new educational techniques, compared to the family as a whole and its tradition. An eccentric artist who leads a bohemian life will cause some anxiety to his children if he educates them at a school that inflicts rigid middle-class value systems upon them; a family that is out of touch with its own inner world has problems when its children are exposed to a creative and imaginative educational experience. This does not mean that parents ought to try to bring up their children so that they are not different, but the effect of differences and, in particular, how these influence mutual attitudes and communication between parent and child, should be considered.

Not all parental uncertainty is due to a difference between the parents' upbringing and the way they rear their children, nor is all adolescent uncertainty due to a conflict between the way parents live and how they try to educate their own children.

Some people, because of their own upbringing, may be quite unsure of themselves as people and thus as parents. Nevertheless, neurotic parents do not necessarily have neurotic children. If one parent is emotionally healthier than the other and if fathers and mothers love and care for their children, the resilience of human nature may mean that emotional difficulties are not passed down through the generations nevertheless, sometimes family traits are carried, like the color of a child's hair or the shape of his body, from parent to child.

Effect of Television

A particular developmental stress, brought about by the use of television is perpetuated on today's adolescents. The use of television for many hours a day as a baby-sitter and as a parental entertainer may cut down very significantly the amount of time parents, particularly mothers, spend with their children. As young children, therefore, today's teenagers may have had insufficient meaningful emotional contacts with people and things. If a family group is watching television, there is little direct interaction between parents and children. They are all observers artificially stimulated by action on a screen with little talk one to the other. The attempt of children to play out aggressively the violence they have seen on the screen may, however, be controlled in an aggressive way by parents. Thus, screen violence is reinforced by an intrafamilial aggression. If there is no television set, the infant spends a great deal of time under its mother's feet. Household tasks may be more difficult; the child interrupts, imitates, and in a whole variety of ways clamors for his mother's attention. The presence of a television set may make things apparently very much easier. The child is put in front of the screen and watches—sometimes for hours. Television shows children a distortion of reality; all actions have an instant, instead of a long-term, effect; time in terms of years is meaningless; objects are easily acquired; violence is really meaningless or clean and neat. Apart from all this, and as important, is that television implicitly puts children in an extremely passive position (Stein and Frederick, 1971). They experience constant stimulation from outside with little activity from themselves (Murray, 1971). This may mean that, when adolescence is reached, young people may expect their "needs" to be met with little effort on their part, a difficulty that may be increased because of the confusion in adolescence of needs and wants. Even if this confusion is not present, it is unrealistic for individuals to expect that their needs will necessarily be met; society does not automatically do this. Thus adolescents develop an implicitly passive approach to life, in which they expect to be entertained by it. There is a remarkable similarity between those adolescents who take drugs for their vivid visual impressions, which they inertly and passively watch within the picture frame of their own minds, and those who sat as small children in equivalent positions watching a television screen.

Television offers many distortions of reality: Goods are desirable and easy to acquire, and there is no need to work for them. Youth is crudely exploited. The anxiety of many young people about their sexual attractiveness is supposedly to be relieved by the application of one or another skin lotion. All this may cause as much difficulty as the amount of violence seen by children on television, which has caused so much public concern. Children acquire the imprint of violence as being a rather distant, clean mechanism. People may be punched, kicked, and knocked unconscious, and shortly afterwards rise to their feet with a polite trickle of blood coming from the corner of their mouths. Clean fighting, using only bare fists, is now almost unknown among young people who watch numerous violent episodes on television. In the United States the knife and the gun are glorified on TV. There is no proof that television alone has contributed to the spread of violence, although it is difficult to believe that it does not have something to do with it. Children are very imitative, and it may well be that violence seen on the screen may encourage some disturbed adolescents to express their own feelings violently (Arkin *et al.*, 1968). But most psychiatrists cannot find clinical evidence of this, although reports of sadism in newspapers and on television can produce a crop of imitators (Miller, 1969).

There has been some public discussion as to the effects of television on the reading habits of the population-at-large but little about its effects on educational techniques or human relationships in general. But television also affects personality development because it exposes the private lives and behavior of well-known people.

Mass Media and Heroes

If they are to develop mature personalities themselves, adolescents need to have hero figures, preferably real people whom they can genuinely admire. The use of the press, television, and radio, with their easy exposé of the flaws in people's personalities and their often superficial approach to problems, may mean that the adolescent's need for distant people to admire cannot be met. Even those young people whom they erect as potential heroes for themselves, are often rapidly exposed as having feet of clay. The failures, deficiencies, and sometimes dishonesty of public figures become available for all to watch, so there is little possibility of young people idealizing anyone.

Heroes ultimately undergo a symbolic death and with the present generation's preoccupation with youthfulness, this death may be associated with aging. Paul McCartney, one of the Beatles, was rumored to have died in late 1969. The excessive mourning of many adolescents signified his departure as their hero figure.

Adolescent Guilt and Isolation

Information given by the mass media in many other ways can enhance the problems of young people. The division of the world into rich and poor nations poses particular problems for perceptive youth in the West. They are made aware, if they use their eyes at all, that they are members of a generally rich society in which most people do not die of starvation. However, even if there were no pictures on a television screen, it would be difficult to deny the presence of the poor. In America the ghetto is just a block down the street in large cities; in Britain starvation stares at well-fed young people from numerous posters advertising famine relief in Africa. Affluent adolescents in the West are uneasily aware that they are envied by the less privileged; they may guiltily feel they have done nothing to deserve their own worldly goods. Some, perhaps as a result of the conflict about this, feel that the appropriate response is either to drop out of a society that they see as alienating and selfish or, alternately, to look deprived and decrepit. In the way they attack society, such young people may unconsciously behave in a similar arbitrary, brutal, and uncaring fashion to the adults they criticize.

Social isolation is one of the major pressures that twentieth-century living inflicts on the young. It is also relevant to the parental world, which is not as uncaring as angry frustrated youth often suggest. A particular problem may develop for both parents and children in large cities and in areas where rapid social change is occurring. These are societies that often have a few built-in techniques by which people outside the immediate family circle can care for each other. In the United States, which has had to cope with mobility for a longer period than has Europe, society has developed ritualized ways of having newcomers to a society meet others. These rituals are relatively meaningless, however, as people do not really become involved with each other until they are sure that separation is not imminent. American children are, thus, in much the same situation as those in societies that have not even developed informal routines to make relationships possible. The isolation of families can mean that parents may not have friends with whom they can discuss the growth and maturation of their children. As a result, parents can become overinvolved with them.

Parental Isolation

Social isolation also means that parents are vulnerable to what their children say happens in other families. Parents may not have sufficient contact themselves to know whether or not this is true. The effect of this lack of parental knowledge is shown by adolescents' demanding that parents stay away from home when they are having a party. Adolescents insist that this is what their friends' parents do and claim that they will be humiliated if their fathers or mothers behave differently. Parents isolated from other family groups are likely to give in to the request; if their relationships with other families are tenuous, parents will not be able to get support from friends when they stand out against their children's pressures. Finally, the isolation of the nuclear family puts individual marriages under greater stress than otherwise might be the case. Fathers seek the phony intimacy of the bar, the pub, or the golf course—clubcar situations in which people appear to care about each other but where the interest does not extend beyond the confines of the activity. Mothers who become unemployed in their homemaking role when their children reach adolescence may go out to work, watch television, or become depressed. The effect of the isolation of individual families is to make them less comfortable family units.

Most parents intuitively understand a good deal about adolescence and often convey this understanding by a series of complaints; their children are difficult, rude, impossible to please, untidy, careless, and unappreciative. It is less usual for parents to talk of the way their adolescent children are expanding their interests in life and becoming more involved in the world. The excitement of youth is less often noted although many are well aware of this. In a larger social network, some of the assets of adolescence, as well as liabilities, will be discussed.

It would appear that society is polarizing the development of its young people. On the one hand, many adolescents, weathering the numerous stresses placed upon them, are healthier, more mature, more outgoing, and more giving perhaps than any previous generation. On the other, a minority who become disturbed are exposed to so much stress and are offered so little in the way of community and other supports that they tend to become more obviously destructive than in the past. These adolescents are in need of specific psychological and other help. Most young people would be considerably assisted by changes in our social organizations, schools, colleges, universities, and community agencies. Almost all psychological help for the disturbed young requires assistance from the people within the institutions in which adolescents spend most of the day. Unless nonpsychologically trained people who are in constant contact with youth improve their skill in forming and keeping relationships with adolescents, expert help for the disturbed is attenuated in its usefulness; psychological growth is impeded.

References

Arkin, G. C., et al. (1968), *The Effects of Television in Children and Youth; A Review of Theory and Research*. Rev. ed. Vol. 6 of *Television and Social Behavior*. Washington, D.C.: Government Printing Office.

Block, H., and Neiderhoffer, A. (1958), *The Gang*. New York: Philosophical Library.

Bott, E. J. (1957), *Family and Social Network*. London: Tavistock Publications.

Fox, R. (1967), *Kinship and Marriage*. Harmondsworth: Penguin.

Gesell, A., and Ilg, F. L. (1943), *Infant and Child in the Culture of Today*. New York: Harper.

Ginott, H. (1965), *Between Parent and Child*. New York: Macmillan.

Group for Advancement of Psychiatry (1963), *Normal Adolescence*. Report No. 68. New York: American Psychiatry Association.

James, C. (1968), *Young Lives at Stake*. London: Collins.

Kandel, D., *et al.* (1968), *Adolescents in Two Societies*. Cambridge: Harvard University Laboratory of Human Development.

Masterson, J. F. (1967), *The Psychiatric Dilemma of Adolescence*. Boston: Little, Brown.

Menninger, K. A. (1963), *The Vital Balance*. New York: Viking.

Miller, D. (1969), *The Age Between*. London: Hutchinson.

———— (1970), Adolescents and the high school system. *J. Community Ment. Health,* 66: 483–491.

———— (1973), Adolescent crisis: Challenge for patient, parent, and internist. *Ann. Intern. Med.,* 79: 435–440.

Murray, J. P. (1971), Television in inner city homes: Viewing behavior in young boys. In *Television in Day to Day Life Patterns of Use,* Vol. 4 of *Television and Social Behavior,* ed. E. A. Rubenstein *et al.* Washington, D.C.: Government Printing Office.

Offer, D. (1969), *The Psychological World of the Teenager*. New York: Basic Books.

Riesman, D. (1950), *The Lonely Crowd*. New Haven: Yale University Press.

Spock, B. (1945), *Baby and Child Care*. New York: Cardinal.

Stein, A. H., and Frederick, L. K. (1971), Television and content and young children's behavior. In *Television and Social Learning,* Vol. 2 of *Television and Social Behavior,* ed. J. P. Murray *et al.* Washington, D.C.: Government Printing Office.

7

The World of School

Problems of Creativity

Although the generation gap is not necessarily the chasm that some publicists imply, there is, nevertheless, at present an alienation between the generations. Although it does not apply to everyone, the isolation of youth from adults is common in all societies of the West. This difficulty has been created by the inability of society to offer emotional anchor points to adolescents, especially in the breakdown of the extended family and tribal-type relationships. Furthermore, it is increasingly difficult for society to give young people an opportunity to be creative. In the past the failure of society to provide for the adequate education of young people was covered mostly by physical deprivation or the absence of awareness that more appropriate education was possible. Now well-fed youth often appear to be increasingly aware of inner feelings of emptiness and desolation; deprived young people angrily demand equal treatment for themselves. With the view that the present generation should pay for the misdeeds of the past, the underprivileged often demand "reparations." This insistence on meeting personal and group needs at whatever cost to others with a pseudointellectual justification is the same attitude that led to the creation of the out-group. Young people project onto their parents' generation a boring, dull,

complacent, self-centered, unimaginative, and materialistic image. This projection may have some accuracy, but it is also a
projection of the anxiety of many young people that this is what
they are themselves. The organization of education can lead to
an inhibition of creativity and an enhancement of passivity. Over-
obedience to a highly rigid system leads to alternation between
passive compliance, alienated conformity, hostile projection onto
minority groups and ideas, and intermittent rebellious violence.

Many intelligence tests have been standardized to measure
cognitive functions, retention, reasoning capacity, and the ability
to make abstractions (Torrance, 1962). The lack of interest in
creativity and imagination is evident in that these cannot be
assessed by any standard tests that are easily and accurately
applied to large numbers (Getzels and Jackson, 1960). Tests of
creativity do have validity, but it is apparent that standardized
tests of IQ are given much more weight as an indication of ability.

Children brought up in a reasonably optimum way—loved,
fed, nurtured, and respected for their sexuality as boys and
girls—are able to be creative, the extent of this depending on
a mixture of genetic endowment, nurture, and personality development (Speigal, 1958). In grade school the child's enjoy-
ment in its capacity to be creative in play, in imagination, painting, building, and games begins to plateau at about the age of
nine. However, after only one to two years of standard closed-
system, classroom teaching in grades one and two, many children
are already somewhat unsure of themselves and unwilling to take
intellectual chances without the permission of the teacher. A
grade-five teacher commented to a group of parents that if she
told the children to follow the written instructions in a book,
most of them felt obligated to check that this is what really was
wanted. British grade schools have used the so-called open classroom for many years, but until recently, and still in many situations, there was a change in classroom structure at age nine
from small-group teaching to a standard checkerboard of desks

with teachers isolated at the front of the room. At this point creativity declines and children start to talk of their teachers as "they."

In the United States grade school teaching has rarely been as highly imaginative as in good British primary schools. Until very recently group teaching had not caught the imagination of American primary school teachers, who have been preoccupied with teaching by reinforcement and tend to put themselves at the end of an oblong classroom. Many still do not understand, furthermore, that the open classroom does not mean permissive abandonment of control.

Americans are generally concerned about the need of people to get on with each other; it is remarkable, then, that the social environment of the school system even in grade school, makes this difficult, because consistent interpersonal relationships are insufficiently valued. Although grade schools are concerned with the child's use of its creative imagination, stress is placed on a high degree of conformity, being obedient, and keeping up with certain age norm standards.

The necessity to achieve in an academic field is given particular status by most schools. When school taxation is not passed, vocational subjects tend to be rapidly erased. In any case, an either–or situation, creative and imaginative against academic and and intellectual achievement, is implicitly assumed. In one affluent school system that was economizing, for example, children in grade ten who took academic subjects could not, if they wanted a balance of science and humanities, also take a vocational subject. The preoccupation with academic achievement for intellectual adolescents is partly based on the demands made by society But creative learning requires teachers who are able to make meaningful, positive emotional relationships with their pupils; it is no accident that it is in the art room of many schools that teachers are felt and seen to be real people. Art teachers do not normally hide behind status and desks.

The maximum problems of creative inhibition seem to ap-

pear when the child becomes pubertal at the beginning of adolescence. There are many reasons for this, some in the psychology
of this age period, some in the organization of the school. The
process of puberty produces a situation in which adolescents
seem able to be creative in fits and starts; many of their imaginative resources appear to be drained off into daydreaming.
When puberty is over, boys and girls are psychologically more
free to be creative. Creativity at the end of the pubertal period
also assists in the mastery of emotional conflicts (Blos, 1962, p.
181), as is obvious both from the poetry of fifteen-to-seventeen-
year-olds and from their paintings and sculpture. But in most
Western countries the right to pursue higher education depends
almost totally on intellectual, rather than on social or physical
achievement. Many potentially academic young people have creative talent, and the overconcentration on examinations, aptitude
tests, and grades does not destroy this. In many, however, an artificial peak of creativity may appear before individuals get enmeshed in the conformity of society. This peak often occurs at
the end of early adolescence, a period of maximum sexual potency
and rebelliousness (Bernfield, 1924).

School as an Interference with Personality Growth

Some junior high schools remove adolescents at the peak of
pubertal turmoil, usually at twelve to thirteen from the grade
school. Children are moved to new environments at the same
time they are coping with the inner turmoil of puberty; so internal and external confusion occur together. Another change at
fifteen also interferes with personality growth. Children in early
adolescence need to test out the personality strengths of the
adults in their environment whom they might hope to use later
as models for personality development. Change to high school
at the beginning of a period of identity consolidation means that
adolescents have to go through another period of testing the

adults in their environment. Even if consistent relationships with teachers were possible, scheduling usually negates this. Finally, in grades eleven and twelve, the pressure is to produce high grades to assist in college entry. So the potential creativity of the midadolescent age period tends to be inhibited by both the arrangement of the educational system and its teaching techniques. The decline of creativity reported by psychologists (Wolfenstein, 1956) as a function of "the adolescent process" may well be due to the negative reinforcement of the educational system.

In Britain the potentially academic student might expect to have five years in the same school from the age of thirteen. There is a greater likelihood of retaining some teachers for two to three years' time. There is an inappropriate push toward taking entrance examinations at fifteen or sixteen and then a further examination two years later. This system, which produces emotional stability, still impedes creativity by a demand for convergent thinking (Blos, 1962, p. 125).

In the British system the essential demand of examinations, with essay-type questions lasting about thirty minutes, is for conformity and a willingness on the part of the adolescent to forego a creative interest in one particular aspect of a subject in order to answer all the questions on the examination paper. A highly imaginative, creative adolescent may find it almost intolerable to abandon the proper study of a subject; such young people may feel that they must answer one question in depth. These individuals are likely to be discarded by the British system. Examination failure due to reluctance to answer all the questions on the paper may be related to a refusal to compromise. It is necessary to answer all the questions because the first 50 percent of the mark on any one question is easier to obtain than the next 30 percent. The multiple-choice examination of American education uses a different technique, but, except for the especially able, creativity is inhibited. Because of technology and increasing leisure time this inhibition is a luxury society can no longer afford.

There are many forms of creativity, some associated with genius and talent, others with less dramatic forms of imaginative productions. Some types of creativity are highly agreeable to society: Obviously masculine creativity in adolescent boys is very acceptable when it involves activity and competitiveness in groups; a boy's need for more feminine, tender creativity, also part of manhood, causes anxiety to some adults and then to adolescents themselves. Cooking and baby-caring may be temporary, if important, creative activities for adolescent boys. Men are allowed to work at a camp-out, with an outdoor barbecue, and this is not seen as effeminate. But a boy cooking in his mother's kitchen is not often felt to be generally desirable. In a British school for delinquent boys the toughest youngsters chose, as a preferred activity, a cooking class. Initially, only sweet cakes and cookies were made, then the boys began to bake, make preserves, and work for others, not just themselves.

Problems of Talent

Talented adolescents of both sexes are likely to have particular problems. Talent makes those who possess it feel unique, and they may never quite know whether they are loved for themselves or their talent. Apart from the stress of not being sure that his activity will be economically viable, the potential artist, during adolescence, is perceived by many peers and adults as being insufficiently manly (Guildford, 1959). In midadolescence when identity is being consolidated, it is difficult for adolescents to decide that their talent will be their life's work. Many wish to keep a foot in the routine academic camp, but a budding violinist has to practice for four to five hours daily. It is impossible for such young people to have full lives and concentrate on academic grades. A ballet dancer is not normally also a mathematician. Those adolescents whose primary emotional involvement is in their creative talent have unique problems

(Wilson, 1956). Many artists appear to take longer to develop a firm feeling of self than those without such talents. When they seek higher education, however, the talented are more fortunate than others: Admission to good art schools depends on the quality of work produced over a period of time rather than on grades and SAT's. Still, art students often face particular emotional problems in colleges; it is difficult with a particular field of talent, for example, painting, sculpture, or singing, to be involved in the routine studies of those academic courses that may be required for graduation. The jury system may expose vulnerable students to intense pain particularly if staff are insensitive:

> Karl, a nineteen-year-old was being treated for severe depression. This had followed the death by suicide of his alcoholic father when the boy was twelve. Slowly in the course of therapy the young man developed a sense of his own worth. As with many talented people this always depended on his feeling that his artistic productions were valued. He held a one-man show in his home town during a vacation and the selling of some pictures was immensely supportive. When he returned to school, his professor told him at a jury that a picture of which he was particularly proud was "shallow and pretentious and showed a lack of masculinity." Two weeks later the boy killed himself by covering his face in a plastic bag and suffocating.

Modern painting techniques, with which young students wish to identify themselves, do not offer much in the way of personality support. Apart from Karl's particular experience, art teachers often comment about the personality of their students in a pseudopsychologizing way on the basis of artistic productions.

Vulnerability is the hallmark of the talented. Both artists and musicians tend to see what they produce as direct extensions of themselves. To criticize a flautist's playing may be a severe personal criticism; to tear a painting apart is to shatter the artist.

Those who study the fine arts, as distinct from the practical arts, find it difficult to establish a role for themselves in society. They are often told that they must know how to express themselves in their chosen media, but it is difficult for them to see how they can produce works that will be sold. Because of economic fear some adolescents abandon their wish to use their talent in order to comply with the system that values less artistic endeavors. Creative impulses may be channeled into socially acceptable paths or abandoned.

> Hillel was the eighteen-year-old son of a rather passive, distant accountant and a swamping, overpowering mother. He sought treatment because of a fear of homosexuality, but actually he was unable to get close to anyone, male or female. His homosexual wishes, which he felt as forbidden, made it possible for him to refuse to involve himself with anyone. With economic motives in mind, he was taking advertising because he felt that if he committed himself to art he could never be successful. After therapy he abandoned both his homosexual fantasies and his advertising goal; he became a heterosexual struggling artist.

Some talented adolescents have an intense creative drive and resist the conformist pressures of the educational system, but the sheer volume of work required in some fields may spoil their efforts. If talented youngsters are to be assisted they almost certainly need special schools such as the one founded in England by Yehudi Menuhin.

Problems of Genius

Another group of adolescents with particular problems are those who may be considered geniuses. A genius who has extraordinary intellectual power may also be talented and possess a special artistic aptitude; however, there is no reason why a genius should be talented or vice versa. The problem for the genius is that advancement in the educational system beyond the usual age norms does not allow boys or girls to make satisfactory comparisons about nonacademic achievement with age-group peers. On the other hand, when such children are held back to their age norm in school they become restless, bored, and difficult to handle (Hollingworth, 1939). If genius is not to be wasted, there is probably no alternative but to opt for a situation that allows an adolescent to advance at his or her academic pace. By adolescence, however, the genius is less mature, as measured by a capacity to tolerate frustration in nonacademic fields, than the less-able peer. Similarly, a genius is likely to be chronologically older than peers before developing a capacity either for an active sexual life or a tender loving relationship with a member of the opposite sex.

> Robert, age twenty-two, entered college at sixteen and medical school at nineteen. He sought counseling help at twenty-two because, "I have never had a girl, whoever heard of a virgin of twenty-two." He showed no marked evidence of emotional disturbance but in his sexual relationships was more like the usual somewhat diffident sixteen- or seventeen-year-old. A year later he was involved in a passionate love affair with a girl he later married. He had been seen three times in all by a psychiatrist.

Teachers as Significant Adults

The more society fails to cope with the problems of adolescence, or even hinders adolescent growth, the greater is the responsibility for personality development placed on schools. As teachers may be unprepared for the role that is thrust upon them, it can be quite frightening; it is not surprising, then, that many teachers tend to project the blame for pupil disturbance on to the youngsters themselves or their parents.

Many teachers are overwhelmed by the demands of parents and children for help; they feel unable to assist because of their lack of training. They say their job is to teach, not to look after disturbed children; it is for social workers to cope with difficult families. Unfortunately, teachers often manage to escape from responsibility for such children in their care. Though they are present in the classroom every day, schedules that expose teachers to 120 different children each day allow many not to notice those who are disturbed, unless their behavior is grossly disruptive. The teacher's probable failure is, of course, not restricted to disturbed children. Schools are social organizations that can influence in a significant way the psychological development and behavior of all their pupils throughout their lives.

There is confusion about the appropriate goals for a school (Silberman, 1970). It is generally felt that schools should provide children with a formal education according to their ability. Society has devised ways in which young people with academic ability can be recognized, but those young people who do not have the ability should not leave school feeling that they are inadequate, that they have not successfully graduated into life. Adolescents often leave high school crushed by sterile competition—labeled as failures because they are not academic or because they develop slowly. Teachers know now that if they track groups of children according to their academic ability or place them in subject sets of differing standards, the results tend to be a faithful reflection of the teacher's original opinions (James, 1968, pp. 181–185). It is recognized that schools should not categorize children as successes or failures. An overpreoccupation with grade-point averages for adolescents means that adolescents are labeled as they leave school.

Effects of Emotional Deprivation on Adolescence

Confused notions of human intelligence have led to the apparent belief in some circles that all human beings have the potential to be highly academic, if only the school and social environment would behave in a sensible manner. This, of course, is a fantasy. There *are* innate differences of intelligence.

There is no doubt, however, that emotional and intellectual deprivation in early childhood impairs human potential at all levels. Emotionally deprived children are most often found among the very rich and the very poor, since neither group of children gets consistent parental handling. The rich tend to be looked after by nannies who are likely to change, the poor are farmed out to a succession of friends, baby-minders, and elderly relatives.

Deprived children brought up in poverty are likely to have their intelligence impaired by physical and emotional deprivation. Often they cannot play satisfactorily with toys that stimulate their intelligence and imagination because these cannot be afforded. The situation is compounded by bad schools, but these only reinforce the inadequacy; they do not create it. The myth is then propounded that special academic enrichment in the late teens may reverse this process. This may work for some, but it fails for many; just as bussing children from neighborhood stability may help a few but clearly disturbs others. This solution, however, offers a deceptive simplicity. It is relatively inexpensive, and failure can be blamed on black and white racism.

The answer lies not just in raising the economic level of the poor, although this is crucial, nor in providing work for fathers, so their sense of worth can be reinforced. Enrichment is needed in the lives of impoverished children in infancy and childhood. The current fad is to try to provide this through day-care centers. The great disadvantage of these, however, is the rapid staff turnover. Children are overwhelmed by multiple handling and the instability of adult–child relationships. A better technique is to teach mothers how to play creatively with blocks and toys with their children, rather than having them watch television. Then, from the age of two-and-a-half, approximately, when separation from parents becomes acceptable, children can go to day-care centers for about two hours daily, hopefully leading to an excellent grade-school experience. Many experts are unaware that this is the successful technique that the Israelis applied to the deprived ghetto children of North African immigrants. It was noticed that these children seemed unable to make the adjustments necessary for them to learn to read. As children, they played only with sand, never with blocks. When the mothers were taught to show their children how to play with building blocks, reading skills at age six markedly improved in the children who had been taught this at three, compared to those who had not been taught to play in this way.

How Schools Can Help Personality Growth

Art, music, expressive drama, and topic and project teaching all assist schoolchildren with the development of academic and imaginative potential. Along with this, a major goal of a good school should be the development of a mutual caring relationship between the children. To make this possible, the structure of a school should allow for constancy in teacher–pupil relationships; many staff will need to be taught how to relate to children in a way that will be felt as meaningful and caring. In a crowded conurbation this is more important than fostering personalities capable of living in isolation. Another goal should be to develop the personalities of young people, so that they are capable of personal initiative and flexible enough to envisage at least one major occupational change in their lives as desirable, as well as inevitable. These goals make many arbitrary demands of adults look quite irrelevant. A preoccupation with hair length and saluting the flag is still seen as the answer to the malaise of the young. Written disciplinary codes with tariffs of punishment and a legislative preoccupation with the form of prosecution are considered a substitute for caring.

Those schools that attack adolescents on side issues may inculcate a senseless and dangerous arbitrariness; the young may identify with the approach, which so often accompanies a preoccupation with the petty, unimportant superficialities of existence. They may come to believe that because a man is short haired and well groomed he is necessarily a better person than someone less well-turned-out. Alternatively, the young may appear to give in and show a bland passivity in their approach to the world. This makes learning more difficult: the assent demanded by the school may force pupils to use emotional energies in trying to maintain personal integrity with a hidden "no." Such a conflict is most evident in those countries where schools are particularly rigid and where questioning teachers is traditionally seen as currying favor. It is extraordinarily difficult for young adults from such backgrounds to ask questions later on, at a university lecture or with politicians. Those who get round to questioning often fail to wait for answers.

Some adults still behave towards adolescents as if all that is needed to produce personality growth is telling children what to do. If repeated orders fail, they then apply a variety of punishments, as if all the school wants is passive compliance. The complexities of relationships are understood intuitively by many teachers, but they are not taught satisfactorily to the rest.

The adolescent personality is in many ways very plastic. A judicious placing of children in particular classes and subjects can assist the resolution of anxieties and conflicts. The example below was taken from a British high school. It is most improbable that this technique could be used in America, where, although classes can be hand scheduled, this is usually done by a computer. The changeover of teachers is also more rapid than in the average English school, and drama is not used routinely as part of the teaching of English.

An inhibited boy in a boys' school found it quite impossible to express normal aggressive impulses in a constructive way. John was shy and withdrawn and not as academically successful as his level of intelligence would have led one to expect, although he was not a total academic failure. John was considerably helped by his environment. Instead of being put in an art class and allowed to do the rather meticulous compulsive paintings that he liked, he was directed by his art teacher toward a more slapdash dramatic form of expressive art. In school plays, instead of being typecast as a weak, inadequate person, he was put in the position of having to play out a more aggressive, more definite role. The school avoided any temptation to use a carping tone in his school reports that would only have made his parents worried. John reacted by becoming more at ease, and there was some improvement in his academic work.

Except in cities with a private school system, the overall conformity of the high school system makes the recommendation for a helpful school transfer unlikely. This is, however, changing. In some junior high schools a small house system is being devised with continuity of teacher–pupil relationships; some large high schools have created "free schools" within their walls, along with a more conformist type of education. If a school cannot provide a wide-enough range of subjects to meet a pupil's needs, it may be possible to recommend that the youngster change schools.

Tom, who had a bossy, anxious mother and a father who was often away on business had always been difficult at school. His mother nagged him and demanded that he do many household tasks such as cooking and housecleaning. When he became angry she beat him with a riding crop. Although potentially academic, his school achievement was lamentable. His school was preoccupied with grades, valued only very good athletic players and conformist behavior, which, because of his family, Tom found impossible.

Tom was moved to a school that provided many varieties of nonconformist physical activity and the opportunity to construct furniture and play music. These gave Tom outlets for his pent-up aggression, and they also allowed him to feel acceptably masculine. Within a year, there was also a dramatic improvement in his academic work.

Those children who are so damaged in infancy that they cannot make meaningful human relationships will probably not be helped by a normal school environment. Special classes in the average high school may contain them, but these are the individuals who become runaways, academic drop-outs, drug dependent, or juvenile and, later, adult delinquents. Young people who are capable only of a dependent childlike relationship because their capacity for further maturation has been damaged may remain emotionally tied to their school, which at least makes these relationships possible. The least inadequate may make an apparently satisfactory social adjustment but will, if they go to college, often remain intensively involved in alumni associations. Others may make an apparently good adjustment at school but become inert and unable to function independently when they leave. They sometimes find a solution by living and working in highly structured schoollike environments such as the army or in highly bureaucratized administrations typical at some large industries, universities, hospitals, and government. In a sense they never grow out of school.

Emotionally vulnerable girls in particular may find it difficult to free themselves from the relationships established in sororities. They may remain emotionally involved with their adolescent friends for the rest of their lives, not by choice but because of their psychological rigidity.

The Small House To Promote Emotional Growth

There are a number of relatively inexpensive changes that can be made that should make possible a happier and more tension-free educational environment. Even if this does not solve all the problems created by adolescent tension, it must create situations in which different sexes, ethnic, and social groups become more aware of each other as people. The separation of teachers from their pupils appears to be built into the educational system. Scheduling of classes seems to ensure that teachers will not know their pupils. Worse, no effort is made to ensure that children can be in classes with their friends, although it is perfectly possible to schedule a youngster's day so that at least half the classes are taken with the same people. Traditional classroom design symbolizes the educational system's unawareness of what makes for easy and comfortable human relations. Putting a teacher at one end of a rectangular room, with pupils arranged in serried rows in front of him makes it very difficult for him to relate to any of the class at any one time. Teachers with powerful personalities can conquer this type of room arrangement, but many teachers cannot project themselves in this way. Customarily the class divides implicitly into a group of children who sit by the window, whose attention wanders to what goes on outside; a group who sleep at the back and do their best not to be noticed; and, finally, difficult children at the front, often those who seek attention or who want the approval of the teachers. The typical classroom may allow isolated children to be virtually ignored for years by their teachers, providing they hand in passable work. This setup enables some children to go through school without talking in any meaningful way to their teachers.

Group relationships are generally insufficiently considered in the typical school, and opportunities to make emotionally meaningful contacts are thus lost. The maximum number of people to whom one other person can easily relate at one time in one place is eight. If a teacher is to have a class of thirty children, classrooms should be arranged so that the teacher can relate to four groups of eight children and is not faced with the impossible task of relating perpetually to the larger whole. In very large classes so much discipline is required from the average teacher that a warm pupil–teacher relationship is practically impossible. In the classroom arranged in groups the teacher can have a central, rather than peripheral, relationship to the children.

Ironically, there are well-designed primary school classrooms in Britain or the United States where children are taught

around tables or in small groups, and there are similarly conceived science laboratories for adolescents. Tradition alone, perhaps based on the image of the preacher or the poor law overseer,
has made for the typical classroom. If the logic of small-group
teaching is inescapable for infants and scientists, it is equally
inescapable through all parts of the school curriculum and for all
ages. If furniture and classrooms were designed to make this
possible, the effectiveness of teachers would improve, for it would
be harder for staff and pupils to hide behind their status and their
desks.

The development of particularly large high schools has
made many wonder what arrangements can best promote secure
relationships. It is recognized that one teacher can only relate
satisfactorily to a certain number of pupils. But a pupil needs to
relate to teachers over periods of time *longer than a semester or
a year.* There is no reason why half a school day should not be
spent with the same two or three teachers and the other half in
modular classes. It may be argued that one of the three teachers
could be less than satisfactory, but children also have to learn
that all human relationships are not satisfactory, and techniques
of dealing with this are necessary as well.

The concept of a small house, essentially a subdivision of
the larger unit with a viable social group of its own, has never
been widespread in the United States. Yet a study of morale in
the British Royal Air Force clearly showed that men do not get
emotional support from identification with a larger unit, and can
only identify with relatively small groups (Ministry of Defense,
1966). The homeroom teacher with a primary task of being
particularly helpful to a group of pupils in their psychological,
social, and educational needs for one year seemed to be an attempt to provide the equivalent support to the small-house unit.
The fact that in many schools homerooms disappeared with a
reduction of budgets indicates that this role failed or was not
understood by either teachers or administrators. The problem is
partly, that homerooms often offered the only sense of stability

in a pupil's schoolday that was not highly structured; therefore, much tension was relieved there. Not understanding this, many teachers responded with a sterile repression. Furthermore, teachers often do not understand the need for group stability and adult–adolescent relationships that last more than one year; usually the homeroom teacher changed as the grade ended.

A number of alternatives to the small house are possible. If a year teacher travels up the school with pupils, a group of adolescents will have the same form teacher for a number of years. This is sometimes called a "social form" organization. In some European schools a change of form teacher takes place after the children have moved up a grade, one change taking place in September, the other after Christmas. Breaking with teachers each year is not helpful—particularly for children in the mid-adolescent period of development who need to keep the same relationship for three or four years in order to make satisfactory identifications.

In the house system a given number of pupils stay in one house for their school career and have one or two staff members who have a teaching role but who also act as their personal and educational counselors. This system does not allow the splitting of pedagogic, disciplinary, administrative, and personal counseling roles. When this split is made, adolescents tend to see people only in their subidentities, they are not provided with whole personalities upon whom they can model themselves. The same applies to teachers. In one high school, if a pupil missed a number of classes, the teacher did not ask why or say he was missed, the pupil was sent to a counselor to be disciplined. If it was thought the individual had personal problems, he was then directed to the school social worker. Adolescents communicate in actions as well as in words, and to turn difficult behavior, a possible request for personal help, into a communication as an end in itself is not helpful to the pupil or the school.

A house system only produces a possible structure for human relations. When house staff fail to understand the needs of children, the house may then become only a means of promoting intramural competitiveness. It is probable that even a perceptive man or woman cannot know more than forty children well. If houses contain more, other staff members must take special responsibility for different youngsters. It then becomes important that the school hierarchy does not conspicuously esteem one such staff member above another.

Whichever system is used, the key factors are that nonparental adult relationships and peer-group attachments are essential for the development of adolescents and one adult can only relate satisfactorily to a certain given number of other human beings at any one time. It is also important to young people that they be able to keep emotionally meaningful relationships that are significant to them through a large part of their school careers. If some teachers who teach academic subjects are to change, then other teachers involved in the more personal side of pupil's lives should be available to them continuously over a period of years.

Just as forty children to a class are too many for a teacher so are forty staff to a principal. Since a school usually has a staff over ten, it will clearly be necessary for a principal to put himself in a position akin to that of managing director: Ultimately he will find himself relating to heads of departments, each of which will break down into groups of eight to ten. The heads of departments will be his "managers" and his main relationship will be to them, rather than to the people on the factory floor, in this case the other teachers and then the pupils themselves.

Large high schools of 1,000 to 2,000 children require a high degree of autonomy for different parts of the organization and probably do not need the overcentralization created by a principal. In most schools academic and vocational departments receive a high degree of autonomy, but there is no recognition that small social units with stability and autonomy are equally necessary. Each huge school could be a collection of smaller units of two to three hundred, each sharing common educational facilities. Otherwise, there is no viable possibility of creating a helpful relationship between staff and pupils. At Eton College in England a relatively large school of 1,200 pupils is broken up into houses of approximately 100 each. The pupils see themselves as belonging to the larger school, but their first and most important emotional attachment is to the smaller house. It is this type of emotional belonging that helps adolescents to identify with the way of life of organizations.

Teacher-Pupil Relationships in the Etiology of Disturbance

The relationship between school boards and management, administrative and teaching staff sets the stage for the relationship between teachers and pupils. When a group of pupils become disurbed, the staff should look at their own social organization and their relationship to the youngsters instead of projecting all the responsibility onto the pupils, their ethnic and social subgroups, or parents and society. All behavior is multidetermined, but it is remarkable how when there is, for example, racial tension, usually everything is considered except staff relationships, social system structure, and the possible psychological needs of the individual young people concerned.

If schools are to fulfill the role given to them by society, teachers must be seen as valued. Perhaps, in unconscious revenge for the errors of past pedagogues, society refuses to pay teachers properly. If this interpretation is accurate, society's neurotic reaction is highly expensive. But the devaluation of teachers may not be just a matter of low pay. Educational authorities who publicly overrule teachers on issues of school reorganization may devalue their staff. On the other hand, the conservatism of many teachers means that sophisticated techniques of social change are necessary to help schools.

The responsibility of the community is to develop people

who fulfill their personal potential; this responsibility the community largely passes on to schools. Adolescents normally identify with the way of life that they perceive in their environment. But the qualities they acquire most easily are those possessed by their parents and the circle in which they have always lived. If their school has a way of life that is totally unlike that of their family, they will find it difficult to identify with it. For this reason schools should consider the needs of the local community; they should not unthinkingly expose children to cultural shock by imposing a way of life quite unlike that learned in their homes and primary schools (Bernstein, 1967). This is a major issue in school integration problems. Teaching white or black children black history may be desirable; it is no solution to the problems caused by an impersonal social organization weighing on individual adolescents. When the significance of personal relationships is really incorporated into the American high school, then the communication problems of differing ethnic and social groups can genuinely be taken into account.

The secondary school cannot widen the horizons of all its pupils. But it can be the catalyst for future change with many of them. The school alone cannot reverse all the damage inflicted on an adolescent who has suffered severe emotional deprivation in the first year of life. But for those children who had a good early experience but were damaged by painful happenings a little later, schools can provide the essential link in repair by offering the good emotional experiences which they are uniquely able to give. This remains a hopeful potential.

References

Bernfeld, S. (1924), Vom dischtenschen Schaffer der Jugend. *Int. Psych. Verlug. Wein.*

Bernstein, B. (1967), Social structure, language and learning. In

Education of the Disadvantaged, ed. A. H. Pasow *et al.* New York: Holt, Rinehart and Winston.

Blos, P. (1962), *On Adolescence.* Glencoe, Ill.: Free Press.

Getzels, J. W., and Jackson, P. W. (1960), *The Study of Giftedness, A Multidimensional Approach.* Washington, D.C.: U.S. Office of Education (Co-op Research Monographs No. 2).

Guildford, J. P. (1959), Three faces of intellect. *Am. Psychol.,* 14: 469–479.

Hollingworth, L. S. (1939), What we know about the early selection and training of leaders. *Teach. Coll. Rec.,* 40: 575–592.

James, C. (1968), *Young Lives at Stake.* London: Collins.

Ministry of Defense (1966), *The Benson Experiment.* Science 4 (RAF), Memo 50, Appendix H. London.

Silberman, C. E. (1970), *Crisis in the Classroom: The Remaking of American Education.* New York: Random House.

Speigal, L. A. (1958), Comments on the psychoanalytic psychology of adolescence. *Psychoanalytic Study of the Child,* 13: 296–309. New York: International Universities Press.

Torrance, E. P. (1962), *Guiding Creative Talent.* Englewood Cliffs, N.J.: Prentice-Hall.

Wilson, C. (1956), *The Outsider.* Boston: Houghton Mifflin.

Wolfenstein, M. (1956), Analysis of a juvenile poem. *Psychoanalytic Study of the Child,* 11: 450–473. New York: International Universities Press.

8

School Integration: Familial, Racial, and Sexual

Home and School

The interaction between home and school and the effect of this on maturation and integration is poorly understood. Even if schools were able to offer positive emotional support to their pupils, they would regularly face turmoil in some of their charges because of the intense struggle between the dependent and independent needs of adolescents, their inability to contain their own internal conflicts, and the need to project distaste for a part of themselves onto others. Meeting dependent needs, because of the threat this poses to a sense of autonomy, particularly in those adolescents who are psychologically troubled, may cause rebellious behavior. Since no social system is perfect, some degree of in- and out-group prejudice is inevitable in adolescence.

Adults are, in a sense, in a no-win situation in relationship to youth; even good schools are likely to experience turmoil among their adolescent pupils. Because parents do not understand the causes of this, teachers can often get little help from the home. Parents are often as bewildered as the teachers. If there is no understanding between parents and staff before the upsets, they are unlikely to be of mutual help. In a difficult situation parents and teachers tend to blame each other or their children. Many school systems seem to have a fantasy that calling

161

parents when their children have been difficult, or suspending the children from school, will offer an automatic solution to misbehavior. The latter may temporarily relieve the school system of responsibility, but it does not provide an answer. Suspension is often based on a middle-class assumption that parents will want their adolescent children to go to school. Obviously referral of the child to its parents to provide a solution often pushes the problem back to the environment that caused the difficulty. Suspension is an immoral act (Ann Arbor School Board, 1970) and the result of a policy of despair that often believes that control is possible only by a punitive action. What is needed is real cooperation between home and school and an understanding of the etiology of disturbed behavior. When this is antisocial, it is rarely recognized that this may be a symptom not only of individual emotional upset, even if it is only temporary; but also of tension within the social system. The low rate of referral of black children and poor whites to psychiatric clinics is partly caused by the failure to recognize the etiology of the antisocial activity of such individuals. Teachers, school administrators, or parents may not understand that repeated misbehavior is one way in which adolescents communicate a need for help. The appropriate action is thought to be only to control antisocial action; referral to the juvenile courts is the likely suggestion. Parents of white, middle-class children often seek psychological assistance for their children themselves; working-class parents either do not know how to do this, are afraid of the expense, or are filled with shame at their failure. Their children are less likely to be offered psychological assistance.

Before real cooperation between home and school is possible, various problems need to be understood: First, the goals of the adolescent, the parent, and the school may all differ. The adolescent may, deliberately or not, play off the parent against the teacher or the teacher against the parent. The adults may, in their turn, withdraw from or become angry with each other. The adolescent may then see school as a refuge from home or vice versa. Even when parent and teacher are full of good will towards each other, if they are unaware of their differing goals and have no way of communicating, good will is not enough. Often parents of adolescents over the age of fifteen do not understand that a good teacher will not automatically tell them about difficulties their child may have; a teacher's respect for his pupils' striving for autonomy may cause parental anxiety.

Another problem may result from a conflict between the structure and atmosphere of the parent's work situation and that of his child's school. In some sociologically sophisticated environments the world outside home and school—the world of industry—is gradually becoming less coercive (McGregor, 1960). It is being recognized that, if workers are really involved and interested in what they produce, they are far more apt to be effective than if they see themselves as being exploited by assembly lines. This change in industry is taking place more rapidly in countries outside the United States, but it is already recognized here that the threat of unemployment will not solve the problem of poor quality control in, say, the automobile industry. However, the parents who are in jobs that offer emotional satisfaction may either have the bewildering experience of seeing their children fail to get satisfaction in school—and it may not occur to them that anything can be done—or they may fail to notice that their children are having an alienating educational experience:

> A group of parents of thirteen-year-olds, many of whom were on a university staff, attended a "capsule night" at a local junior high school. They made no complaint about the fact that their children had but twenty minutes to eat lunch. The parents were apparently not distressed by the absence of recess and did not seem to register the effect of the barren, tiled lavatory-like walls of the school. Even when a homeroom teacher boasted of the fact that she would not let the children move from their seats (after a day of being educationally harried), the parents sat in silence.

When there is a change in the type of teaching that is offered to some children they find abundant interest and fulfillment at school; on the other hand, their parents may get no real emotional satisfaction at work. These parents may be attacked by their children for being dull and uninteresting, or the children may find themselves quite unable to communicate with them. What is still most usual in society, is that parents and children find themselves in a similar work situation. The parents may work in a factory that treats them as automatons; their children may go to schools they perceive as equally impersonal and authoritarian. Just as many managing directors see the well being of their workers as secondary to profits, some principals and administrators see their individual pupils as secondary to other goals—for example, apparently successful integration, academic achievement, or conformist behavior. Some principals are still convinced that only they have the understanding, the commitment, and the authority to run a school and insist that all decision making must flow from them. The authoritarian school contains the seeds of its own destruction in that it has no way of listening to its pupils. Their words may be heard, but their teachers are not encouraged to respond. Adolescents give up trying to communicate with many staff members, who in turn, resent being given a controlling function with children they do not know. The pupils are, therefore, often seen by teachers as indifferent, unwilling to attend, or needing a high degree of control. Adolescents in such a setting do not have their whole personality engaged; they are given the role of pupils with specific tasks, attending school as if it were a factory, for a given number of hours a day. Parents have the role of coercing their children to conform to the school's requirements. The parent may reject this—and come into conflict with the school—or he may accept it—and clash with his child. Furthermore, groups of children are given and accept labels—blacks, greasers, jocks, freaks, straight—and treated according to this label rather than as special and unique individuals. Schools that have a freer form of organization and staff who involve the whole personality of their pupils in an enjoyable learning experience do their best to avoid parent–child and parent–teacher conflict. Pupils are more likely to enjoy learning when parents are told by schools about their educational goals and techniques.

The pressure for change is on schools insofar as social organization, educational methods, and curriculum are concerned. This may mean that many parents find it difficult to grasp what schools do with their children. If proper cooperation between home and school means anything, schools will then have to show parents what their aims are. School systems can avoid change by playing democratic games, pretending that parents are educational experts; no change can take place without the latter's approval. Community participation can become an excuse for administrative inertia. Local control of school systems via budgetary restraints and school board elections may make innovative changes in education much more difficult. Every layman feels himself to be an expert in education and psychology. Even if a school system wishes to change, this may be stopped as the aims of parents for their children may differ from those of educationalists. Parents often want schools to prepare the children for life only as they have known it. A school that gives a child an education too different from the one the parents had, can cause difficulties. A school may develop the artistic sensitivities of the children of a rigid accountant or give an academic education to the children of an unskilled laborer. Both these enrichments may hinder communication between generations, not just because their interests differ but because different types of communication techniques are used. The staff members of schools need to recognize the nature of the community in which they are placed and the quality of life in the children's homes and social environment. All too often they fail to understand this, particularly with less privileged pupils:

A junior high school's staff were preoccupied with the acutely aggressive behavior of six black girls age thirteen to fourteen. The black staff were as concerned as the white and both tended to project blame, although in different places. Neither took notice of the following simple facts. The disturbances almost always took place after the lunchtime break, in which the children, after lining up in an inadequate dining area, had about fifteen to twenty minutes to eat lunch and return to classes. Most upsets took place at about noon. The girls' day began at 6:30 a.m., when they went to the local community center for breakfast. As well as looking after smaller grade school children, they had to clear up after them. At 7:10 a.m. they caught the bus to school and, having traveled across town from the ghetto area they reached the school at 7:30 a.m. Since the building was not yet officially open, they then waited in a vestibule between two sets of doors if the weather was inclement. After starting classes, they were allowed ten minutes between class periods to move across the school and only at 11:30 a.m. did they get lunch.

School systems are apparently unaware of the developmental needs of adolescents; fifty-minute class periods are too long, but a five-hour stretch without a satisfactory break period for free physical movement and play is a torment for the pubertal age period. Not surprisingly, these girls projected their hostility onto the weaker group of the white establishment, which they felt as oppressing them; they terrorized the middle-class pupils but stood off from the children of blue-collar workers whom they knew would fight back.

Most parents do not realize that the schools their children attend are more impersonal than they were a generation ago. The computer schedules classes, and personal needs as regards friendship, liked teachers, the need for group stability are not data that are fed into the machines. A class in physical education, which may disappear as budgets are cut, is thought to take the place of the unstructured free play of a recess period, which adolescents need at about two-hour intervals. Teachers' breaks occur every one-and-one-half to two hours; children are not given this. At conferences teachers rarely start on time; pupils are harried for being tardy.

Schools should have roots in the community in which they exist, those children who are bussed into school are at a disadvantage compared to those who are from the immediate neighborhood and who can play and socialize together on the way home. Communication in a bus is not the same as free interchange on a walk home or with a small group on bicycles or in a parental automobile.

Although home and school should cooperate with each other, the need of adolescents, and indeed all children, to separate themselves from their immediate home environment means that it is important for them to feel that home and school are separate institutions. This is first demonstrated by kindergarten children who will not tell their parents what happened at school; later some adolescents may resent special parental visits to their school, seeing it as an interference. To avoid this, parents' visits to schools should be made routine; a parental visit is not then felt as unusual. School and home should be considered by adolescents as separate places with common aims: the less conflict there is between them the better. To use parents to help in schools that their own children attend is less appropriate than having them in other schools.

Schools should treat parents with respect and vice versa. It is the responsibility of parents to see that their children go to school, the responsibility of the teacher to see that the children learn to enjoy academic and vocational work. Parents should not feel that it is their responsibility to see that homework is done, though they should, of course, try to provide opportunities for children to do it. Adolescents need to feel that parents are interested in the type and quality of the work they do, but it is the teacher's responsibility to ensure that it is done. If parents are unable to provide the conditions in which homework can be done —for practical or emotional reasons—it becomes the responsibility of the school to provide both space and time. On the other hand. parents who nag their child to work may create resentment. Those adolescents who underachieve are particularly unlikely to be helped by this parental prompting, often because they consciously or unconsciously resent their parents' action.

The school report, before it became a computer printout of grades, was one link between parent and teacher. It could give the teacher the opportunity to assess a youngster's progress and make suggestions on what he *ought* to be doing. It could also be an invitation to parents to talk with their children's teachers. The absence of a school report that describes the child in his life space means that communication is mostly with the parents of children in quite severe difficulty who have demonstrated unusual academic failure or conspicuous disturbed or antisocial behavior. The parents of difficult pupils, however, may feel completely helpless when they continually receive complaints about their child. Having told their child about the complaints and listened to the youngster's explanation of causes, most parents can do remarkably little—especially when the pupil's lack of success stems from immediate domestic pressure the parents do not know how to change or personality problems they can neither recognize nor alter. Further, the relationship between parents and these young people has often broken down, and parental control has been effectively lost.

From the primary stage onwards, defensive and inconsiderate behavior by teachers can destroy communication between home and school. On the other hand, a sympathetic attitude on the child's first day can set the tone for years of good parent–teacher relationships. In one large English high school, the parents of newcomers are summoned to a meeting by the principal, told how they should behave, and then asked if they have any questions.

Usually children's communication techniques are consonant with those of the nuclear family, even allowing for the action-oriented communication of the adolescent. However, by mid-adolescence academically educated pupils begin to put a high value on the use of words and attach less importance to action: In those families in which action communication remains highly significant, techniques of parent–child communication may be lost (Bernstein, 1961). Sometimes an adolescent is worried that too much is being learned for the parents to bear or begins to believe that they are stupid. Some nonacademic parents may find it very difficult to tolerate the educational chance that their child may be having; they are not prepared to face the inevitable loneliness when their child seems different from themselves. Parents may envy their child's opportunities and in subtle ways attempt to sabotage their achievement because they fear the break in the family relationships. Their children may find difficulty in doing homework not just because there is little room in the house or because there is no tradition of reading but because of the active opposition of their parents. If grade-school children are to be academically enriched, the school must not only encourage a pride that children may have in their racial and ethnic origins, it must involve parents in such a project (Silberman, 1970, pp. 110–111), otherwise unconscious or conscious sabotage occurs.

By adolescence active involvement of parents is of less help because of the drive of youth for autonomy, but many adolescents are still susceptible to implicit, if not explicit, parental wishes. It is self-evident at this stage that socially isolated parents are more likely to seek ways of hanging on to their children, even if these are unconscious. Those techniques—asking for obedience to implicit expectations, which adolescents grant— may retard academic growth. In nonacademic families lip service may be paid to the concept of a university education as a way of progressing socially, but the threatened father will constantly criticize the "long hairs" at the local university. Parents may tell their daughters that a little education is all right, being a nurse for example, but a postgraduate course such as medicine will be "too much for you."

Socially deprived adolescents may be highly imaginative and creative, but their thinking may be highly concrete. They thus find it difficult to deal with the abstractions that are required for an academic education. Furthermore, they may sense the anti-intellectual attitudes of their parents and find it hard to accept a way of life that values education. Such young people may also wish to leave school at the earliest possible moment because the school is inadequate and does not understand their special talents and problems. Often these points are not consciously appreciated by the adolescent, the school, or the parents. The adolescent may try to solve the conflict by working less well; the teacher may respond to this inability by rigid instructions and punishments; the parents may not understand why they want their son or daughter to leave school and get a job.

Many grade schools ask parents to come to the school to discuss their child's progress with individual teachers, and they enlist the help of the parents. This excellent practice is less common in high schools. Unfortunately, the parents of children who worry teachers most are least likely to come to the school even when asked. The anxiety of parents about the education of their children might be somewhat allayed if they knew their children's teachers. But teachers in the United States and Western Europe are usually unwilling to go to their pupil's homes and think that group contact in a capsule night is enough. There is an excellent tradition in parts of Eastern Europe that a teacher is expected to call on a child's family three times a year.

Adolescents learn most easily from people whom they, society, and their family esteem. It is easier for pupils to see that their teachers are valued by their parents when the school has been specially chosen, for example, when parents move into a neighborhood so their children may enter the local high school or when they send their children to private schools. The latter through individual consultation, annual parents' days, and the like manage to keep a relationship with parents that gives the teachers a certain mystique in the eyes of both parents and children. In good high schools that are neighborhood based, parents will be less likely to devalue staff in the eyes of their children; teachers will be likely to lose respect only through personal inadequacy.

The adolescent who grows up as part of a large family in a stable social environment may look on adults with mixed feelings, but clearly the big network of adults is valued by his immediate family if only because they are part of it. If there is no such network available, school teachers and all youth workers need to be valued by parents as though they were members of an extended family and social group. Where they are not, society can, to some extent, compensate by valuing them as conspicously as possible. If the staff are not so supported, the school cannot replace the missing networks and anchor points that are necessary for adolescents to mature.

Schools that are not chosen by parents, especially those that children are directed to attend, have a particular problem. When children are bussed across town in the interest of integration, it becomes difficult for the parents to value teachers, and the teachers often do not show respect for the parents. Black and white parents tend to view teachers of the opposite race with suspicion, black parents feel exploited and middle-class white parents, whose children are bussed to lower socioeconomic-class neighborhoods, feel their children are being offered second-rate education at the behest of impersonal administrators.

The typical campus plan of high schools symbolizes architecturally the isolation of schools from the neighborhoods in which they are placed. Surrounded by massive car parks such schools all too often appear cut off from their communities. Older schools that are physically a part of the area are allowed to deteriorate, and the isolation of the school from local life is apparent.

Parent–teacher associations may perform many valuable tasks for a school as a whole, but many do not necessarily improve the relationship between the school and the local community. Quite often they will be preoccupied with such topics as whether to provide a Coca-Cola machine in the school corridor or new curtains for a classroom rather than with an evaluation of the essential work of the school. As a potential threat to some school administrators, the groups may be manuevered into becoming rather sterile; alternately, they may be used to block change. Sometimes a visiting speaker once a semester talks to a group of parents and is introduced by the school principal or his deputy; this may be the only function of a PTA.

The best schools and neighborhoods tend to get the most effective parent–teacher organizations. The sterilized PTA has its equivalent in Britain and other European countries where there is often resistance among teachers even to the setting up of parent–teacher associations; the more rigid the school, the more likely does this appear to be the case. It may well be that teachers in such schools are so defensive about their role that they are fearful of the criticism they may meet from parents.

The breakdown in communication between teachers and parents means that usually, unless there is a crisis, teachers may not tell parents what is happening to their youngsters; sometimes the parents only know that something has gone wrong when a child is suddenly sent home for misbehavior. Many teachers see themselves as having a purely academic or vocational role in their relationship with the child; they do not consider themselves responsible for total personality development. Not surprisingly, many teachers are fervent believers in behavior-modification techniques, in which they do not have to take note of the dynamic subtleties of interpersonal relationships. The unalterable boredom of much of the high school curriculum is justified by the necessity to reinforce factual knowledge. Hence, the American high school is almost internationally alone in teaching the same subject at the same hour every day.

The impersonality of high school—with most parents having no knowledge as to what individual within it, if any, has any special knowledge of their child—makes it possible for parents to fail to inform teachers not merely of a child's current circumstances but even of events which could seriously affect other children:

A fifteen-year-old boy who had taken repeated doses of LSD

was sent to a psychiatrist by his parents. John had managed to do reasonably well at school because he had abstained from tripping while he was taking important tests. But he and a group of other boys had taken LSD intermittently during the year and in quantity since the end of the school year.

When his problem was discussed with the parents, they were reluctant to take the matter further. It had never occurred to them that they had any responsibility to inform the school or the parents of the other children.

Adolescents will often act out at school the tensions resulting from family conflicts; for example, parental separation can lead to a dramatic decline in the quality of school work:

Peter had a brilliant academic record at school until his mother took him to a motel room when he was thirteen and told him that she and his father had separated. Peter seemed to take this in a very matter-of-fact way; it was four years before he was referred to a psychiatrist for help because of his poor academic performance. He began to function again only when he understood his own rage and grief.

The tensions resulting from school conflict may also be acted out at home:

Kenneth was a sixteen-year-old pupil at a rigid, religious school at which boys were beaten for poor work. He was rude to his mother and physically assaulted his father. After six months at a co-educational school with few formal rules but a high morale, his parents talked about him as if he were a different person.

The structure of the school may, in itself, cause quite severe emotional problems:

Jane was a thirteen-year-old girl who was referred to a psychiatrist because of lack of appetite, sleeplessness, and isolation from her peers. Her parents said that she had "no friends," withdrew from the family, and seemed "angry" all the time. They had moved to a new location some nine months earlier, and Jane did not seem to settle in. They had taken her back to her old home the previous Christmas, and Jane had appeared to enjoy herself. However, she had refused to go again.

Jane was a small, postpubertal girl whose menarche had appeared when she was twelve. She said that she had "lots of friends" at her last school but "here no one wants to know me." She then described how on her first day at school, she found it impossible to get to know anyone. She knew the names of no children or teachers, all of whom "seemed to know each other." Jane was in six classes a day with six separate groups of children. She had no special talents but was an average, bright child. She was driven to school by her father daily, and the move to the school had taken place in the fall.

It is easy to see how Jane could become isolated. She was offered no stable peer group against which she could be tested. To each teacher she was one of 120 children to whom they were exposed each day, and none felt particularly responsible or interested in her. Since she dealt with anxiety by depression and withdrawal, they never noticed her; and because Jane's family had moved in bad weather there was no available neighborhood social life. Her depression and isolation were a function of a highly insensitive social organization, the school she attended. If Jane had been with the same children for a considerable part of each day in academic and nonacademic situations, the peer group available to her would have put her through a variety of unconscious initiation rites, but she would have been isolated for a much shorter time period (Bettleheim, 1956).

If there is a breakdown in communication between school and home, or if such communication has never existed, neither parents nor teachers will appreciate the importance of each other in cases of difficult behavior. When children misbehave, many schools are still far too likely to send for parents and order them to make their children conform. Teachers may prefer to blame parents for a child's difficulties and unconsciously treat them just as they were treated by their own parents in childhood. Similarly, parents may project fantasies from their own childhood onto the schools of their own children and look on teachers with awe, fear, or ill-disguised contempt. Parents may see teachers as policemen to control antisocial behavior, as knowing nothing, or as complete experts in the bringing up of children. At a previously mentioned capsule night run by a PTO, a parent obsequiously told the homeroom teacher who boasted of making the children sit still that she knew more about child rearing than the parent herself.

Much is made of the rebellious nature of adolescents but not enough of their conformity, to implicit expectations in particular. Nowhere is this more evident than in the relationship between parent and child. There is an important interplay between the wishes of a parent, stated openly or not, and the wishes and actions of the adolescent. This applies to healthy as well as unhealthy behavior. The emotional disabilities of children often meet the unconscious needs of their parents. The mothers of boys with homosexual difficulties often seem very reluctant to have their sons seek help; they seem to accept a situation in which normal masculinity is not valued. The mothers of promiscuous girls, although they may apparently disagree with their daughter's actions, sometimes appear to obtain satisfaction from hearing the details of their sexual behavior. The fathers of aggressive boys often seem to get satisfaction from talking about their sons' exploits (Miller, 1965). The mothers of boys who wet their beds have been known to become severely depressed when their sons recovered: The wish of an adolescent to remain an irresponsible child may meet the parents' wish to keep him in that state. In these cases it is difficult to help the youngster unless expert assistance is being given to the whole family.

The adults within the adolescent's network of relationships should be able to communicate with one another freely. It is quite unreal to expect that they will always agree with each other, and it would not help young people learn about the complexities of life if they did. But if the adults who are the important inhabitants of the adolescent's world respect each other's integrity and do not allow themselves to be manipulated, one against the other, home and school can assist the young to develop into caring adults. If adolescents need the extrafamilial world to mature into adulthood and if this world consists of peers and adults, the microcosm of school should provide a range of potential relationships for individuals. Even though adolescents are likely to stay within their in-groups, if the school is neither overrigid nor overpermissive and if it plans the childrens' day appropriately, some mutual understanding across racial, ethnic, and class barriers is possible. It is not enough to deposit white children in black schools or vice versa, rich white children with poor Appalachians; a complex social mix requires a sophisticated social system to produce a tolerant integrated society. Nowhere is this more evident than in the failure of schools to provide an adequate system to educate together children of two sexes.

Sexual Integration in High Schools

There are remarkable similarities between the problems of educating boys and girls in the same school and those of educating children of different ethnic groups together. Just as segregation is tolerable when ethnic groups have a strong sense of identity and the opportunities for advancement are almost equal with a host population—the story of Jewish and Chinese immigration into the United States—so it may well be that single-sex schools were tolerable when any boy or girl could spend the rest of the time in a stable mixed environment. But when a wide range of other people is no longer available outside, single-sex education is a psychologically harmful setting likely to damage personality development. Similarly, if a population is a victim of prejudice, has lost its ethnic identity, and lives in severely deprived ghettos, segregation of the black American from his white peer becomes a national tragedy.

Deprivation in all-male societies leads to certain specific types of social pathology. In closed male societies like boarding schools boys may be morbidly preoccupied with sexuality up to sixteen or seventeen. If adolescents in these circumstances are tense and unhappy, those who are least able to tolerate anxiety and loneliness may turn for solace to homosexual activity. Particularly toward the end of early adolescence masturbation between boys is common when they are members of all-male societies. This would appear to have several causes: if a boy has made, no firm identification, if girls are not present for any type of relationship, if the boy feels lonely and isolated and needs *emotional* contact, he may need to experience *physical* contact with another boy. Boys are often taught to masturbate by others, and in unhappy schools physically bigger boys may use smaller ones sexually. In boarding schools there is rarely any physical violence in homosexuality, although in the delinquent groups threats may be part of the seduction. The more harshly boys are treated by the staff, the more likely it is that bullying homosexual behavior will occur.

In a penal system for offenders in the teens, even where there is no formal physical beating by the staff, homosexual behavior is likely. If the staff members are at loggerheads with each other, this more probably will reach a peak of intensity. In one such section of a youth prison, a woman social worker dominated the male staff and talked to the boys in such a way that they felt she was contemptuous of all men. In the living quarters controlled by those staff members in conflict with each other, small boys were being assaulted by bigger boys. This situation is typical of highly deprived and depriving youth prisons.

Homosexual conflicts that are not expressed may be tormenting for individuals. In schools for boys in which the environment is too rigid or overacademic, boys can often be terrified of showing any sign of affectionate feelings towards each other; they are afraid other boys will label them as "queer":

> A seventeen-year-old school boy, academically successful and a football player, was referred to a psychiatrist because he had an acute episode of withdrawal from everybody. For five months previously he had been tormenting himself with the idea that he was going to be "queer" because he had felt fond of another boy six months younger than he. He had no feelings of sexual attraction toward this boy but was afraid to show he liked him because of what others might say.

Closed male societies also produce physical bullying, and verbal abuse is usual, but the deprived school in an underprivileged neighborhood produces similar social pathology. Release of tension is sought by early heterosexual or homosexual experiences, bullying, verbal backbiting, and massive projection of anger onto the larger society. When children in such settings are from ethnic minorities they either project hatred onto other racial groups or internalize it. When rage is internalized, in recent decades drug taking, principally cheap alcohol, amphetamines, and then opium derivatives have become common. If drugs are not used other types of self-destructive behavior including adolescent suicide is not rare.

In single-sex schools for girls in which the children are unhappy, in- and out-groups of girls are formed. The girls who see themselves as most select will treat other girls with verbal cruelty; there tends to be an atmosphere of bitchiness. It is rare in girls' schools, however, to get any degree of physical bullying, fighting, or homosexual behavior, although these appear in penal institutions. Girls in deprived segregated schools see themselves as sexual objects and are filled with unresolved hostility toward men.

An unsatisfactory school environment for boys helps to produce antisocial behavior and self-destructive activity, and it prevents some from developing their full emotional and intellectual potential. The equivalent situation for girls is likely to produce many depressed, isolated women whose sexual and intellectual adjustment is never really satisfactory to themselves or their families.

A genuinely co-educational school is better educationally and psychosocially than a single-sex school; similarly, a truly desegregated school provides a better education for all children, underprivileged or not. However, just as having girls and boys in the same school is not necessarily co-educational (Miller, 1969), mixing ethnic groups and social classes in the similar setting is not in itself integrated education.

True co-education is rare because of the failure of most schools to recognize the special educational needs of girls. If girls in early adolescence are to establish a firm feeling of femininity they need affectionate, essentially platonic relationships with males other than their fathers and brothers. They also need shifting one-to-one relationships with other girls and with boys, initially without sexual activity. Girls in isolated families who are not members of a "tribal" environment find it difficult to mature satisfactorily if they are educated in schools that often have a high percentage of women staff, and the assumption is often implicitly made that they will automatically relate better to women than they would to men. For example, in one school system male social work students may not work with adolescent girls; it is thought that seduction is too likely. This is similar to, if an exaggeration of, the system in most high schools where lack of stable relationships with extraparental adult males can hinder the maturation of girls. Neither is there the opportunity to make stable asexual relationships with older boys. Age segregation because of junior high school–high school separation cuts off any possibility of such relationships between younger and older adolescents. With these deficiencies it can follow that the social and academic capacity of girls will be impaired, for example:

A junior high school that was bedeviled with typical institutional tensions was overwhelmed by the notorious behavior of a group of angrily destructive black girls. A black social worker saw that the effects of control made by the staff were disintegrating into a sterile confrontation. She called the local high school, got in touch with the president of the black students' association, and a group of grade eleven and twelve male students came over to the school. They told the girls of thirteen or so to cool it and behave like ladies. The trouble immediately subsided.

These girls were deprived by the structure of the school system of the opportunity to feel valued by older boys, neither could they worship them from afar or project with some safety sexual fantasies onto these young men. The effect of the isolation of girls from stable, older, peer-group and adult attachments is to force feelings of alienation with an increased likelihood of early promiscuity, drug involvement, or just general unhappiness. The frenetic attitudes of some women's groups who parade their hostility to men under a political umbrella may well be a reaction formation against feeling, from an early age, grossly devalued as women.

It is well known that after puberty, girls tend to become less academically successful than boys (Abelson, 1972). Too few able women use their talents in the community and take up occupations that demand intellectual training. The reason often given is that this is a result of a male-dominated society or that women are too involved with the process of mothering. Whether or not this is true, the higher education of girls is unsatisfactory. Clinical evidence shows that they tolerate unimaginative education less well than boys and are more likely to be damaged by the grade-point-average rat-race. Girls have a greater need than boys to develop their imaginative and emotional potential; as a result they cannot easily tolerate an educational system that puts cognitive achievement at a premium and that greatly undervalues esthetic and emotional expression. Girls are more future-oriented than boys of the equivalent chronological age; they have a greater capacity to empathize with the feelings of others and have a much greater need for emotional sensitivity (Undeutsch, 1959).

Since boys in early adolescence are considerably less effective in height, intellectual efficiency, and imaginative potential than the equivalent-age girl they find competitive situations with girls intolerable. It is thus no accident that the honor rolls of junior high schools are occupied mostly by girls; apart from their greater effectiveness boys would rather not compete, preferring to believe that they could, if they wanted. The early adolescent boy usually hates to be beaten by a girl at any activity in which he expresses interest; when there is a danger of this occurring, he tends not to try. Then he can claim to himself that the situation was always within his control: "If I had wanted to, I would have won." On the other hand, girls who want to be attractive to boys and know that boys have this feeling, are themselves likely to do less well; they do not wish boys to frown on them. Girls who cannot tolerate their own sexuality or the sexuality of boys are more likely to retreat to an academic hole.

In a co-educational setting it is, of course, desirable that the boys and girls should treat each other with mutual respect. This means that they have to feel respected by their teachers. Under such circumstances the use of arbitrary punishment should be inconceivable for boys or girls. If the teachers do not respect the integrity of their charges, it is unlikely the pupils will respect each other. The proper education of girls is not the same as for boys with domestic science as an optional extra. Their need for groups is different, their sense of privacy is not the same as boys, and their need for physical activity is not the same as that of the male.

"Therapeutic" Role of Co-educational Boarding Schools

American schools differ from those in England, with some exceptions, in their overall conformity and in the absence of different types of schooling, which the British private schools system provides. Even in state education, there is a shortage of special schools, both day and boarding, for emotionally disturbed children. The shortage is of good co-educational boarding schools available to all children as well as to those in emotional difficulties. These are not panaceas for disturbed adolescents from broken homes, but they can at least provide a framework and support. At its best, the boarding sector of the educational system shows that stability for a number of years can be provided for boys and girls within an environment that they can perceive as valuable and that values them. They can then successfully identify with the people in it and its way of life (Atherton, 1966).

Although co-education is preferable, it is still possible for the all-male boarding school that is not isolated from the community-at-large, to educate boys satisfactorily if they stay until seventeen or eighteen: Through this age period, the development of a satisfactory male identity in a boy depends to a great extent on his being able to relate to other young males. Compared with other countries Britain has a large number of single-sex boarding schools and very few co-educational ones. Of course, those single-sex schools are attacked for perpetuating class barriers. Nonetheless, their boarding facilities enable them to hold and support the more disturbed with the more stable. On the one hand, this has lessened the burdens on the already strained state system; on the other, it has allowed the British health services to "neglect" to provide hospital beds for disturbed adolescents more than most Western nations. "Progressives" in England often demand that today's boarding schools for privileged children be added to the state system. This might be democratic and egalitarian, but it would certainly cause disturbance. Their society would then be confronted suddenly with many more intractable adolescents than it had imagined existed. It would have to try to find new resources to cope. An alternative which is much needed in the United States, is to create new co-educational boarding schools that could be helpful to disturbed youngsters and do more than merely contain them:

> Thirteen-year-old Clive kept absconding from a large all-male boarding school. He was a big, overgrown, early developer who was, in many ways, severely disturbed. He had fantasies of being beaten and homosexually attacked. He was also dependent on taking barbiturates that had originally been prescribed as a sedative. His parents lived in the country, and they had no network of relationships to assist Clive. For such an isolated youth, boarding education had many advantages, but the restricted male environment of his school increased the homosexual pressure that he was experiencing. A psychiatrist recommended that he go to a co-educational boarding school with some 300 pupils. A school much larger than this might have been overwhelming for him, and he would then have gained little from such an environment. The school to which Clive was moved was not a school for maladjusted children. The presence of too many disturbed children in one setting might well have made it useless in this case. Within six weeks, Clive was getting on well with three members of the school staff and, in particular, his housemaster. For the first time in his life, he had made friends with both sexes. For this boy, a new environment did not in itself mean that no more help was needed. However, the school did provide a network of people and a way of life for him.

Such a boy in the United States would almost certainly require treatment on an adolescent service of a psychiatric unit, if one could be found. This would not keep him for two or three years and is more expensive than a boarding school.

Academically, good co-educational schools have been shown to produce better results than single-sex schools. Though there is a mass of research (Dale, 1966) on this topic, controversy about it continues. Even those educationists with no prejudice on the subject tend to feel that they are being influenced by the results of the comparatively small proportion of outstanding single-sex schools. However, when the major surveys of academic achievement in Britain since 1921 are brought together, the evidence is unequivocally in favor of co-education. This should be more widely known; the adherents of co-education themselves are often unaware of it and quote only the social nonscholastic advantages of co-education. Many parents who have academic ambitions for their sons send them to single-sex schools. In parts of Europe where parents can choose between both types of education, there tends to be a massive premature withdrawal of boys from the co-educational schools when they reach puberty.

In boarding education school staff members sometimes are exceedingly anxious in case seventeen- or eighteen-year-olds have an occasional drink or use marijuana. It would appear that the staff feel that alcohol or pot in small quantities may so release sexual inhibition that there will be an orgy. There is little evidence that bacchanalia take place more frequently among co-educational schoolchildren than others. It appears that if the limits of sexual exploration are implicitly laid down in a co-educational school, intercourse between the pupils is less likely than homosexual behavior in an all-male environment.

It is probable that the issue of sexual behavior in co-educational settings whether school, hospital, or group home causes more anxiety to teachers and parents than the adolescents' conduct merits. Co-educational living situations do not force physical intimacy between the sexes. In a well-designed, co-educational setting, when children are shy of their bodily development, they should be able to withdraw from contact with the other sex. Since co-educational living is a healthier environment and more likely to meet youngsters' needs than a single-sex setting, promiscuous behavior is likely to be less common.

Promiscuous behavior in all-female living environments may be fairly usual, if the girls need to prove their femininity to other girls. In one girls' day school in London, it is usual on Monday morning for the girls to boast to the other girls of their sexual prowess over the weekend.

The same type of conversation occurs in girls' group homes

in the United States and in penal settings for girls. In such places, after a leave, girls find it necessary to talk of their conquests to their friends. The talk in such settings is not just in terms of boys being "in love" with them but of boys having had intercourse with them. The need to prove femininity through this type of mutual boasting does not appear to be necessary for the adolescents in co-educational environments that meet their psychological needs.

The clinical evidence from Britain seems to indicate that children from co-educational boarding schools are more likely to care about each other than those from single-sex schools. It would suggest that their moral standards are higher. As long as emotional needs of their pupils are met, they are clearly very much happier schools. A study (Atherton, 1966) shows that children who attend co-educational schools describe their school experience afterwards as happier than children who attend single-sex schools. This is hardly surprising, as the unconscious message of the single-sex school is that relationships with the opposite sex are wrong and are to be feared.

The same concepts must apply to the American penal and therapeutic systems for disturbed and delinquent youth. Many private schools that have been specially created to treat emotionally disturbed youth often appear too ready to send their difficult pupils away because of staff worries or because students run away or fail to respond fast enough to, for example, behavior-modification techniques. It would appear that those schools that are more rational in their general disciplinary approach are often more reluctant to accept irrationality and disturbed behavior in their pupils. They are overanxious about the effect of individual disturbed behavior, which is only contagious if a school is unhappy because of tensions among staff and pupils. They also tend, when they exist, to be unaware of the importance of physical surroundings to their pupils. The environment in which children live gives a clear message to them as to how adults care about them. For example, for years the adolescent service of a well-known university hospital had furniture built by the prison service, brown tile walls, inadequate lighting, and toilets with no privacy. The patients' eating area was drab and often dirty. That this situation was allowed to exist is perhaps a measure of the ambivalence of society towards its youth.

Problems of Racial Integration

The most important recent development in secondary education in the United States is the introduction of widespread attempts at racial integration in schools. The argument for ethnic integration is that it can provide a better all-around education for the children than can be provided by schools that try to concentrate on the needs of one particular group. It has also been suggested that schools automatically will break down social barriers and improve the quality of the education of the underprivileged. This view is extremely naive (Silberman, 1970, Part II), as there was no evidence prior to the racial integration of the school system that it produced social integration, although clearly the availability of general high school education produces social mobility among some members from nonacademic groups. The children of a blue-collar worker, however, whatever their innate intelligence, are statistically less likely to go to college than middle-class children. In a large high school those children whose parents go to the country club rarely mix socially with children from the "wrong side of the tracks." Since there are many differences in the behavior and communication techniques of different social classes in the same society, merely dumping children of these groups together increases their tendency to isolate themselves from each other. The ethnic and social subgroups of society are likely to huddle together behind a barrier against others.

An unthinking mixture of academic and nonacademic, black and white children from different social backgrounds—with staff whose experience is restricted to children of one particular group or who are unaware of how the difficulties involved in such a mixture may be resolved—may create serious problems. The two following examples are taken from English schools that were attempting to become socially comprehensive. In that type of education little attempt is made to understand the differences, needs, communication techniques, and social attitudes of children from different social groups. The third example comes from an American high school where the same problems, compounded by skin color and ethnic group, apply.

A bright middle-class boy of fourteen was referred to a psychiatric clinic for help because he had outbursts of temper, could not bear to have any of his things touched, and spent long periods of time arranging everything meticulously or obsessionally doing his homework. His school had no complaints about him and was surprised when his general physician sought a psychiatrist's opinion. Some of this boy's trouble was due to the emotional instability in his home, but it also stemmed from his school life. He was in an accelerated academic track in a large comprehensive school. The intention was that he should complete his schooling by the age of sixteen-and-a-half, then be ready for college. The boy was very small and said that his friends in his form were about his size. He said they were looked on as being square, sissy, and so on by bigger, less academic boys. He felt that he and his friends were envied by these other boys, because "they feel the teachers prefer us." When asked about the unnecessary time spent on homework, he said that he was terrified of losing his place in the academic track. If this were to happen, he felt that he would be placed with the larger boys: They would bully him; he would be helpless. He accurately detected a very real feature of the school. He felt rather like a Jew expected to leave the safety of the ghetto in the Middle Ages.

Jenny, a middle-class girl of thirteen, was attacked after school; she was kicked and beaten by a group of boys from a different social class at the school they all attended. She had previously told her teacher that this group had been responsible for bullying her brother. In doing this Jenny broke the code of the boys who saw the adult group as a hostile authority; they were a bad "they" against a good "we." The boys felt that the girl must be taught a lesson. Just as Jenny had felt that she had acted properly in reporting the previous bullying of her brother, the boys felt justified in attacking her.

Carla was the sixteen-year-old daughter of an automobile assembly-line worker. Although she was very light, she was black. She was bussed into a high school that had little or no feeling of social solidarity, although it was reported to be one of the most expensive buildings in the state. Carla made no mention of her racial origins, although she did not deny them; but she was sexually teasing and provocative to some of the black boys, although much of this behavior was unconscious. She sought help from the school social worker because she had been threatened with knifing by a group of black girls for "trying to take their men" away from them. Because she had not defended herself to the group by announcing her own black origins, she was referred to a psychiatric clinic for an opinion as to what was to be done. She talked there of being tired of being thought of by her black brothers and sisters as a "white nigger," while she lived elsewhere in the state. She had decided, when her parents moved, to make no mention of her racial origin to see if that would be any better.

It would be wrong to assume that the only causes of the attack on Jenny were differing class attitudes or of that on Carla, racial tensions. The English school was so unable to cope with the tensions in its children and its staff that six members of the top form were taking LSD for many months without being noticed, even though they were in a small class taught by the same teachers over a long period of time. These youngsters were appearing in the school in clothes grotesque even for young people. They were obviously toxic and spaced out and showed scant ability to concentrate on their work. Similarly, with Carla racial tensions were, to a considerable extent, a result of the children's projection of anger onto each other because of the overall tensions in the school. No effort was made by the staff to produce any sort of social cohesiveness around life at school. The teachers who taught 120 children a day rarely knew them. After six weeks of one semester some fifteen-year-olds did not know the names of many children in one of their math classes. The only educational technique of which the teachers talked was reinforcement.

The various social and ethnic groups will only learn to understand one another if there is considerable effort and understanding on the part of teachers. Even then there is as yet no evidence that young people from different backgrounds will wish to be friendly outside the classroom. It certainly cannot be argued that comprehensive education automatically breaks down the barriers of social class.

It is self-evident that gross physical deprivation of both children in the school and the school itself need to be resolved, but it is also true that money is not enough. Tension, despair, and violence exist in affluent middle-class suburbs as well as in the ghetto.

Mixing social and ethnic groups in childhood and adolescence thus does not automatically increase understanding. The best that often occurs is that children from different social groups in the same school may appear to relate to each other, but meaningful positive emotional contacts may not be present. There is some evidence that a social mix may raise the standards of academic education available to underprivileged children and adolescents, but the absorption of greater academic capacity requires more sophistication in teaching techniques and the organization of social systems than is currently usual. At the present time the best that seems to occur, often, is that some pupils may discover that a difference of appearance does not change common humanity. Integrated education in which the school staff do not understand the effect of social and ethnic difference is likely to fail. The best that may occur is separate and equal in the same local system. On the other hand, the failure of the average high school to recognize the special needs of the physically and emotionally deprived, and the different sexes, leads to a total failure of the educational system for some. But a continued inability to provide a satisfactory socially and ethnically integrated school environment can lead to a national tragedy. The black children who are deposited in white schools with a fantasy that this will produce significant racial integration must project their anger onto nonblacks, and each other, in order to keep any sense of identity. The former projection, which is thought to be necessary by many authors (Pinderhughes, 1968), inevitably exists with the latter and must enhance school tensions. This impairs the stability that a school system ought to have if it is to provide a social field against which children might grow.

Despite the wishes of some, there is no absolute norm for behavior in any one society. What is acceptable to one subcultural group and family unit is not allowable for another. Therefore, any description of adolescent behavior must take note of the social class and ethnic group from which the youngster originates. In any one school teachers should be aware that normative behavior for one group may be aberrant to another. If this is not understood, instead of pupil–teacher relationships offering emotional support to vulnerable adolescents, stress may be increased. Mistakes may be made by assuming that color is more significant than it actually is; as we have shown in other societies, too, social-class differences are most significant. In the United States these are sometimes thought to be covered by the color of an individual's skin; but aristocratic blacks and those who attempt to be socially mobile to that group have more in common with aristocratic whites than with their black working-class brothers. The common experience of prejudice is often all they share. In England, where immigrant groups still retain their cultural identity, this is less true. Thus, the black adolescent in Britain still grows up with a sense of cultural identity that protects him from prejudice to some extent. The black young in America have no such defense either against prejudice or the attempt of some well-intentioned adults to inflict a false value system. When ethnic groups and social classes return into themselves because the social environment cannot meet their needs, they project onto each other, attack each other, and end a school career with prejudice and dislike reinforced. The preexisting relative failure of the high school to understand the differing psychosocial development of boys and girls and to understand the problems of mixing different maturational age and social groups adds to the problem faced in ethnic integration. Different subgroups can live amicably together if they share a common sense of identity; all need to feel a member of the same "club."

The need for individuals to identify with the larger group of the school as a whole is paramount if, in early adolescence, in particular, the different groups are not to attack each other or, at best, isolate themselves from each other. The small-house system with a core of permanent staff available to the children over the years is necessary to make this possible, as is continuity of relationships within a school from age thirteen to eighteen. As well as identifying with the institution as whole children, if integration is to be meaningful, adolescents need to be able to model themselves on teachers who are themselves of different ethnic groups; they also need to identify with the mode of interaction between teacher and taught. Further, individuals need to be treated as such and not be made special because of ethnic group or social class. Special permissiveness to any one subgroup is taken by adolescents as a rejection. The concrete thinking of nonacademic middle-stage adolescents poses a particular problem, if attempts at creating mutual tolerance on the basis of educational techniques alone are made. With a social mix of pupils, if individuals of one social class are allowed to be more impulsively aggressive than another, a victim of such behavior will decide that all people are like that. No novels, films, or teaching seminars will change a belief based on a concrete experience in such adolescents. A nonacademic blue-collar white boy who is harried by a group of blacks, or vice versa, will then generalize about a whole ethnic group. Of the more inhibited middle-class group who have conflicts about aggression, because of an internal process or family attitudes, some will become more aggressive; others will withdraw completely.

Some of the differences between black and white children are really differences between social groups. For example, it has already been noted that working-class adolescents are more sexually experimental than their middle-class peers. Views on politeness between boys and girls also vary between social classes. Middle-class children in socially mixed schools are likely to find the impulsive behavior of other groups highly attractive on the one hand and yet slightly shocking on the other. A middle-class boy talked about his shock at discovering that boys would quite happily push the girls as they were rushing upstairs. Conflict can also occur between job-directed, working-class youth and more academic middle-class pupils and teachers. If the teachers are made anxious by the behavior of working-class groups, they are likely to try to inflict upon them a middle-class conformity. It may well be that teachers, in demanding middle-class behavior from children, can start a process of alienating them from their own families and ethnic groups. Sometimes behavior that is unacceptable to teachers on a class basis is falsely labeled as belonging to an ethnic group.

If teachers are to be acceptable models for children they will be tested as to their worth as adults. An effective way of doing this is for adolescents to use different ethnic status as an attack. A black teacher may find written on his chalkboard "Up the KKK." The response to this provocation will indicate to the whole group, black and white, something of the individual's personality strength. As the children as a group try to establish an identity with their teacher, some will accuse others not just of "sucking up" to teacher but of selling out their race. Given the necessity of adolescents being able to work out their tensions in relationship to a stable peer group, and a known adult, over a period of two to three years, it is not surprising that the failure to provide these makes for difficulties. Finally, teachers need a level of personality training that is rarely offered.

Apart from providing anchor points and a wider network of friends, a real integrated educational environment, in which children learn together rather than happen to attend the same school, is socially realistic. For all disadvantaged adolescents, from single-parent families (particularly if the parent and child are the same sex) to deprived black youngsters in ghetto areas, it is clearly an advantage that the children attend such schools, especially if they are enriched by what different cultures have to offer. If children and adolescents have been exposed to bereavement through the death or separation of their parents, it is self-evident that boys who are missing their mothers will be more likely to be helped in co-educational settings with women as teachers, just as girls who lose fathers have a need for male teachers. The ethnic group of such an individual can be irrelevant if they are well trained. The opportunity for perceptive, skilled, and long-lasting adult relationships makes true integration possible. Apart from the pupils, it appears reasonable to suppose that well-adjusted teachers would prefer such a situation, and to shift the social system of schools to provide this would not be more expensive than present educational costs.

Those human relationships in schools that are necessary for real integration, whether co-educational, ethnic, or social class, are clearly not easy to introduce. Because human beings are conservative in many things, it is possibly unrealistic to expect many individuals to want change. Integration requires an active cooperation between schools and parents, a real relationship between home and school. Since most parents love their children, if parents and schools really worked together, some interracial and social class suspiciousness would also break down. Nevertheless, if the educational system is to meet the demands that are put upon it by the changes in society, particularly in large cities, there should be a planned and widespread change to a genuinely integrated school, not created by bussing children across cities and merely dumping them together. The co-educational errors of the past that still persist should not be reinforced with social-class and ethnically vulnerable groups.

References

Abelson, P. H. (1972), Women in Academia. *Science* 175: 4018.
Ann Arbor School Board (1970), Minority Report of Citizens Committee on School Disciplinary Policy. Ann Arbor, Mich. (Mimeo).
Atherton, B. (1966), Co-education in marriage. *Where,* November: 25–26.
Bernstein, B. (1961), Social class and linguistic development: A theory of social learning. In *Education, Economy and Society,* ed. A. H. Halsey, J. Floud, and C. A. Anderson, 288–314. Glencoe, Ill.: Free Press.
Bettelheim, B. (1956), *Symbolic Wounds.* Glencoe, Ill.: Free Press.
Dale, R. R. (1966), The happiness of pupils in co-educational and single-sex grammar schools. *Br. J. Educ. Psychol.,* 36: 39–47.
McGregor, D. (1960), *The Human Side of Enterprise.* New York: McGraw-Hill.
Miller, D. (1965), *Growth to Freedom, The Psycho-Social Treatment of Delinquent Youth.* Bloomington: Indiana University Press.
———— (1969), *The Age Between.* London: Hutchinson.
Pinderhughes, C. (1968), *Unconscious Factors Affecting Black Youth Today.* Symposium on Contemporary Issues of Youth.
Silberman, C. E. (1970), *Crisis in the Classroom.* New York: Random House.
Undeutsch, U. (1959), Neueu Untergudengen zur Altersgestalt der Pubeszens. *Z. Esp. Ang. Psychol.,* 6: 578–588.

9

Student Conformity, Alienation, and Aggression

Etiology of Student Alienation

Students in higher education are exposed to particular stresses over and above those of younger students. For middle-class students, in particular, the current difficulties of the educational system in high school and college can be partially understood if a comparison is made between the way of life of the nuclear family and the expectations of the schools. Child-rearing practices in the West have increasingly become preoccupied with meeting children's needs. Some parents have tried to conceive of their children as special unique individuals, but, since few parents were brought up in this way, this has led in these families to a great deal of parental uncertainty. Children learn in such family groups not only that they themselves have the capacity to make value judgments but that authority figures are often unsure of themselves and often wrong.

Teaching staff, at the high school, undergraduate, and graduate level are rarely prepared to allow these attitudes to be conveyed to students. Some faculty resolve their anxiety about their role by overidentifying with the young, but, if anything, doubts teachers might feel are projected into the student group, who are often made to feel that they are wrong to question the way they are taught. Alternately, they may apparently be listened to, but nothing seems to happen. The aim of education up to graduate level, whatever overt statements are made, appears to be conformity; the reverse seems true nowadays in many family groups. The inconsistency between family attitudes and the educational system as a whole gradually percolates up to the latter. For example, grade schools particularly responsive to psychosocial pressures move to a concept of more creative education, but the change does not occur as children grow older so there is inconsistency between their attitudes and those of junior high and high. Even if high schools become more able to personalize the educational needs of children, consistency between school and places of work or higher education would be unlikely in the immediate future.

In Britain the emphasis in schools with a high reputation has always been on the intellectual achievements of an elite group. More recently, such schools have become more sensitive to the emotional, creative, and imaginative needs of their pupils. Although often strait-jacketed by an anachronistic examination system, a large number of British schools are trying to encourage the fine arts and creative activities such as music and drama, as well as academic performance and sport. In this way they are ahead of the American educational system, which often seems unaware of the values of imaginative creativity.

> In one junior high school, an art teacher would not allow the children to put pictures on the walls of the corridors in case they got "spoiled." In another, a child who refused to draw in exactly the way she told was isolated from the rest of the class.

The distinction between creative and imaginative as against cognitive achievement is largely unnecessary, as is shown by modern educational techniques. Those schools that are themselves creative in their teaching do not inhibit the creativity of their pupils. French as a living language, science in relationship to life, the new mathematics and project teaching, learning about topics rather than being taught subjects, all allow young people both to feel and be creative while acquiring conventional knowledge.

A particular problem of the higher educational system for those students who do not conform to their families' wishes is that they are exposed to a demand for conformist responses often before they develop a firm feeling of self. Similarly, difficulties may exist for overconformist youth who have never been able to deny parental wishes. Such students are likely to be educated in a high school environment that demands conformity in behavior and rarely values nonacademic imaginative and creative outlets. Individuals like these, who have been forced to play the academic game prematurely, may persevere with it while they have the emotional support of their families or of their known environment in high school; not uncommonly, they break down in their first year of university. Such individuals often have an acute feeling of uncertainty about themselves; they internalize their anger and see themselves as worthless:

> Timothy, an eighteen-year-old student was suspended from one of the universities for failing grades at the end of his first year. He had attended a rigidly academic school and had obained entry to college when he was just over seventeen. Shortly thereafter, he began to feel depressed, but this feeling was for a time relieved by the onset of the summer vacation. Then he began to feel he had taken the wrong path, "I spent all my days daydreaming or living vicariously by going to the movies. I have too much imagination but I have never known what to do creatively. I have tried to do some paintings but they are not much good. At school all they cared about was that I behaved like a jock, got good grades, and did not express unpopular opinions."

As secondary education attempts to become more creative, more and more young people and their teachers will find that standard tests spoil learning experiences. Students are likely to find these increasingly intolerable. However, given the circumstances of society most schools prefer to ensure that their more able students obtain a university place at almost any cost: The schools maintain the teaching standards demanded by the universities. Nevertheless, because it is important that late adolescents be as cooperative as possible, if they complain about the quality of high school education, schools often try to obtain their compliance by agreeing with their complaints. Good teachers tend to explain away the fact that they have to teach in a rigid fashion by blaming the admissions office of universities; the necessity for good grades and high SAT scores as a measure of academic excellence is stressed. The insistence on the former is likely to inhibit creativity. If this blame is directed toward the university, students are likely to have very mixed feelings about admission even before they enter university. Many see a degree as a necessary ticket to an economically viable life; others arrive with a guarded "wait-and-see" attitude. Some are apparently highly motivated, but this may change dramatically toward the end of their first year.

Among the many other reasons for the projection of blame by the young onto the educational system is that society has not yet learned to handle the long moratorium before adulthood is reached. Students often do not feel valued; they are not paid either with status or money for their work, and yet they have to tolerate a dependence at a social level long past their psychological or physical need for this (Bettelheim, 1971). Furthermore, American society has incompletely developed some of those techniques devised by other societies to make the late-adolescent moratorium more creative and exciting.

The uninterrupted nature of American educational systems that was only partly a result of selective service, is a particular problem. In a routine pattern, for example, a medical student will have twenty years of continuous education prior to graduation. Summer vacations are often needed to earn money to help pay for a further educational year. Thus, there is not time to explore the self in relation to the world as part of a general play experience. Other countries make longer time periods available for such "play." For example, in Britain, many students finish high school at Christmas and expect to enter the university in the following fall. This allows time for the late adolescent to explore the larger world. This is of particular help to those students unsure of their own identity or whether they will be acceptable, who would have been likely to arrive at a university feeling anxious, wary, and hostile. Without the transitional experience available to their European colleagues, many American students arrive at higher education feeling like this. Back-packing through Europe later, or membership in the Peace Corps may change this, but these are outlets for the few.

In large universities the student is immediately exposed to an alienating impersonal system. Sometimes registration for classes resembles the Chicago stockyards at their worst. Classes are full; courses are often obtained by what seem to many the underhanded means of seeing professors directly rather than through course counselors who often appear to students to be confused, overwhelmed, or disinterested. Students may have been admitted only on the basis of SAT scores and a grade-point average; they know no member of the staff and no effort is made to get to know them.

A further area of stress and, hence, alienation for freshman students in particular is that the universities appear to have abandoned all concern for their emotional and moral well-being. Dormitory living no longer provides a social structure with significant adult input within which students might grow. The decline of the Greek societies has led to the absence of tight peer-group support as an alternative to faculty interest. Many freshmen with permission to live off campus feel lost in isolated apartments.

Social Response of Students

These stresses placed on students produce a variety of responses: Many, particularly those who conform to the wishes
of their nuclear family and who plan to take up postgraduate
training for well-developed roles such as the law, engineering,
or medicine, pass the hurdles of the system and are apparently
satisfied with themselves and their society. They know that they
can expect consistency from the world. Late adolescents, just as
those who are younger, have a psychological need to be conformist as well as to rebel, to be dependent as well as independent. For these individuals, their sense of inner security depends
upon their taking up roles that society values, both economically
and socially. They obtain satisfaction in their lives because the
work they do is valued and gives them economic satisfaction.
The issues connected with their work tend to be ignored. Such
people, essentially obedient and conformist, are looked on with
favor by the authority structures of a bureaucratic social organization. Unless they encounter inefficiency, consider themselves
badly paid, or are made redundant by economic game plans or
technical change, they do not challenge the authority structure
that has given them security. For them radical change is unnecessary as conformity pays social and economic dividends.

Those individuals who are unsure of their ultimate role in
society are under greater personal stress than those who know
what their place is to be. The pattern of education for fine arts
students, for example, is not generally as alienating from their
creativity and imagination as for others. Often they do not need
to conform to an alienating experience in high school when
they wish to go to art school. Their admission to higher education may depend on their talent, as measured by the work they
have produced over a period of time, not just on their grades.
These students do not suffer so much from the feeling that the
right to obtain such an education depends on a grade-point average. Unfortunately, once undergraduate status is reached, many

art students find that universities are preoccupied with this even for those in art, music, and drama. Furthermore, once art students have entered colleges of art, it may be very difficult for those with a particular talent in, say, painting or sculpture, to involve themselves in the routine distribution of studies demanded for a degree. A particular additional stress for those who study fine arts, as opposed to those whose vocational interest is more economically viable, is that they often find it extremely difficult to see a role for themselves in society. Partly because of this and partly because they tend to see what they produce as an extension of themselves, such students are very vulnerable to staff criticism. Some may protect themselves by projecting blame onto the staff, which is not difficult because the hierarchical authority structure of many art schools has led to the alienation of students and junior staff from senior staff and administration.

It is not surprising that nonconformist student behavior should appear most obviously in many art schools. The inability of art students to assess whether society will value their productivity is one reason why they have not conformed to usual social demands since Victorian days. As art schools become bureaucratized, diffuse nonconformity for many becomes focused on the school staff in an open rebellion against the system; thus, many art students drop out of college.

Students of the arts, such as English and languages, have always had more difficulty in establishing their final adult roles than science students, though until the last decade they were looked upon as an intellectual elite. However, the change in the economic climate of the seventies has begun to create a semi-educated professional class of BA students. In the West, a situation that has long been a problem in India could be reproduced. It seems that this burgeoning group, if forced into a menial job or, as an alternative, unemployment will be likely to threaten the present tenuous fabric of organized society.

Arts students tend to be in a much more conflict-ridden situation than students of technology, for their courses appear to demand more use of imaginative and creative abilities and to be more involved with the personal individual life experience of the student. It is much easier for an adolescent to identify with historical and fictional characters and live imaginatively and vicariously through a novel than through Boyle's law. Poetry and the written word are more likely to arouse the creative imagination of the reader, at an early stage in the study of such subjects, than are the sciences. In arts courses the student's imagination and creative impulses in school are inevitably stimulated by subjects when they are well taught.

Social science students are particularly likely to be critical of the established order of society. The rigidity of the general social systems they study is likely to make them turn their attention to the organization of their own departments. Thus, they, like students of political science, tend to direct criticism at their teachers.

Students' Perception of the University

When those students who feel alienated from the way of life of the educational system reach the university, nevertheless having made the necessary grades, they are likely to feel confirmed in their opinions. The university is often perceived by them as a hostile authority structure. Staff, particularly at higher levels, are seen as arrogant and privileged, often because they are so distant from meaningful emotional relationships with either junior staff or students. University administration and faculty are sometimes involved with in-group power struggles over what seem to some, esoteric issues. Much time may be spent in meetings. Students may be present at these as token participants but usually seem to feel overwhelmed.

University power is despotic, but it attempts to be benevolent. Universities try to assist their students by providing a counseling service for academic affairs, and often personal counseling and mental health services for those who seek them are available. However, even if staff are appointed who are either good teachers or capable of making significant interpersonal relationships with the students, in a large university the structure of the undergraduate educational system makes interpersonal relationships between the average student and adult staff almost impossible. This is not just a problem at an undergraduate level:

> A university medical school had 225 students in the class of 1975. In the first semester, the structure of the education was such that the students had no opportunity for significant interpersonal contact with even one teacher. In ten weeks no less than 30 students referred themselves for personal help to the school's psychiatrist with anxiety symptoms that they felt to be crippling.

A whole variety of student services proliferate to meet student's needs for human relationships; attending the mental health clinics, becoming a member of the student newspaper or marching band, joining an organization such as the Gay Liberation Movement are ways of belonging. The failure of the structure of undergraduate education to enable each student to have significant emotional relationships with at least one faculty member, who is interested in him as a total person leads to an expensive proliferation of systems designed to be helpful. Too many are found to seek technical help when all that is really needed is an involved, interested adult.

Anxiety and Aggression in the Alienated

The social system of universities is likely to produce alienation at both a graduate and undergraduate level. Alienated individuals are particularly likely to respond to stress with anxiety and then aggression, which may be internalized, leading to a

variety of symptoms that are more or less self-destructive, or
may be directed outwards. Until recently, the bureaucratic establishment of universities needed to offer only a most trivial or
seemingly irrelevant pretext to students for troubles to begin.
The etiology of this was multiple: Any potentially angry person
may have his rage triggered by events that seem trivial to the
outsider but are felt as significant because of idiosyncratic or
unconscious meaning. Isolated individuals often have a frantic
need to belong to a group of peers. Some students may join
organizations that offer them a feeling of security, hence the
success for some religious groups such as the Children of God
which almost totally submerge the individual identity of some,
or, in the past, such organizations as SDS. The last five years
have shown a variation in the reported response to alienation
among students; self-destructive drug taking, alcoholism, and
academic dropping-out; the creation of so-called alternate lifestyles; violently aggressive behavior, which culminated in the
tragedy of Kent State; more recently, the seeking of surcease
in the fields of orthodox and unorthodox religion. The large mass
of students resolve some of their conflicts by intense engagement
in none of these but rather by living vicariously through identification at a distance with the reported activities of a few. No
repetition of group violence is possible, unless the large mass
of students collude in its presence (Redl, 1949).

Understanding Student Aggression

The aggressive behavior of students can be understood in
many ways. Riotous behavior by students is not new; in England
the night of the Oxford and Cambridge boat race and rugby
matches between medical students from teaching hospitals offered
opportunities for policemen to have their helmets knocked off.
Only in recent years in the United States and Britain did student

riots become student revolt, although this has been common for three decades in the Middle and Far East.

There were many general social reasons for this: More than in any other decade there were conflicts between young and old, and youth felt itself to be a victim of gross inconsistency on the part of society. Having given their children opportunities they never had themselves, parents of the class of 1969 to 1971, who were adolescents in war and depression, envied the freedom they watched their children enjoy; having taught them to think for themselves, they were anxious about their unwillingness to conform. Experiencing doubt about their abilities as parents, they were baffled by the apparent reluctance of their adolescent children to take notice of them. When a comparatively small number of students took revolutionary action, all the anxieties of adults in authority, particularly some politicians, became focused on them. Actions were blown up into great significance by communication media and a halo effect was created. Students began to think that revolt was expected of them, just as some still feel that they ought to smoke marijuana.

> One English university student spent a summer vacation in the United States and visited other students in California. For the first time in his life, he began to use pot and his justification was "all the students at Berkeley smoke; I would have felt a fool if I had not turned on."

The same argument was used as a justification for taking part in demonstrations and sit-ins.

Nevertheless, there are many specific reasons why students should have been more than rebellious for a time and may be so again. Students who enter universities in Britain and the United States have to bear a unique burden of guilt. They know that many equally qualified have been rejected because of insufficient places; students know that admission based on grades is educational roulette. They are also acutely aware of the divisions in society between rich and poor. As with all those who are rich—and compared to the poor and underprivileged of this world, students are rich—they have to bear the burden of being envied. One way of denying their own affluence is to attack the affluence of others; their own privilege is negated by their attack on the privileged. Another technique is to demand fair quotas for minority admissions irrespective of whether supporting services for such students are provided—what is sought by the affluent majority is a magical expiation of guilt.

Universities ask their students to accept that their role is to acquire specific skills. An inquiring mind is rightly felt to be important, but the university system tends not to direct the inquiry toward its own social organization; the motto might be "study everything but us."

Violence is likely to appear when adolescents feel an absence of structure. In the last decades universities have been rapidly dismantling the social supports that their previously rather rigid rules provided; they have not replaced these with the controls that are implicit in mutually caring human relationships. In high schools the absence of these controls is one of the determinants of racial violence and wanton property destruction; in universities the violence was directed at the establishment.

The shift away from violence at universities appears to be due to several factors: Parents who were adolescents after the last war envy their children less. Society has become a little more consistent in its attitudes to violence; more and more of the adult population began to disapprove of the wanton slaughter of the Vietnam war, which led to American withdrawal. Just as parents who behave violently provoke this in their children, so a society is identified within its openly condoned behavior. On the other hand, some people, by their attitude to the Kent State slaughter, indicated they were prepared to collude with the murder of their own young. This took place against a background of atomic destruction in which a balance of terror, if it is disturbed, will lead to death of all young people at the hands of their elders (Beloff, 1968). Thus, by threatening the life of young people society shifted the focus of the former's aggression. Economic pressure was also brought to bear by threatening some university funds and by making it more difficult to find work for many after graduation. This was all doubtlessly unplanned, but the "elders of the tribe" became dangerously punitive to the young. Finally, the social demands of young people were to some extent met, in the letter, if not the spirit (Louis, 1971). The quota admission of minority groups and women to universities can be prejudice at its worst and a potential rejection of academic standards, but it is a cheap way of propitiation and helps society expiate its guilt relatively inexpensively. Of other demands of students, which appeared to be of two types, some were rejected. The naive insistence that all authority structures be dismantled was ignored. This anarchic concept ignored the nature of the human animal to seek emotional safety in some type of power structure. The demands for representation on the governing bodies of the universities were granted in a token fashion. This does not seem to be a demand for a change in the form of the institutional structure: The students merely wanted to sit with adult authority at the triangular apex of power that inevitably alienated those at the base. As they participate in administrative committees, student representatives are often considered by their peers as having gone over to the "they"; the institutional weight of the system hangs heavily on those students who are not then able to produce real social change.

None of the changes associated with the relative cessation of overt violence have resolved the problems of late-adolescent alienation. The presence of small terrorist groups and a relatively large secret police force means that in some ways students are in a similar social system to that which existed in Czarist Russia at the end of the nineteenth century (Pares, 1960). Aberration now shows itself more in individual self destruction with some flirtation with social denial of autonomy and self:

Lionel was a twenty-year-old student who had a stormy relationship with the university in his first three years. He provoked his professors; involved himself with pot, pills, and acid; dressed in a bizarre fashion; and made barely acceptable grades. He was persuaded by his parents to consult a psychiatrist just before the summer vacation. He complained of emptiness and an inability to form any goals for himself, and he felt that only radical violence was the solution, "but they shoot you for that."

He returned after the vacation to continue his psychiatric consultations wearing a large cross but dressed neatly with relatively short hair. He announced that he had been saved, was now in communion with the Lord who wanted him to save people. He joined the Children of God. The following week, he left the university and spoke only to his parents and old friends in the presence of other disciples.

The solution to problems of alienation rests largely with a change in the structure of universities, just as an equivalent change is necessary in high schools. Only when human relationships between adults and late adolescents are restored can true learning begin to take place for most.

The answer is to look closely at the present power structure of the universities, decide where and how change is wanted, and then face the enormous problems involved. Social change is impossible unless it is desired by the senior authorities of a system. They will only want this if the system, by its failure to function, makes them sufficiently uncomfortable.

It is argued by some that far from producing an alienation from the self, the present social system as it impinges on the late adolescent produces a valid counterculture. Reich (1970, p. 352) believes that there is a new consciousness developing that "seeks restoration of the non-material elements of man's existence . . . since machines can take care of our material wants, why should not man develop aesthetic and spiritual sides of his nature." There is no doubt that many young people have been exposed to just enough stimulation of their creativity so that they yearn to get in touch with their own and other's imaginative sensibility.

Regrettably, most members of the human race when they are starved of imaginative and creative outlets as young people, are likely to become apparently dull, conformist, and rigid, living in a private world of their own. Or they become openly rebellious and destructive. Repressive inhibition without removing the causes of rebellion ensures that the next bout is more destructive, although in the meantime a nihilist and callous intolerance may cover both sloth and an antirationalist approach to life (President's Commission on Campus Unrest, 1970). There is, perhaps then, a general disinclination to use man's capacity to be reflective. The argument is used that only the ability to experience sensations matters; sometimes this is elevated to a therapy that, it is believed, will heal magically the alienating discontents of humanity.

Man cannot get in touch with himself unless he has significant emotional contact with others. Social systems that produce a distance from the other people also produce a distance from oneself.

Change as a Social Necessity

Just as high schools have to learn to produce viable small social units, so must universities. The logical structure is the collegiate system, with academic staff having the ability to relate to students. The demand for student power is also a demand for human contact with others. It is a slogan that implies omnipotent solutions. The real demand is for human contact and respect for human dignity.

A change in family relationships has pressured the lifestyle of schools and universities so the inevitable changes in the latter will force changes in industry. If creativity is valued as the norm in places of higher education, even the boy or girl who leaves school at sixteen will find the present structure of industry intolerable.

Those adolescents who are exposed to imaginative teaching and who are given the opportunity for creative expression in schools, already have particular conflicts when they leave school. They tend to find themselves teased by the society in which they are to live and work. A good school attempts to give the child status as a person, so that he or she will develop talents and a sense of self as valuable and worthwhile. The nonacademic students who attend good high schools find that employers are not interested in the creative imagination that the schools may have fostered. One manager of a successful business said at a parent–teacher's meeting of a fairly conformist school: "I find the boys from this school excellent employees. They may not be too bright but they work hard and do what I ask them to do."

All too often the jobs that nonacademic late adolescents obtain are dull and boring; they demand only a part of their attention, and there is often a basic assumption on the part of their bosses that they need to be coerced to work effectively. Outside their work experience, nonacademic adolescents find that life has little to offer them. If they are fortunate, they are able to find fulfilling interpersonal relationships with young people of the opposite sex. But social existence for most of them offers either the passivity of television watching, with its vicarious living, or a degree of somewhat frenetic excitement in discotheques, clubs, and commercial entertainment centers. It is no accident that drug pushers often find a happy hunting ground in such places of recreation.

In Vietnam the draft has shown the violent alienation of nonacademic late adolescents, both black and white. The assumption that the cessation of that war will resolve the problems that are hidden by "fragging" and pure heroin in Southeast Asia is naive. The war highlights the problems of youth, it does not create them in the first place. Well-fed youth becomes increasingly aware of an experience of emptiness and desolation. In a panic young people may attack the middle-aged for being dull, complacent, and unimaginative. This may be true, but it is a projection of the late adolescent's anxious feeling that society is making *him* dull, complacent, and unimaginative.

Evidently many people are waiting for a hero figure they can follow. Most vocal at the present time are members of the student Left whose heroes are Guevara, Castro, and Mao. But there is another mass of young people—inarticulate, often highly prejudiced, usually semieducated—waiting to be stirred to an activity that will make them feel valuable and worthwhile.

The most bitter and disaffected are among the eighteen-plus failures—those students who fail to gain admission to the higher education of their choice. Some start work unwillingly. Others go to a college they have not chosen to be treated as second-class citizens. Others drop out, and an unknown proportion become hippies and the like. An equivalent group is being created in the twenty-one- or twenty-two-year-olds who graduated from college, cannot find jobs and go to work as janitors. A catalytic force that exists in the United States, and hardly exists elsewhere in the world is the disaffected black young. (An equivalent group in Northern Ireland is the Roman Catholic young who are the "blacks" of Ulster.) Led by disaffected intelligentsia, they light a violent fire whose coals are also present in American society.

Among these groups there is an unresolved rage that is often internalized because the individual tends to feel impotent and helpless. It is pertinent to ask whether any society can produce large numbers of disaffected young, offer no constructive solution, and survive; the evidence from history is that it cannot.

References

Beloff, M. (1968), October for the rebels. *Encounter,* 31 (October): 48–56.

Bettelheim, B. (1971), Obsolete youth. Toward a psychograph of adolescent rebellion. In *Adolescent Psychiatry,* Vol. 1, ed. S. C. Feinstein, P. Giovacchini, and A. Miller, 14–39. New York: Basic Books.

Louis, G. F. (1971), The slow road to student liberation. *Am. Assoc. Univ. Professors Bull.*, 57: 495–499.

Pares, B. (1960), *A History of Russia.* New York: Knopf.

President's Commission on Campus Unrest. (1970), *Report.* Washington, D.C.: Government Printing Office.

Redl, F. (1949), The phenomenon of contagion and shock effect in group therapy. In *Searchlights on Delinquency,* ed. K. R. Eissler, 315–328. New York: International Universities Press.

Reich, C. A. (1970), *The Greening of America.* New York: Random House.

10

The Etiology of Adolescent Stress

Homeostatic Shifts at Adolescence

The personality strength an individual brings to the adolescent age period is clearly the result of genetic endowment, interpersonal relationships within the nuclear family, and that family's relationships with its total environment. The latter provides children with economic and social stress or support and the opportunity for peer-group and extraparental adult attachments. If parental relationships, peer-group attachments (Bowlby, 1969) and meaningful emotional contact with nonparental adults are thought of as significant in personality growth, in childhood parents are probably most important; in adolescence peers and adults most needed (Miller, 1970). The loss of one of these supports throws particular stresses into the relationship with others, but in both childhood and adolescence the nuclear family alone cannot successfully rear its offspring. In adolescence the absence of peers makes successful personality development almost impossible; the absence of significant extraparental adults is almost as bad.

Adolescence can appropriately be called the age of anxiety. Young human beings have to cope psychologically with anatomical and physiological change; the drive to autonomy leads to changes in family relationships; new demands are made by the world, and adolescents have new expectations of society (Freud,

1958). The success of adolescents in dealing with stress helps create the ultimate capacity of the adult personality to cope with psychic pain. The capacity to cope with frustration should be firmly developed during adolescence.

Behind all adolescent behavior that causes environmental stress is a level of tension and anxiety the youngster cannot contain within himself. There is a spillover to activity that either relieves or avoids *Angst*, the experience of tension. The behavior may alter the environmental situation so that the precipitant of the tension is automatically removed—when the adolescent is seeking external controls and gets them—or the situation may be worsened. For example, anxiety caused by rejection may cause behavior that leads to further rejection (Miller, 1966).

Anxiety, which is a tension awareness, can be understood as the result of the balance between stressful and supportive factors that play on the personality of the individual. The individual's physical development, environment, family, and perception of the world offer either emotional support or emotional stress; these interact with each other. The goal is for the individual to experience minimum anxiety, either by the production of a series of coping devices (Menninger, 1963, pp. 125–152), or by acting to alter an external situation directly and consciously. If normal coping devices fail, the threatened disorganization evokes tension that produces special devices to maintain equilibrium, a variety of symptoms are produced, aspects of the conflict are repressed, or there is a misperception of the situation. Unconsciously, attempts are made to alter the situation. Thus, a homeostatic balance with environment is reestablished (Cannon, 1939).

Early adolescents in particular have a difficult task. At a period of maximum internal turmoil, they are likely to face maximum external confusion; the applied pressure comes both from the school system and from the social-environment-at-large. For both girls and boys, adolescence introduces an element of extreme peer-group competitiveness. Boys, by comparison with agemates, make important assessments of masculinity, which are stressful if the individual perceives that he is inadequate. In a relationship with a particular friend, or a closely knit peer group, the adolescent may also get general emotional support.

> Jim, a sixteen-year-old boy who did extremely well academically and was perceived by his family and their friends as extremely well adjusted, sought help because of his anxiety about "excessive masturbation." Just prior to puberty, his best friend had left town, and he had not found another. He masturbated about once or twice daily but had no way of discovering that other boys "beat off" with the same frequency. He did not feel able to ask his father because he was striving to free himself from the dependent feelings of childhood.

Thus, a social lack exposed Jim to particular stress; this made him feel more isolated and increased the frequency of the masturbatory act. His family attitudes also added to this stress. Apart from his struggle for autonomy, the parent's overmoral attitude towards sexuality made him feel that he himself was unduly interested in pornography because he liked looking at pictures in *Playboy Magazine*.

Jim's difficulties were compounded by a usual adolescent family struggle; the absence of psychosocial support from a close friend with whom he could talk intimately, compounded his difficulty. Furthermore, his anxiety was enhanced by his criticism of his own bodily self. During a physical examination, which should be routine in all adolescents who seek psychological help, a medical student examining Jim noted that he had a very mild indentation in his lower sternum. The student's inquiry about this led Jim to talk of how uncomfortable it made him feel. Jim said that his body was unsatisfactory, his head was too large, and his walk ungainly.

This bodily preoccupation and self-criticism is typical. Jim felt, however, that his muscles were good, and he thought his penis was as large as that of the other boys; he especially noted this when he showered with them. Thus, his bodily perceptions offered him both stress and support.

To an extent, Jim's masturbation could be understood as an

attempt to gain control over his bodily anxieties, which is one of the uses of this act in the male. It was a regressive act due to the stress he experienced. On the other hand, it was also a way in which sexual fantasies became associated consciously with the genital experience of tumescence and detumescence (Reich, 1951). Finally, it was a way in which control over a bodily experience was reinforced, and it reduced the anxiety associated with loneliness and sexual tension.

Place of the Nuclear Family

Within the family, pubertal striving for freedom from dependent feelings of childhood is a confusing process both for adolescents and their parents. The adolescent may become over-aggressive and overassertive. Parental reactions may enhance the stress, provide support for the adolescent in the autonomy struggle, or both. The testing behavior of children around the issue of parental controls is an obvious example. Parents may respond to their children's difficult behavior with feelings of obvious dislike. Because of their own uncertainty, they may be overpermissive or overcontrolling relative to the new differing needs of their child. An individual's "adolescent" reaction may worsen the situation. Parents may find that they do not know how to talk to their children; simple remarks are felt as intense criticism because of adolescent hypersensitivity. Doors may be slammed over trivia; loss of face may be experienced by the young adolescent if a younger brother or sister is given what is sensed as priority. The physiological state of the adolescent may enhance stress. The intense lability of the blood supply to the skin may cause some obvious psychic pain, blushing exposes inner conflicts to the whole world. If parents comment about this, more discomfort can be caused. Pleasant family experiences, such as meal times, in which the equation of food and a warm loving atmosphere should be apparent, can become miserable periods of stress. Food fads may develop; individuals are likely to feel overwhelmed by a chance remark and rush dramatically from the table. Mixed feelings about mothering may be demonstrated by food refusal.

Often adolescents seem to stop talking to their parents in an agreeable way, they only argue, and the parents may find themselves doing the same. It is as if adolescents feel themselves to be alive by being oppositional. When friends visit, some adolescents find this a major trauma and withdraw to their rooms at once. Others run out of the house with minimal provocation. "Now what's the matter?" is a typical parental cry. During the early adolescent period it becomes extremely difficult to perceive the family as being supportive, so relatively minor stress, due either to personal misperception or reality, may take on major proportions.

Physical Change as a Stress and a Support

The new sense of self acquired in adolescence is associated with changes in bodily shape that lead to a radical reappraisal of the body image. A major anxiety of puberty is produced by adolescents' feeling that their body is out of control. Rapid growth in boys and girls may be supportive to the developing personality as it signifies maturity; if it occurs at a different time from peers, it may be a stress. The uncontrollable menarche, before premonitory warnings due to premenstrual tension occur, is a gratification; real womanhood has arrived. As a stress, bodily substances are inexplicably lost (Klein, 1932). The bewildering increase in frequency of penile erections relative to earlier years, apparently unrelated to any psychic experience of sexual excitement, means adulthood is arriving. It also gives rise to anxiety. In the balance of support and stress in adolescence, anxiety will depend on the individual's perception of the situation, which is based on interactions with the parents about loving, controls, sexual feelings, guilt, and shame.

Children whose bodily play has been respected by their parents are less likely to be troubled than those who have been handled with parental anxiety; parents who seductively parade their own nudity to their children cause problems at adolescence. Mothers who appear half-dressed may imply to their sons that they have no significant male sexuality. Exhibitionistically nude fathers both stimulate and ignore their children's sexuality and may lead to adolescent sons' anxiety that their genitals are too small.

Late development to puberty demonstrates the effect of physical impairment on the homeostatic balance that makes for a feeling of security in early adolescence. From a social viewpoint, a boy who develops late to puberty, in comparison with other boys of his own age, sees himself as smaller and weaker and his penis as considerably inferior to those of his friends. This makes him feel inadequate as a male (Schoenfeld, 1950). Adolescents have little sense of time; what is not happening today will not happen tomorrow. Direct and indirect reassurances, including those of doctors, are not believed. A distant event is not meaningful, since it has not happened.

Cultural Factors Influencing Stress

Cultural factors may also enhance the tension experienced by adolescents. Because of concern about loss of control and a fear of regression to infantile dependence, the difficulty that adolescents may have in controlling the expression of their feelings often gives rise to feelings of tension and discomfort. This control is socially reinforced in some cultures in males. But, in these, the denial of the expression of feeling that is considered a virtue may lead to the suppression of feeling and create additional stress. Pubertal adolescents are particularly likely to find themselves suddenly overwhelmed with feelings of happiness, sorrow, or anger, and these they may anxiously fight to control. Boys are likely to see the expression of sorrow, particularly if it leads to crying, as an indication of weakness and femininity.

Helplessness as a Major Trauma

Adolescents may act to alter the situation in which they find themselves, and both boys and girls use emotional energy trying to change both their social environment and the way it is experienced. The particular aim is to avoid an intolerable experience of helplessness. For example, overrestrictive family situations that deny to adolescents the responsibilities they are able to handle may lead to a projection of a sense of unfairness onto society-at-large. The complaints about the latter may be realistic. However, the intensity of the adolescent's response may be partially due to their own internal conflicts created within the nuclear family in the past as well as to present familial tensions. That such attacks may be overdetermined does not mean that adolescents who negate the values of an established social system should be labeled as emotionally disturbed.

Activity and Inactivity in the Etiology of Stress

Physical activity is an important way of sublimating feelings of tension and consequent anxiety and aggression. It can provide socially acceptable outlets for the latter, especially for boys with competitive sports and general athletic activity. In addition, this also helps such adolescents develop a feeling that they are in control of their own bodies. Diffuse muscular activity is used to drain off tension, and the restlessness of adolescence is so important as an anxiety-relieving mechanism that the immobilization of adolescents due to illness may not only cause nursing problems but create severe emotional difficulties.

John was a nineteen-year-old college football player. He was
the older son of a highly overcontrolling business tycoon and a
brilliant, beautiful, emotionally cold mother. In prep school he
had a brilliant academic and social career and was actively
engaged in all competitive sports.

A leg injury necessitated his immobilization in a cast. For
the first five days of his hospitalization, he was an excessively
good patient. On the next two days he was withdrawn when his
family visited him. He then told them that he was in direct
communication with Christ and he described vivid visual hallucinations. In his personal history he had been a head-banging child
who was extremely hyperactive. His school career was stormy
until he began to engage in sports such as ice-skating and
hockey, thus he became a highly successful athlete.

The adolescent confined to bed has many techniques of
coping with an anxiety that may be reinforced by anything from
excessive parental concern to inappropriate placement of a
youngster with a good prognosis for an illness next to a dying
patient. The regressive experience of physically sick adults in a
general hospital, that all unheard professional conversations are
about them, is enhanced in the adolescent age period because of
the extreme sensitivity of adolescents. The unease of the age leads
to a certain inevitable paranoia. To reassure themselves about
their more mature identity, adolescents in hospitals may also
be overtly sexual with staff and other patients; girls may forget
to put on their robes and wear flimsy nightgowns; boys may repeatedly ask for a urine bottle or "pat the butt" of passing nurses.

Within the nuclear family, the techniques sick adolescents
use to contain anxiety may enhance parental concern, and a
circular state of tension may then be created. An adolescent boy
may attempt to resolve his anxiety by regression with infantile
and demanding behavior; alternately, psychic withdrawal may
occur and the youngster becomes passive, obedient, but essentially
noninvolved. Some adolescents may be extremely difficult; they
may refuse to follow physician's orders to stay in bed, take medi-

cation, abstain from exercise, and so on. Immobility leads to tension, but in some adolescents the implicit dependence associated with illness is felt to be intolerable. The adolescent responses may lead to parental over solicitousness, anger or withdrawal.

Death as an Adolescent Stress

In hospitals anxiety created by the presence of dying or physical disintegration in adults may be denied by adolescents; angry feelings about the age of adults are expressed or the adolescent isolates himself from the experience by insisting that only the old die. Confrontation with death always arouses great anxiety within everyone but particularly in adolescents.

Dying patients initially deny the imminence of death, feeling that there has been a mistake; they are angry with doctors and nurses, their families, and fate because death is going to occur. Often such people withdraw into themselves, and only at the point of death do they become accepting. Sometimes both the patient and his relatives enter into a conspiracy of silence, each to protect the other. These natural psychological processes are present in all those who are dying, although sedation by doctors and nurses and the presence of pain varies the visibility to others of these responses.

Death in others arouses such anxiety that even young adults are unwilling to face the issue. This is obvious from the behavior of young medical and nursing staff in general hospitals. They often withdraw emotionally from the dying and may criticize and sometimes neglect them. The emotional difficulties of young adults are compounded in adolescents, who are not yet ready to face their own mortality. Denial is the typical response of both adolescents and young adults when those near to them, either physically or emotionally, die (Kubler-Ross, 1970). Beneath this is the same human variety of psychological defense mechan-

isms seen in older adults, but typically young people may show
their anxiety many months after the episode of death:

> An eighteen-year-old, British medical student, abruptly decided
> to withdraw from school shortly after starting in the anatomy
> laboratory. He said, "When they began to strip the corpse, I
> began to think of a favorite cousin who died a year ago, and I
> could not stand it. It's strange because, when she died, I didn't
> think it troubled me too much."

Social Pathology as a Producer of Stress

Social causes of midadolescent anxiety are most commonly
due to the absence of an extended network of people with whom
they can relate, extraparental adults or peers. This is now at
least as usual clinically as when the adolescent suffers from a
personality disturbance such that an available extended network
of people cannot be used. The anxiety may be defended against
by projection: The angry feelings that are a consequence of
anxiety are projected onto others who are seen as bad. Thus,
individuals create scapegoats—the establishment, the older generation, adolescents who are seen as different. Sometimes these
and other defensive manuevers fail to work, and a pervasive,
empty anxiety is felt. An absent feeling of self creates general
despair that may be sedated by drug dependence.

Sometimes the constrictions of the society may cause an
otherwise healthy adolescent to experience diffuse anxiety attacks:

> Kenneth, a seventeen-year-old boy was a satisfactory scholar at
> school until an unsuccessful foot operation temporarily made it
> impossible for him to play games, thus cutting off a necessary
> outlet for his anxiety and aggression. His work fell off precipi-
> tously, and he was diagnosed as suffering from depression. He
> appeared withdrawn, was unwilling to talk, and isolated himself

from others. When he saw a psychiatrist, he said, "I knew what I was thinking but I could not bring myself to say anything as I felt too nervous." When talking of his life, he said, "We live miles from anywhere and when other boys get a social life or girlfriends, I cannot. My father suggests we fish, but I don't want to do this. In any case he is too old for me. At night I feel terribly lonely and envy boys who talk about their girlfriends. I don't know what I want to do and my parents don't seem to be able to help. My teachers don't seem to care."

The apparent depression covered an acute anxiety state and was really acute withdrawal. The anxiety was held at bay by competitive physical activity. When this was no longer available to relieve tension and anxiety, he was confronted with inner loneliness. He had been unable to find a girlfriend; he was also acutely uncertain as to his life goals. The failure on the part of his environment to meet his needs created a deficiency in his capacity to use this environment at all. A circle of inadequacy was created, the world had nothing to offer.

Adolescent girls, who find themselves unable to find suitable boyfriends because none are available, may become anxious, depressed, or aggressive. Such girls may spend a great deal of their time fantasizing the love relationships they cannot find in reality. This is a particular problem for minority-group female students. Ethnic prejudice is often intense among black students who see themselves in a hostile, racist world. For many psychological reasons barriers of overt, if not covert, prejudice are ignored by men who often have white girlfriends. However, apart from many black women refusing to have white boyfriends because of ethnic pride, black males are felt by black women to refuse to allow them to do this. As a result, many black girls cannot find boyfriends. Not only do they suffer severe emotional deprivation, many of them become violently aggressively militant, sometimes storing guns for revolution against white society.

Midadolescent boys who cannot find girlfriends usually do not fantasize love relationships with imaginary girls, but rather sexual intercourse, often with older women. Hence, the interest of this age group in either magazines such as *Playboy* or in more obviously pornographic pictures.

In the wider social context, there is no doubt that the gap between the generations is responsible in many ways for the current malaise of youth: the atom bomb, the bureaucratic society that loses touch more and more with individual needs, the loss of social stability, and the breakdown of tribal networks in large cities.

Space Needs of Youth: The Place of Architecture

Architecture and town planning are among the most powerful forces available in creating or destroying communities and family structure. The typical modern house or apartment—with a small kitchen, a communal living space, a hall, and bedrooms—does not meet the basic needs of the nuclear family. For example, adolescents cannot get away from their parents unless they go out or to their bedrooms, if they have bedrooms of their own.

A large amount of space is often wasted on bedrooms; with the same space better provision could be made for psychological needs, which include in a typical family, a large eating area in the kitchen, because of the equation of food and love, and space for passive isolation or intimate talk. Children and adolescents need an area for activity away from parents where they can be noisy. The basement may provide this need, but all too often it has become, for the middle classes and the more affluent workers, the symbolic space to which children are banished when guests arrive. The typical open-plan modern house with inadequate soundproofing fails to meet the needs of different generations.

In the community-at-large children and adolescents also require space to be both constructive and safely destructive outside their home; they need to roam about and to test themselves physically. They also need to feel safe. The destruction of the core of cities is creating a social problem that is worsening in a geometrically progressive fashion, particularly as social organizations of society are allowed to decline.

Paul was an eighteen-year-old black youth from the inner city of Detroit. He entered a state hospital because of a toxic psychosis, almost certainly due to a combination of alcohol and drugs.

He was a well-built, pleasant young man, whose father had died when he was ten. He had dropped out of school at fifteen and had never worked for more than one or two weeks. He had shown some flicker of interest in girls at fifteen and at seventeen had attached himself to an older woman of twenty-two from whom he apparently caught gonorrhea. He then took many drugs, in particular, amphetamines and wine. He settled quickly into the hospital, showed obvious evidence of unresolved mourning for his father in that he wept when discussing him, and he was capable of making meaningful emotional relationships with others.

It was thought that a treatment program should contain the following: he needed an opportunity to work through some of his feelings about his dead father. He needed an activity program that would help him resolve his sense of guilt, enhance his masculine identity, and train him for a gainful occupation. Not one of the physicians in the hospital were of American birth or had English as a native language; their case load was high, and they had little or no psychotherapeutic training. The occupational therapy area of the hospital was understaffed and underequipped, and Paul had two hours of activity, other than ward cleaning a week. The vocational area of the hospital could take forty patients and was not prepared to keep patients who could not at once work a full day in a productive way.

Paul returned to the inner city, disenchanted with the effects of the white establishment and presumably, was ultimately lost in the black drug scene. In his turn, he is likely to breed more damaged human beings whose deprivation will be ignored until they attack the outer suburbs.

If society makes a determined effort to rebuild the inner city, neighborhoods, homes, schools, and youth-club facilities, which cater to our urban adolescents, are more necessary than tower blocks. If new homes are built, it should not be beyond the wit of man to organize them so that no one is too far away from natural countryside or the means of getting there. From the young adolescents' point of view, it is unfortunate that the bicycle cannot be used safely in many large cities.

When families move into new districts human relationships can be created between them if their small children can play together. Adolescents with no extended family often relate well to the parents of their friends, particularly if they have made these friendships before the age of puberty. All this has implications for the way family units should be housed. It is now generally accepted that the high-rise building is an unsatisfactory social organism because of its effect on the family. If small children play a long distance away from their mothers, they manage well, unless there is a crisis; then they need the solace of mother's presence. In this situation they begin to learn that mother is not to be trusted because she is not there if she is needed. Alternatively, they are deprived of the experience of playing with others unless their mothers are able to accompany them. If high buildings were wide enough to allow several familes to live on one floor with enough space for the children to play with each other, these buildings might be less damaging.

School architecture should take note of emotional needs, particularly those of developing personalities. Primary schools tend to be small in size and numbers. But the large complex of buildings found in many secondary schools can be overwhelming, arousing anxiety in both parents and children. If adolescents feel dwarfed by bricks, mortar, steel, or glass, they can enter a new school for the first time with unnecessarily increased anxiety. This does not help their later relationships with each other or the staff.

We do not really know how large schools should be, yet

relationships are certainly distorted by distance and inaccessibility. The interdepartmental memo is no substitute for relationships. It is also a mistake for schools to be isolated from the local population: The educational campus˙ is outside the main stream of community living.

Tall buildings also create problems. Human beings do not communicate if they have to go up too many stairs, and elevators do not help communications. As in high blocks of flats where families become isolated from each other, tall school buildings mar the formation of a coherent social structure. The furniture arrangement of a typical classroom creates distance between teacher and pupil. Similarly, architecture may separate teachers from pupils. Even those whose primary task is the emotional care of pupils may have their offices in a corridor away from the main stream of school activities. This makes it much more difficult for the pupils to contact them. The isolation that pupils in emotional difficulty are likely to feel is reinforced. Many high schools, in addition, socially isolate social workers from the mainstream of school life, thus children have to make direct efforts to reach such staff: Little free, unscheduled contact is possible.

It often seems that those who plan and design school buildings have not considered the needs of the organization: Buildings should be the servants of the school not their masters. The answers to some of these problems may be to have relatively small school units of a few hundred pupils. Four or five of these could be placed within easy walking distance of a central core of buildings for specialized and technical subjects.

There has been very little consideration of the effect of architectural styles on the school's ethos: Will its buildings enhance or inhibit a child's appreciation of beauty as it grows?

A girl was moved from a very beautiful contemporary high school to one that was more likely in other ways to fit her special needs, an excellent private, co-educational boarding school. Her parents, acutely aware of the effects of environment, said: "We can't believe she can be helped in the scruffy buildings to which you want us to send her. However, the staff really seemed interested and the principal spent a great deal of time with her when we went to be interviewed."

Bricks and mortar do not in themselves make the character of the school, and the beautiful, contemporary high school repeated its architectural arrangement so all corridors looked similar. But these parents were making a valid point. The girl's new school, which especially prided itself on its ability to meet human needs and to be helpful in personal relationships, was a very ugly place. This made the work of the school much more difficult.

Anxiety is, then, the result of an obvious interplay between physical, psychological, intrafamilial, and social forces. Within each of these, there is a capacity for support for the individual but also a possibility of the individual being put in a state of stress. It is the balance of these factors that creates an effective human being or an anxious, dependent, inadequate, or over-aggressive personality.

References

Bowlby, J. (1969), *Attachment,* Vol. 1 of *Attachment and Loss.* London: Hogarth Press.

Cannon, W. B. (1939), *The Wisdom of the Body.* New York: Norton.

Freud, A. (1958), Adolescence. In *Psychoanalytic Study of the Child,* 13: 255–277. New York: International Universities Press.

Klein, M. (1932), *Introduction to Child Analysis.* London: Hogarth Press.

Kubler-Ross, E. (1970), *On Death and Dying.* New York: Macmillan.

Menniger, K. A. (1963), *The Vital Balance.* New York: Viking.

Miller, D. (1966), A model of an institution for treating delinquent adolescent boys. In *Changing Concepts of Crime and Its Treatment,* ed. H. Klare, 99. Oxford: Pergamon Press.

———— (1970), Parental responsibility for adolescent maturity. In *The Family and Its Future,* ed. K. Elliott, 23–38. London: Churchill.

Reich, A. (1951), The discussion of 1912 on masturbation and our present day views. In *Psychoanalytic Study of the Child,* 6: 80–95. New York: International Universities Press.

Schoenfeld, W. A. (1950), Inadequate masculine physique in the personality development of adolescent boys. *Psychosom. Med.,* 12: 49–56.

11

Verbal and Physical Aggression in Adolescence

Need for Aggression

Aggressive behavior is at the root of man's success or failure in coping with his environment (Lorenz, 1966, pp. 208–236). It is associated with physical changes that prepare the body for fighting, and it may or may not be associated with subjective feelings of anger. It is both an enjoyable and an emotionally disintegrating experience, depending on its intensity. Behind every aggressive act of mankind is an attempt to cope with a potentially unpleasant experience of tension that is externally provoked (Scott, 1958). There is a gradation in the expression of human aggression from the more or less controlled use of language and physical activity to an uncontrollable or barely handled turning of destructive aggression against the self or others. Aggression may also be projected by fantasizing the other person as aggressive, actually creating this, and then controlling it.

Language as a Vehicle for Aggression

Language is one way of expressing and beginning to relieve angry feelings. The English-speaking world is fortunate; as a language, English is particularly rich because accent, intonation, and word forms carry implications not only about the role and status of the user but they also convey shades of anger (Johnson, 1948). Furthermore, language has always been used to show group cohesion, often against an outside aggressor. The Welsh and Israelis revived their ancient tongue. The black American, whose language is remarkably like the eighteenth-century English of the indentured servants of the South and whose use of swear words is almost similar in color and frequency to that of the London Cockney, uses language to try to create a sense of ethnic pride.

The generation gap and subgroupings within the youth culture are reinforced by the use of special language. Slang words may have an idiosyncratic meaning to an in-group, when translated they become aggressive; adolescents do not see "panhandle" as being pejorative; "begging," however, is deplorable. It is acceptable to be "stoned," not to be "drunk." The language of adolescence changes regularly, the phrases of the fifties are now obsolete. Adolescent language is taken over by the adult world, and new words are then introduced by youth. Apart from private language within their family group, adolescents, particularly among the middle classes, often deliberately use words both to shock as well as to assert autonomy. An adolescent, using the language dissonance between himself and his parents, told them in the late 1960s to "keep their cool" and to "get themselves together." Language, as an attempt to reinforce feelings of separateness and autonomy may also be used to show defiance. Mixing rebellion with independence, employing language similarly to clothes and hair styles, adolescents attempt to demonstrate the gap between themselves and the world of adults. Since language, like all fashions, seems to be taken over by adults, adolescents then have to devise new techniques of communication.

Use of Accents

The use of a special language for certain groups, prevalent throughout all societies, means that accent may be used aggressively. Superior groups in the social scale use one sort of language to show their dominance over those whom they consider inferiors. In recent years in Britain the use of working-class English has come to be thought of as acceptable in association with the aggressive needs of some of the present generation to reverse many traditionally held beliefs; a similar process occurs with middle-class black Americans, whose youth now goes out of its way to use the language of the black ghetto.

Language as a Reinforcer of Group Cohesion

Conformity to the demands of a peer group is obvious among adolescents, particularly as they try to free themselves from dependence on parents and are involved in the world outside the family. However, long before adolescence, language may be part both of the technique of self-assertion and of peer-group acceptability. This becomes obvious as soon as children, who are highly imitative, begin to make special friends. When they play outside their own immediate social groups, especially in socially and ethnically integrated grade schools, they may acquire a language that is unacceptable to their nuclear family. Correction may follow, and the children may then learn to speak with two tongues: one at home and one at school. Initially, in an unthinking way, they may bring the unacceptable language to the family table. Later this may be used aggressively against parents. Thus, developmental behavior can once again be used as a rebellious way of establishing autonomy.

The success or failure for the individual in an aggressive use of language depends on the codes of the individual's nuclear family. It is a concern of many parents when their children go to grade school that they will learn bad manners and language, the definition of bad being determined by the individual family. Bad language does not just consist of swear words and vulgarities; it also involves grammatical construction. The use of special words, as in dialect, may carry an aggressive connotation with some. A West Riding, Yorkshire, joke demonstrates the point that bad language, like beauty, is in the eye of the beholder:

A Yorkshire farmer was walking down a lane with his son when they passed two dogs copulating. The boy was highly intrigued and, pointing to the dogs, said, "Sithee father, two dogs fucking." The father immediately hit the boy across the face saying, "I told you not to use bad language; if I hear you say "sithee" again I will clout you."

Swearing

Some swear words are common in Britain and not in the United States and vice versa. "Son of a bitch" is unknown in England, and "mother-fucker" is extremely rare; "bloody" and "bugger" are not significantly used in the United States. Just as aggression and sexuality are clearly mixed behaviorally (Kinsey *et al.*, p. 269), so many aggressive words are sexual. Literally a bugger is a sodomist; the swear word has lost this meaning. Some words acquire a sexual meaning in one culture, not another. In Lancashire, to be "knocked up" means to be awakened in the morning. "Keep your pecker up" is northern English colloquial slang to keep cheerful.

Just as parents may perceive the language of their children as aggressive, the reverse may also be true. Sometimes proper language is felt by children to be aggressively obtuse:

A nine-year-old boy reproached his mother saying that he thought that she never lied to him. His mother, who prided herself on her honesty with her son, was more than a little offended. She asked him what he meant. He told her that she had not told him the truth about the word "penis." The mother wondered what on earth he meant. She was told that the proper name of it was "prick."

At the age of nine this boy was beginning to feel that the language of his age group was more personally appropriate than that of his parents. Having established its nonacceptability to his parents, the word can now be used in the service of aggression; "you prick" will be said to his agemates.

Bad language may be disapproved of on moral or religious grounds; it may also be considered poor taste. The dictionary definition of "vulgar" shows the class bias associated with swearing; it is "course, impolite, common, of the people."

The use of swear words develops in all societies around subjects that arouse special anxiety (Montague, 1961, pp. 182–201). Words that are associated with conscious or unconscious conflicts are used to express anger. In Tudor England expletives were especially associated with religion. The absence of concern about doctrinal questions of religious belief now means that swear words associated with them are no longer bad. The British swear word "bloody," originally associated with the idea of God's Blood and the wounds of Christ, is a diminutive of Shakespearean England's "Od's Blood." It no longer arouses a frisson in polite circles.

Anxiety about maternal chastity is more significant in some cultures than others. It is particularly likely to be an emotionally laden issue for adolescents. The stronger the unconscious maternal tie and the younger looking the mother, the greater is the unconscious incestuous threat to the male. A mother known by her adolescent son to be sexually promiscuous makes for more intense oedipal conflicts because of her obvious availability. "Whoreson" was freely used in Elizabethan England; nowadays in the United States "son of a bitch" is in aggressive use (Ross, 1961). An even more angrily abusive term for one young man to howl at another is to call him a "mother-fucker."

The constant repetition of swear words in books, plays, television, and the movies has much the same effect on young people as the use of their adolescent language by their parents. The four-letter words eventually cease to have meaning as terms of abuse and they have to be replaced by something else. The need to swear does not change; the actual words used may. Furthermore, if the forbidden conflicts behind the swear words change, new words have to be used that express what the culture then finds unacceptable.

Most cultures have many individuals within them who suffer from sexual anxieties. Until recently, in the United States, these were mostly about normal sexuality, so sexual words describing genital organs became thought of as swear words. These are often acceptable between men or boys in their own groups but are considered unacceptable in family circles. Despite the aggressive identification of some women's political groups with apparent masculine norms this remains true between men and women or boys and girls. However, words that boys might be unprepared to use to their mothers may now be said to girlfriends. A late-adolescent boy may comfortably use "fuck" to his girlfriend; he is less likely to say it to his mother. So societies that are particularly conflict-ridden over normal sexuality use the vulgar words for sexual organs and sexual activities as swear words. Angry boys will call each other "prick"; to be particularly offensive they use colorful words for the female genitalia, "you cunt." Boys will tell each other to "fuck off." Such swear words are particularly likely to occur in all male groups cut off from female company. In such circumstances the erotic quality of these words that, in normal heterosexual societies tends to be much overlayed by their aggressive connotation, comes to the fore. Thus, men unconsciously express their homosexual anxieties.

As normal sexuality has become less of a source of anxiety to the community-at-large, the sexually abusive words have tended to leave the area of normative sexuality. Some words carry specific derogatory meaning for one socioeconomic or ethnic group or in one part of the country. Sometimes the same social group may change the meaning of a word over a few years. For example, in northern England "queer" means strange, in the south of the country, it is offensive for one boy to angrily call another "queer," for this implies homosexuality. "Queen" and "camp" are two homosexual words that appear to be moving into fashionable and theatrical language and losing their sexual meaning. Adolescent girls in some parts of London who wish to abuse another girl of their own age may call them "lesbians." English boys call other boys "cock suckers"; American boys are aggressive to others by asking if they "suck." Sometimes conflict-ridden individuals, particularly those whose conflicts are associated with sexuality and aggression, may become compulsive swearers and in an ejaculatory way scatter swear words through their conversation (Hollander, 1960).

Anal Aggression with the Use of Language

Until recent years, men and women have been highly prudish over natural excretory functions. A whole euphemistic language grew up around the use of the toilet. Even the formal words are confusing: A "lavatory" really is a place to wash, yet it is used in England to describe a "watercloset," the official description there of a "toilet." A "closet" in America is a "cupboard" and has no bladder or bowel significance. A "toilet" is really a place to adorn oneself. A lavatory in England may be called a "loo," in America a "John." Some middle-class American women refer coyly to "the little girls' room." The vulgar words for urination and defecation are still replaced in many families with a whole variety of apparently innocuous words: "big job," "BM," "wee," and so forth. Only in the last two hundred years has the flight from natural vulgarity over natural functions occurred. It was perfectly acceptable for Chaucer to write of the parson in the *Canterbury Tales:* "What needeth then a shiten shepherd and a clene shepe." In case generations of schoolboys were corrupted, Victorian morality replaced the word with "dirty." Shakespeare freely used the word "piss."

Adolescents today are less liable to need to be imprecise in their use of excretory language: "Piss off" is still abusive, but an almost acceptable description of rainy weather is that it is "pissing down." The relationship between the parental use of language and adolescent aggression is again apparent. If parents use euphemisms for urination, their adolescent sons are more likely to tell each other to "piss off." If "piss" is the parental word, the adolescent will be much less likely to use language in this way.

Aggression as a Function of Personal and Family Lifestyle

Each family and each society decides on its own limits and techniques of control. Physical assault when angry, as from parents to children, is tolerated in some social groups (Miller and Swanson, 1958, p. 221). Some fathers will hit their sons until the latter are big enough to hit back. In other families physical assaultiveness is very rare, if not unknown. Nevertheless, acceptable outlets for anger have to be found. Those parents who believe that they should never show anger convey to their children that anger is very dangerous. Alternately, they may be felt to be dishonest if children know their parents hide angry feelings. Parents who completely repress their own anger either create children who are incapable of self-assertion, those who fear that their anger may spill out dangerously, or both.

If anger is not to be expressed in assaultive behavior, it would then appear inevitable in healthy personalities that the aggression will have to appear in words. Swear words are the safest and least cruel way of showing rage. Personal security can be destroyed more effectively with polite and cutting language than with violent words. Parents may make distinct efforts not to swear in front of their children, adolescent or younger. The justification for this is that parents do not wish to set a bad example, but it is important to give children safe areas for defiant and aggressive behavior and at the same time to convey that parents too may be imperfect.

All parents have secrets into which they do not allow their children to pry, for example, bedroom behavior. Adolescents have inevitably experienced situations over years in which parental language has only been partly understood. Furthermore, most parents swear at each other when they are enraged. In healthy families children know that special words are associated with mutual parental irritation; sometimes these are swear words. Social hyprocrisy still exists about this: An embarrassed mother will pretend that her child's bad language has been picked up at school; no such social games are possible with their own adolescents.

Children have a relatively unchanging language and lore of their own, handed down through the generations (Opie and Opie, 1965). If all swear words were to be banished from all homes, they would still continue in the world of children, just as their games and rhymes are transmitted. The private language of adolescents needs to be seen by them as bad in the eyes of the adult world. This concept is part of their need to in-group with their own generation.

Adolescents have a need for aggressive defiance of the openly stated norms of adult society. To accept bad language is to deny to adolescents a whole area of potential defiance that is relatively safe. If bad language between parents and children is totally forbidden, the probability is that young people will conform as they do in many areas of interfamily functioning (Macoby et al., 1954). Other outlets for aggression will then have to be found. If bad language is disapproved of but implicitly condoned from time to time, it will be used when adolescents wish to show aggressive defiance.

Physical Expression of Aggression

It is possible that ethnic and social groups that do not develop a concept of forbidden language are inevitably beset by greater physical aggression. Almost all people swear and use bad language when they are angry. Some adults may then be tempted to abandon attempts to control the use of bad language. If this is done the effect is the same as overrepression; an area of relatively safe defiance and angry expression is removed from the field of human conflict. If all language is permissible within the family setting, words cease to be a satisfactory vehicle to express feelings of anger. If defiance is taken out of the use of bad language, children and adolescents may then feel forced to act out their anger in physical ways in the world-at-large, rather than by the use of words. The old phrase about sticks and stones breaking bones but words never harming has validity. In spite of Biblical injunctions, it is better to take the name of the Lord in vain than to be physically violent with other human beings.

The physical expression of angry feelings involves the attempt to inflict damage on inanimate objects, the self, or others. In the former, the object is personalized; adolescents suffering an accute loss of ego identity (Erikson, 1968, pp. 9–12) will attack their family furniture as an expression of their rage with their parents whom they perceive as preventing them from developing a sense of autonomy (Miller, 1967).

Bullying

Anger turned against the self is evident in a whole range of self-destructive behavior. but, apart from outbursts of rage directed against others in temper tantrums, physical bullying is the most usual form of outwardly directed personal aggression in the young. "Perhaps, our most unpleasant characteristic as a species is our proclivity for bullying the helpless" (Storr, 1968, p. 92). Beyond this, use of angry and violent behavior toward others is particularly likely to occur during childhood and adolescence. The streets of both the inner city and the schools may be made dangerous by violent and aberrant youth. In England alienated skin heads (greasers) haunt parts of London to "Pak Bash," attack isolated Pakistanis whom they perceive as helpless. Disturbed adolescents are likely to persecute others who are weaker than they are for three reasons: They cannot yet control their anger when frustrated. Bullying and violence is not felt to be wrong because the victim is dehumanized; during violent outbursts the usual awareness of what is felt to be wrong is suspended. Typically, individuals or groups are scapegoated and although weak, are felt to be powerful (Cohn, 1967). Scapegoats are given qualities by individuals that they find intolerable in themselves or in their environment; they are felt not to be the same as the self, but at the same time they possess the powerful inner badness of those who bully.

Adolescent boys may get sexually excited when involved in aggressive behavior. At all ages, particularly in the male, sexual and angry feelings are easily mixed, but in adolescence this mix is enhanced.

Etiology of the Increase in Violence

The increase in violent behavior among young people in the present decade appears to be absolute in the countries of the West, and there is much preoccupation with its causes. It is sometimes thought to be the result of changes in child-rearing techniques, but there are many more positive results from these than otherwise. New ways of bringing up children are thought to be part of a permissive society that is said to have created a moral turpitude in the young. However, society is probably more confused or rejecting than permissive; this has led to adolescents' feeling neglected and not cared about. Some may identify with this and become uncaring adults. Others are raised without the recognition that needs are not the same as wants and should, if possible, be met. Many parents are aware that children are not just extensions of themselves; children who are raised with a recognition that they have valued personal integrity become adolescents who do not value violence and who also feel that respect for the integrity of others is important.

In this respect, the comments from some deans for student affairs in medical schools are pertinent. The class of 1972, generally born in 1947 or 1948 were angry, often impulsive, and had a high withdrawal rate, even if this was only temporary and due to psychological reasons. This was the class that was, as undergradutes, part of the destructive wave of campus violence. The class of 1975, born in 1951 or 1952 are apparently more perceptive, thoughtful, and hypersensitive. Although there may not be a relationship, by 1950 changes in child-rearing techniques, particularly among the middle classes, were firmly under way.

Although most young people have become less inclined to use physical violence, as antiwar demonstrations have shown, crimes of violence have increased. Their increased incidence is present in the deprived and underprivileged and drug-dependent groups of society. It is associated with the polarization of society into haves and have-nots, and is also related to individual alienation, an aspect of human development for which the American school system has apparently some responsibility. Teachers in Britain, where the schools are considerably less alienating, report a general decline in the amount of physical bullying among their pupils. In America the rigidity of school systems that are usually unable to tolerate any physical outlets for aggression that are not planned (thus disrespectful of adolescent needs), along with tension produced by forcible, and from a psychosocial view, unplanned integration has led to excessive tension among underprivileged members of the majority and minority groups. An unthinking ethnic and social-class mix has removed a neighborhood base for many children and placed them too far away from their parents, in social settings where they are not understood. The school counseling system has meant that often the average teacher has opted out of feeling any responsibility for interpersonal relationship with pupils.

> A group of teachers in a discussion session suddenly realized that if an adolescent missed one of their classes they did not usually tell the individual that he or she had been missed. A note was sent to the counselor who would determine whether or not disciplinary action was necessary. If he thought the adolescent was emotionally upset, the child would then be sent to the school social worker. Furthermore, none of these levels of staff, if they were to call the youngster's home, would ask for him, irrespective of age. Parents were always told first.

Parts of the adolescent's personality are thus isolated from each other by a social system. Furthermore, because an intrafamilial striving for autonomy is not recognized, the adolescent is further alienated. In addition, the rigidly organized day means that there is little opportunity for freely permitted social interaction. Middle-class and white adolescents are more prepared to say what they feel rather than act it out, but even they begin to demonstrate a hostile "we–they" attitude between teacher and taught. The obsession with behavioral conformity has led in many places to the use of behaviorist teaching techniques, but these have not resolved the social, educational and psychological problems of the young. Greater classroom freedom is a function of sophisticated and wise teaching, a general improvement in the educational climate dramatically leads to less disturbed behavior.

Physical bullying and its verbal equivalent, teasing, can be understood in two ways: It is related to the capacity to tolerate frustration and handle angry feelings and the degree of inner security an individual might feel. Bullying, a provoked or unprovoked physical assault on a weaker individual, is an idea children develop with the growth of conscience. Without conception of actions as right or wrong, an awareness that one is bullying does not occur. Physical bullying is more usual in boys, verbal teasing in girls. In England, girls rarely bully; boys quite often tease. However, physical violence among girls is much more common in the United States than in Britain. In America it is not unusual for racial violence to break out among girls in school locker-rooms; usually less privileged black girls try to physically intimidate whites whom they perceive as more affluent. The placing of policemen or human relations counselors as an attempt to stop this is not unusual; without control the situation could be worse, but controls alone cannot succeed.

There is less adult concern about taunting behavior than physical bullying, so it takes longer for the adolescent who indulges in verbal assaults to give these up than physical attacks. Adolescents who would not persecute others in a one-to-one setting may do this in a group. The stage performer who disappoints an audience may be given a slow, measured handclap instead of applause; everyone present joins in this behavior.

Conscience around the control of physical assaultiveness first appears about the age of two; parents show disapproval when it is directed at other children. This disapproval is perceived as a loss of love, so the child initially avoids such behavior in sight of his parents. At about three or four recognition that weaker children should not be hit is expected. In nursery schools physical attacks will be controlled and disapproval shown. However, in free play the concept of nonviolence may be honored more in the breach than the observance. It takes many years before the internal image of parental and adult disapproval becomes a well-developed conscience that automatically controls behavior. Kindly behavior is not always consistently present among three-year-olds, nor is it always present in early adolescence. Aggressive behavior in children and adolescents is related to anxiety; the more potentially anxious a child may be, the more he is likely to fight. Violence is therefore more common in environments in which children's needs are not met, in poverty-stricken neighborhoods in the United States and other parts of the Western world.

Social Systems and Violence

Natural violence is present in all men, it is particularly obvious in early adolescent boys. They have a great need for semiaggressive physical contact with each other. The friendly punch and the playful wrestling bout is typical behavior of adolescents to help the control of aggression, the assessment of physical strength, and the provision of a sense of boundaries due to developmental distortion of body image. This may easily spill over to become bad tempered, violent, and bullying.

Rigid social systems that do not respect the individual needs of adolescents are more likely to see violent behavior than those that are able to respect the integrity of the children in their care. A vicious circle tends to be created. The more rigid the system, the more rigid is likely to be the response to violent behavior (Morris and Morris, 1963, pp. 257–261). So a situation can be created in which schools never allow unsupervised activities because of fear of how the children will behave. This is presumably one of the factors that has led to the disappearance of recess in most American high schools.

Parents and Bullying

Small children report bullying to parents and authority adults; adolescent boys consider it antisocial to tell tales. This in-group loyalty can mean that a boy may be bullied and scapegoated for a considerable time before it comes to the attention of adults. A typical site for early adolescent bullying is in school toilet areas, perhaps in a social way confirming analytic observations of the relationship of anality to aggression. It also occurs in poorly supervised school showers. Often those bullied are least physically developed; the sexual implications are obvious.

Most adults do not have optimum control of their own angry feelings, so parents may be unduly defensive when told of their child's bullying behavior. Others, in an attempt to demonstrate that bullying is forbidden, may bully themselves.

A three-year-old boy angrily bit a two-year-old for taking his toy away. The boy's mother, when she learned about this, immediately bit her son.

The intention undoubtedly was to show that biting was wrong. The message probably given was that to bite one should be bigger and better than the opponent.

By school age, after the child enters the latency period, a strong enough conscience to prevent bullying, except under conditions of intrapsychic tension, should have developed. The relationship of cruelty to humanizing and dehumanizing is obvious in children. These children who learn to humanize animals do not behave with cruelty towards them. Cruelty directed towards other children is associated with them having become temporarily dehumanized. Overwhelmed with intrapsychic tension and sadism, the child ceases to see the other individual as a person.

Children try out the strength, both of their own consciences and their own capacity to be impulsive and aggressive, by fighting other children, often in various types of war games, and cowboys and Indians. In the excitement of this activity children are likely to allow the impulsive breakthrough of angry feelings. A similar situation occurs in early adolescence. Smaller children see themselves as having been bullied in games, and an accidental blow can be felt as deliberate. It is not unusual for the ritual of a game to allow bullying under the guise of play. This may be fairly frequent and obvious between brothers and sisters who are jealous of each other.

A group of ten-year-old children, having heard about the Spanish Inquisition, decided that they would have a ceremonial burning at the stake. As their victim for this *auto da fe,* they chose an eight-year-old younger brother of one of the group. The older boy allowed his brother to be tied up but insisted on his release before the pyre was ignited.

Apart from the chance occurrence of bullying in games or its appearance in the roughhousing of early adolescence, children are likely to hit others who are smaller when they feel overcome with frustration and rage. The weaker child may be the victim of the frustration that older individuals feel as a result of their own relative weakness. A boy who feels bullied by his parents is likely to bully others. Often the young thug of the classroom has a bullying father who does not hesitate to beat his child.

Transient emotional disturbance caused by circumstance, a family move, for example, may lead to bullying behavior. Some social and ethnic groups are more prepared to be violent than others. When almost all parental frustration is dealt with by a cuff, children hit others more easily and with less guilt than those who come from families in which the physical expression of anger is controlled. Social class and ethnic behavioral differences can create conflicts between children. Such differences may cause severe social disruption, particularly in early adolescence, because this is the age of projection into out-groups.

Trouble in a high school is often ascribed to conflicts between black and white. Particularly in deprived neighborhoods, this explanation of school riots and violence has some validity; nevertheless, the social organization of the school is highly significant. Children do not destroy school property and attack each other if the adults in their immediate environment are felt as supportive and caring.

Violence as an Intergroup Phenomenon

Small children who are in emotional difficulty easily refer back to the family ethos; although it may be defied, the parental attitude is consciously and unconsciously accepted as correct. Adolescents are more involved with their own age group as a function of emotional withdrawal from parents because of anxiety about childish dependent and incestuous feelings. They become susceptible to the culture of the group of young people with whom they ally themselves. The groups may be quite small, six to eight, but they, in turn, are also influenced by the way of life of the larger society. For example, if most adolescents in a school come from one social class, providing the social environment meets a reasonable number of adolescent needs, the school will be comfortable and productive. Furthermore, any environmental tensions can be dealt with by projection onto groups outside the school with whom there may be little actual contact, although different interest groups are always a fertile field in adolescence for mutual problems. A mix of social class and ethnic groups means that stress may be dealt with by projection onto the other group. At best, groups may withdraw from each other in mutual incomprehension. This has happened in high schools on the basis of religion, social class, or ethnic background. The Jews sat at one table, the WASPs at another. Now the phenomenon is very evident on the basis of ethnic groups, although more subtle withdrawal on the basis of social class is also present. The failure of intergration is apparent in undergraduate and postgraduate schools. There the minority groups may cluster together, often at the back of the room. They may demand separate housing on the pretext that they are harried by whites and see prejudice when it is not there:

> A lecturer in a class of social work students commented in the course of his first hour lecture about a girl who was rather obviously balancing her checkbook. She happened to be black. After the break, every black student had vanished from the class.

Different social and ethnic groups become a convenient vehicle for the exchange of violence. Sometimes one adolescent may behave in a way that fits his social group. A lack of understanding on the part of a member of another can lead to an outburst of aggressive behavior.

Personal Reasons for Violence

Bullying is related to the ability of an adolescent to handle his own angry or envious feelings and to put up with another's teasing or provocation. Adolescents uncertain about their identity and ability to handle feelings of anger and sorrow may be afraid that their own angry feelings will be uncontrollable. They may also have grave, if transient, doubts about the physical effectiveness of their own bodies. Doubt about personal weakness may be resolved by attacking that apparent weakness in others. Adolescents who have problems of personal self-control may provoke a peer to tears or anger, then scorn, mock, reject or hit the playmate. This is similar to the smaller child who, easily provoked to tears, is only too willing to mock another for being a "cry baby." Finally, the adolescent may enhance his own feelings of strength by imagining how he would respond if he were tormented. Adolescents with distressed feelings, whose personal controls are rigid but weak, often respond to teasing with temper outbursts. These adolescents are likely to be bullied. They are ready-made victims for those adolescents who fear loss of control themselves and who can reassure themselves that they would behave differently. So bullies both identify with their victim's torment, projecting onto them in order to make the torment possible and, at the same time, dehumanizing the object of their sadism.

Early adolescents are likely to bully those whom they envy. Young people who make a conspicuous display of their worldly goods, particularly to those who do not have them, are likely to be set upon and tormented. Affluence is not always economic. Those boys who work excessively hard in high schools and make their agemates feel guilty are likely to be pilloried in one way or another.

Some schools develop an ethos among their pupils in which work is always denied. A boy or girl who works hard and enjoys this is likely to deny to others that work is ever done. Jealousy and envy are feelings that most individuals try to avoid (Rosenfeld, 1957). People who are likely to be envied do their best to deny this, since they fear the physical or verbal assault of others. The very rich often try to hide their wealth and pretend to others and themselves that economic bargains are significant. The upper-upper social class groups in the United States often do not drive new cars; in Britain the very rich may take pride in wearing old clothes.

Problems of the Physically Handicapped

Since early adolescent boys are likely to be anxious about physical effectiveness, a physically inadequate early adolescent is a likely victim of bullying. Such an individual may attempt to buy favor by sidling up to teachers with work and to other adolescents with gifts, jokes, or dirty stories. The attempt to buy off bullying is likely to produce bullying; a vicious circle of sadism and inadequacy may then be created. The conflicts of early adolescence pose particular problems for these young people who are physically handicapped. They may be tormented, teased, or bullied, especially at this stage of personality development. Children may be kind to their agemates who suffer from physical disability, providing they do not experience any anxiety about their own physical security. The severely crippled child is not likely to be teased or bullied, partly because sympathy is aroused and partly because the severity of the illness is not a threat to the normally developing youngster, although such crippled children may be victims of the emotionally insecure. The mildly disabled are more likely to be teased and bullied; they are more of a threat, particularly to adolescents somewhat doubtful of their own potency. In schools that overvalue competitive sports early adolescents pick on boys who are physically inadequate; adolescents who show idiosyncratic behavior are bullied by those afraid of their own idiosyncrasies.

Homosexual Anxiety and Bullying

Pubertal adolescents, unsure of their own physical maturity, are likely to tease late developers. Particularly in single-sex institutions, physically immature boys are likely to be tormented by those past puberty, since once puberty is over, boys normally begin seeking heterosexual relationships. If this search is inhibited, particularly if boys are living under emotional stress, the immature boy is thought to be effeminate. Thus, the naturally developed fifteen- to sixteen-year-old becomes anxious about his own homosexuality, and the immature boy is teased for being a fag. This is particularly likely when, in a closed male community, sexual gratification with other boys is a distinct possibility. The perception of a younger male as effeminate is, of course, relative.

In closed penal settings late-developing boys, those who are weak or those who are younger, are likely to be homosexually seduced. Often they accept the homosexual role because they feel that if they do not they will be bullied into homosexual activity and raped. In such environments special rituals and codes develop. Tough boys may take weaker, more effeminate, boys as homosexual partners and look after them. The aggressive boy is not then thought to be queer. In some penal settings boys who are flagrantly homosexual are often rejected because they glory in activities that boys with a heterosexual orientation feel guilty and angry about.

Minority Groups and Persecution

Racial persecution is mass bullying and assultiveness writ large. In adolescence individuals are bullied because they are given the qualities their tormentors fear they might have themselves. This mechanism is also present in the racial persecution of minority groups by the majority: blacks by whites or vice versa, Jews by Gentiles, or Catholics by Protestants. The persecution of minorities is partly related to the belief that they are too clever, cunning, privileged, inferior, or a social and economic threat. The unacceptable bad qualities ascribed to the minority by the majority, qualities that must be controlled, are commonly qualities that the majority group unconsciously fears. If the majority are under pressure—economic, social, or emotional—prejudice, which produces social ostracism, is converted to persecution. This is persecution by the majority of their own sense of internal badness, ascribed to others. It is also an attempt to relieve tension by playing out aggressive feelings on others.

Adolescents may attack minorities for being deceitful, dishonest, dirty, mean, greedy, and sexually unreliable; these are all qualities that they have to deal with inside themselves. But national and ethnic prejudice only becomes persecutory action when the social climate puts people under stress, and often there is a political motive. Those who are responsible for the stress divert the attention of the population onto external enemies, perhaps a minority group within the host population. A psychological need to be prejudiced against certain groups and individuals within the population is then capitalized on. Minority qualities are also used as a scapegoat for other anxieties. When one social group is rehoused with another, the host population that is not prepared to receive the new group may ascribe the inevitably disturbed behavior of those who have been moved to qualities inherent in their ethnic or religious group.

Individuals identify with their tormentors; they both believe they are right and become persecutors themselves, given the opportunity. The boy who is bullied toadies up to the bullier, not just out of fear but also out of admiration. The victims of prejudice may ultimately agree with the attitudes of their tormentors. They become highly prejudiced themselves about their own ethnic group irrationally accepting the negative qualities they have been given. Alternately, they may implicitly agree with prejudice as an attitude by being as prejudiced against the larger population as that group is against them.

Small children who are bullied may often become bullies themselves as they grow into adolescence and become physically more effective. Such adolescents may persecute others for the same reasons for which they themselves suffered. Some social environments bring out the latent bullying qualities that exist in some adolescents; some schools are notorious for the amount of bullying that goes on in them.

The equivalent among girls of the physical bullying of boys is usually verbal backbiting. Just as one boy can become a scapegoat and be physically attacked, so a girl becomes the victim of verbal assaults. In very deprived societies and socially aberrant girls' institutions, bullying among girls is common. Then it is even more usual for one girl to fight another girl than for a group of girls to behave in a bullying manner.

Bullying may be an identification by young people with the behavior of their elders, but any consideration of adolescent aggression has to include the bullying of the old, weak, and helpless by the young. Throughout history, groups of young men have been known to wreak impulsive havoc on these groups; this has always been known in ill-disciplined armed forces. Young, ill-trained, or demoralized troops are exposed to the excessive psychological trauma of murder and brutality on the battlefield. If the social structure of the army unit does not offer enough psychological support, such soldiers are likely to act out their anxieties with sexual and murderous attacks on helpless populations, hence, the massacres in Vietnam (Gault, 1971). A relatively new historical phenomenon arose in the 1930s: the systematic widespread bullying of older people by young adults and late adolescents for ideological reasons. Nazi youth, reinforced by authority, divided the world, both inside themselves and externally, into good and bad. Jews and gypsies were bad and dehumanized; they could be justifiably tormented, bullied, and then murdered. The cruelty of this was partly a function of a group process that gave individuals permission to act out their internal sadism. Also, authority was given the more disturbed sections of the populations to allow them to inflict their own own angry feelings on people who represented to them a bad, uncaring world.

A somewhat similar phenomenon has appeared in the late 1960s with some university students. Small groups bullied and humiliated some of their teachers. Those aggressive and violent students were protesting, among other things, against the agressive violence of society. Unconsciously, these young people identified with the very qualities that they criticized. Many who insisted that they had been alienated by society treated their victims as if they were nonhuman. Adolescents who experience themselves as the repository for the aggressive fantasies of adults may repay the compliment in kind. Often late adolescents, who may complain that the older generation has treated them in an uncaring fashion, appear not to care how they relate to individuals younger than themselves.

Role of the Police

To a great extent in America, and to a lesser degree in Britain, the police are seen by adolescents as bullying symbols of authority. This difference is evident in slang names; in the United States the police are called "pigs," in Britain "the fuzz." Just as the individual who bullies often does this because he feels hated and taunted by his victim, so this may be true for a bullying policeman. Furthermore, as middle-class youth comes more into contact with police forces because of driving and drug offenses, they often provoke the violence they claim to deplore. It is as though the long-haired university student represents to a young policeman all the things he could not be; the violent club-waving policeman is, for the student, a representative of the licensed aggression he craves for himself.

Usually adolescents who treat older people with bullying contempt have unsatisfactory relationships with their own parents. To some extent young bullies are a demonstration of the failure of family and social processes in rearing the young. Fortunately they are a minority. Adult authority may reinforce the whole bullying process by using bullying techniques, behaving like the mother who bit her own child. The message that the important aspect of living is to be bigger and better in aggressive control over others is reinforced, as though the balance of terror that is the official policy of those nations with atomic weapons ultimately corrupts the whole of society. The two atomic super powers both behave in an illiberal way, similar to those young people whom they perceive as defiant. In one country the technique may be more effective than the other; the difference is of degree, not kind.

Problems of Personal Self-Control

The major preoccupation in handling and coping with problems of aggression in the adolescent age period, for young people, their parents, and society, is control of angry feelings. The amount of self-control an adolescent can show in words as well as behavior is assessed as a measure of maturity. However, overcontrolled adolescents are not in touch with their own feelings or their inner world of fantasy and imagination. This overcontrol may be crippling, particularly if adolescents then face additional crises:

Carl, an eighteen-year-old boy, hid from his friends the fact that he had failed to make adequate grades in his first year of college. He was the second son of Roman Catholic parents, his older brother was something of a ne'er do well, and his older sister had disappointed his father by failing to marry by the age of twenty-four. Carl was a friendly, outgoing boy until his failure, and he was referred to a psychiatrist because his parents felt he had become increasingly withdrawn when he came home for the vacation. Carl could not understand his increasing inability to concentrate and found it hard to accept that the necessity for him to hide his failure was an everpresent stress for him. He also denied having time for any sexual interests but sat throughout the whole interview with his hands covering his genitalia.

Despite his denial that he was bothered by any of these aspects of his personality, Carl accepted the offer of psychotherapy to "see if it will help you become freer with yourself and others," with great relief.

The amount of control expected of an individual is not just a function of personality and family style; it is also related to religious, ethnic, and national identity. The British aristocracy is immensely preoccupied with the control of behavior and formal gestures carrying infinite nuances of meaning; the middle class are concerned with the control of the expression of feeling.

Role of the Victim

It is rare for the adolescent who inflicts pain on others to seek consciously to have this controlled; more commonly the victim of aggression seeks assistance from adults. They do this despite the adolescent pressure not to tell tale to grown-ups about their behavior; the peer group may insist this is unmanly. A request by an adolescent boy to parents for help with bullying may therefore be an unconscious question as to how masculine they feel him to be. A too rapid attempt at rescue may imply lack of respect for the boy's manliness, suggesting that he cannot solve the problem himself; no rescue attempt may be neglectful. Adults may perceive some adolescents as being perpetually victims. Such adolescents may have become institutional scapegoats; but, even if they are, they may be in severe psychological difficulties.

> Kenneth was the fourteen-year-old son of a dominant, aggressive businessman and a highly controlling mother. She dealt with his aggression at home by asking how he could hurt her so much. He was regularly scapegoated by his peers, members of an extremely unhappy group who were the victims of gross overpermissiveness in an otherwise academic school. The boy's psychiatrist was so impressed by the scapegoating that he neglected to consider the psychopathology of the victim. He arranged for the boy to move schools and, when all seemed well, he left the matter at that level.
>
> One year later he was asked to see the boy who had made a murderous attack on a younger and weaker boy with minimal provocation. In his former school the patient had been provoking aggressive attacks on himself in an attempt to control his own murderous fantasies.

When adolescents complain that they are being bullied, the usual initial adult response is masterly inactivity with appropriate empathy. As most bullying is quite transient in healthy societies, most young people survive being a passing victim of the difficulties of older and bigger adolescents. If adolescents have felt secure within their family groups, and if their life experience is not that of victim, they have to learn that all life is not fair or kind.

Social Change to Eliminate Bullying

As with all symptomatic behavior, any action taken to eliminate violence should depend on an understanding of the etiology of the situation. Sometimes even the action can be mislabeled and, on occasion, group bullying can become extremely aggressive because of group contagion.

> A race riot was reported in the newspaper as having occurred at a local high school. A group of black girls had verbally tormented a white girl, and, when they began to push her around, she ran away. They ran after her and in the ensuing scuffle she was stabbed.
>
> The etiology of the outburst was multidetermined. The school was a typically structured high school with generally fragile relationships between staff and pupils. The specific event occurred because the white girl had dated a black boy. The black girls were furious with the black boys because they inflicted a double standard: Girls should only go out with black boys, boys could date white girls. Feeling devalued, the girls projected their rage onto the white girl; she, in turn, had been provocative in her dating habits. The stabbing occurred because the black girls felt that carrying a knife was justified because they feared attack.

A relatively simple problem can be solved by appropriate communication with school authorities, but often episodes of bullying behavior require complex social change, otherwise the repression of one incident will only lead to another. It is not generally helpful for a group of adolescents to be told that individuals have complained about the way one of them has been treated. With a complex etiology control is an inadequate answer. Inappropriate physical aggression can almost be eliminated from the life of adolescents if the social climate meets the needs of most of the adolescent group.

References

Cohn, N. (1967), *Warrant for Genocide*. London: Eyre and Spottiswood.

Erikson, E. H. (1968), *Identity, Youth and Crisis*. New York: Norton.

Gault, W. B. (1971), *Some remarks on slaughter. Am. J. Psychiatr.,* 128 (4): 82–86.

Hollander, R. (1960), Compulsive cursing. *Psychiatr. Q.,* 34: 599–622.

Johnson, B. (1948), *The Lost Art of Profanity.* Indianapolis: Bobbs-Merrill.

Kinsey, A. C., *et al.* (1948), *Sexual Behavior in the Human Male.* Philadelphia: W. B. Saunders.

Lorenz, K. (1966), *On Aggression.* London: Methuen.

Macoby, E. E., Mathews, R. S., and Morton, A. S. (1954), Youth and political change. *Public Opin. Q.,* 18: 23–29.

Miller, D. (1967), Family interaction and adolescent therapy. In *The Predicament of the Family,* ed. P. Lomas, 34–57. London: Hogarth Press.

Miller, D. R., and Swanson, G. E. (1958), *The Changing American Parent.* New York: Wiley.

Montague, M. F. A. (1961), On the physiology and psychology of swearing. *Psychiatry,* 5: 189–201.

Morris, P., and Morris, T. (1963), *Pentonville, A Sociological Study of an English Prison.* London: Routledge and Kegan Paul.

Opie, P., and Opie, I. (1965), *The Lore and Language of School Children.* Oxford: Clarendon Press.

Rosenfeld, H. (1957), Psychoanalysis of the super-ego conflict in an acute schizophrenic. In *New Directions in Psychoanalysis,* ed. M. Klein, R. Money-Kyrle, and P. Heimann, 207–216. New York: Basic Books.

Ross, H. E. (1961), Patterns of swearing. *Atlas,* 1: 77–78.

Scott, J. P. (1958), *Aggression.* Chicago: University of Chicago Press.

Storr, A. (1968), *Human Aggression.* London: Penguin.

12

Regression in Adolescence

Flight Mechanisms of Adolescents

One technique of escaping from psychological tension that is felt to be unbearable is to take flight either literally or by emotional withdrawal from the painful reality that provoked the internal conflict. Another is by regression, in an attempt to re-create the omnipotent pleasures of infancy. This is often sought by the use of drugs. This re-experiencing of that emotional level in which tension was not experienced, is attempted as an escape from tension.

Some regressive activity is usual in adolescence and it appears as a part of the normal defensive structure of the personality. The convenient escape mechanisms of adolescents are masturbatory activity and sleep (Bateson and Mead, 1962), idleness, social isolation (Greenson, 1949), or isolation with a group of other young people. A flight into fantasy may be helpful in emotional growth; not only do imagination and fantasy protect the personality from the effects of stress, they may also provide enrichment.

Fantasy and Lying

Youth is a time of vivid imagination in which the world can appear new and startling. Both childhood and adolescence can be ages of fantasy (Murphy, 1947, pp. 391–405). Children up to the age of five find it difficult to separate fantasy from reality: Daydreams and imaginary events are thought to have occurred, principally because this is the age of eidetic (picture) imagery, based on past and present experiences. Adolescents still retain the capacity to distort their perceptions of the real world to avoid the experience of intolerable anxiety; what is false becomes true and vice versa. The awareness of such distortions, perceived by others as lying, varies from time to time in the adolescent. An escape technique that is common to everyone is play, particularly games involving bluff. For some, the game of bluff may become a permanent, deliberate distortion of reality; for others, it becomes an unutterable personal conviction; a lie becomes a way of life.

"Beauty is in the eye of the beholder," and, to an extent, the reality of the world is as individuals see it. Although human beings reach a general consensus as to what the world is really like, there is a margin in which one person may see the world one way, and in a sense be accurate, while someone else sees it differently and is equally correct. Intuitively, all parents know this.

> Jane, age seven, alleges that her brother John, age nine, has tripped her. This is hotly denied. Both children insist they are telling the truth. Jane says that John deliberately attempted to make her fall. John says that his sister got in the way of his foot. The stories may be contradictory, but neither child necessarily lies. John unconsciously wanted to hurt his sister and had no real remorse. Jane wants her brother to be punished by their parents. The declared innocence of the brother has validity, since he feels he was not responsible for hurting his sister.

With adolescence, children are thought by adults to know what is real and what is not. However, early adolescents in particular are experts in making the world as they want it to be; their preoccupation with themselves means that all reality is likely to be thought of in terms of their own needs. A lie can be aggressive as well as being regressive, a deliberate way of alienating and attacking others. It can also be a way of deceiving the self and inferentially making the outside world punitive. The need for this is common in adolescence, as it is easier to assert oneself against a world that is felt as hurtful. Reality that does not meet the perceived needs of the early adolescent is thought to be deliberately persecutory and unfair; it can also be made this way. This reality distortion is enhanced by the needs of early adolescents to distrust the motives of emotionally meaningful adults as part of the conflict over autonomy and dependence. Furthermore, adolescents easily assume the whole world feels as they do. A youngster confronted with a misdemeanor will assume others will be as angry with him as he is with them.

Fantasy is an escape from painful reality (Menninger, 1963, pp. 138–139). This may be perceived as even more persecutory than it actually is, because the adolescent all too easily assumes that the world is a narcissistic extension of the self. If an individual adolescent is filled with anger, he easily assumes that this is the feeling of these around him; young people first may project; then they lie and anxiously distort reality to avoid the punitive response, imaginary or real, of others. Of course, the lie may convert the imaginary to the real. So the adolescent child is often dishonest on the basis of what seems to be irrational anxiety; the other person is thought to be as vengeful and angry as the adolescent might feel in an equivalent situation. As early adolescents have a highly punitive conscience, their attitudes tend to be based on the Old Testament doctrine of "an eye for an eye." On the other hand, tariffs of punishment, based on the needs of social organizations, whether family units or schools, inevitably produces lies in those who feel that this is safer than telling the truth.

By early adolescence most have neither developed a firm idea as to what they would like to be like nor an acceptable social conscience. Particularly if threatened by anxiety, such youngsters may lie as part of an attempt to get away with socially inappropriate ways of meeting individual wants at the expense of others. Adolescents can be honest depending on a number of factors: their inner sense of security, how much honesty has been part of the family's way of life, and how maturation has taken place past the attitude that wishes should be immediately gratified at whatever cost. Sometimes honesty is a way of proving one's own goodness to oneself and others; it is a type of lie as the motive is to seek affection.

Types of Lies

Lies can be of omission—when significant facts about events are deliberately omitted—and of commission—a deliberate distortion of reality. Both these types of lies may have roots in parent–child relationships. The omission lie is a deliberate attempt to protect privacy. Children ask questions and adults may then respond in three different ways: They may refuse to answer and make it clear that they are doing this; they may give a partial answer—for example, parents may decide to answer questions about sex up to the point that they feel the child will understand; finally, many appear to be answering completely, and both they and the child know that this is not the whole truth. The latter is the genesis of the omission lie.

Partial truth is a typical adolescent maneuver to avoid discomfort in interpersonal relationships; it is a sop designed to appease the other person. If further inquiry is not made, the adolescent appeases his own conscience by projection; the omission lie is now the adult's responsibility. The adolescent's attitude is that if the adult had wanted to know more, more should have been asked. Often an adolescent will use this technique to test the sensitivity of adults:

A seventeen-year-old boy was deciding how he wanted to get a battery for his girlfriend's car. He and she had two dollars between them. He said "I was meeting a friend in the school car park who was going to go out at lunchtime and get one for me." The interviewer said "You mean rip one off." At this point the boy who had been evidently tense obviously relaxed and began to talk of how he was still stealing.

Lies of commission, when told by parents to children may be a deliberate attempt to be helpful; in an attempt to avoid emotional discomfort, the predicament is apparently made easier. To run away from unpleasantness is not consciously advocated, but if adults have this attitude, explicit or not, the young identify with it. Money and sex produce adult commission lies. The gooseberry bush story or its equivalent taught many of the present generation of adults to distrust their parents; unconsciously they may repeat similar behavior in their own families. An increased allowance may be refused on grounds of poverty, even when this is inaccurate. The conscious wish is to be helpful with minimal anxiety for adults. Adolescents, because they try to do it so often themselves, easily sense the easy way out in others.

Development of Reality Sense

The developmental reason for lies can be partially understood in the history of each child's relationship to his family. Children inevitably go through a developmental phase in which they feel that their parents are untruthful because they feel promises are made and not kept. This is related to the development of time sense (Friedman, 1944a). In infancy there is obviously no difference between an expectation and a promise. When a baby is picked up by its mother, the expectation of being fed has an automatic promise of fulfillment. The child then learns through experience that expectation does not necessarily mean promise. However, under stress this distinction is blurred. The child sees "I expect" as "I promise," and angry disappointment comes. So just as an adolescent's way of seeing his own actions may mean that he does not consciously lie, so adolescents feel that their parents, who see themselves as being honest, are being unreliable. This is particularly likely because adolescents may still be sufficiently immature to feel that an expectation is a promise. A particular difficulty is that adolescents may still have an uncertain sense of the past (Bradley, 1947) as well as the future (Friedman, 1944b), although adults think they have developed an adequate sense of time. A child may ask for a toy; parents may promise "tomorrow." The child's sense of time may mean that this is felt as a commitment to obtain the gift now. A capacity to consider the future begins to develop, in particular, between the ages of five and ten, but this capacity may disappear under stress. Under psychological pressure, adolescents have a here-and-now expectation that tension will be relieved; tomorrow then becames a relatively meaningless concept. The concept of adult unreliability can thus be reinforced for the tense and anxious adolescent. The adolescent who justifies his own conscious un-reliability on the basis that the whole world behaves that way can feel parents, in particular, as being equally unreliable. It is not until the maturational middle stage of adolescence that young people develop a time sense equivalent to that of adults.

Apart from the problems created by natural development, many parents are not completely truthful with their children. The myth of the white lie may bedevil parent-child relationships. Insofar as the demand for truthfulness is concerned, adolescents may often feel themselves to be in a world of "Do what I say" rather than "Do what I do." The belief that trivial lies that will cause no harm are acceptable further reinforces the same atti-tude in adolescents; inevitably, their definition of trivial differs from that of adults.

The ability to separate fantasy from reality is a quality that is slowly acquired from infancy; education toward reality is a slow process with many reinforcements for reality distortion. The mouthing movements of babies whose hunger has not yet been appeased is the basic model for the fantasy lie designed to relieve inner feelings of discomfort and restore psychic homeostasis. Children may experience fantasies that are so vivid that they speak of them as if they were really so. This type of lying is harmless. A critical confrontation by adults about these lies makes children give up mentioning, but not necessarily experiencing, false beliefs. Adolescents escape from what is perceived as a life of intolerable dullness into unrealistic fantasies. Covert fantasies become overt lies as a way of reinforcing self-esteem; other people believe that the adolescent is important. Thus, the adolescent attempts to get people in the world outside to cancel out personal feelings of inadequacy.

Almost all children go through a period of telling commission lies, usually between the ages of five and seven, because at this time a primitive harsh conscience is projected onto authority figures. The inner expectation of the child is that a bad action will be severely punished. A small girl who chastises her dolls inflicts a punishment more severe than any that her parents have ever applied. This is the retributive fantasy behind her dishonesty.

In adolescence, the fear may not be of physical punishment as such but rather of what adolescents fantasize others may think. When adolescents perform actions of which they know others will disapprove, they may lie because they do not want the disapproval put into words, a situation that leads to humiliation and loss of face. To avoid this, the adolescent may tell lies and justify this by alleging it is done to avoid being nagged. In modern societies adolescents who are trying to free themselves from dependent family ties nevertheless need their parents to make this possible. To enlarge the boundaries of their world, adolescents may depend on their parents to provide either transportation or money. If they are planning to do something they feel their parents will disapprove of, they may lie in advance. Some scorn a lie. If they cannot obtain permission for what they wish, they become openly defiant, in words if parental control is still present, in deeds if this has been lost. Adolescents who have parents who are honest and who are consistently felt to be loving and fair are likely to be honest themselves. Adolescents who do not like themselves (although they may be highly self-involved), who lack self-respect, who often feel hated and unloved, are likely to be consistenly dishonest and deceitful although some may be compulsively and meticulously overhonest. Thus, the occasional lie of development becomes a deceptive facade to cover the anxious feeling of being unloved which is experienced by an inadequate personality.

Character Distortions

The etiology of the adolescent character disorder is as complex as the presentation of symptons. The adolescent who has to distort either the personal perception of reality or manipulate the environment to avoid the experience of psychic tension reaches puberty but may never be psychologically adolescent. Reality distortion, when it is embraced by a child as part of his personality, means that neither valid steps to personal autonomy nor a true sense of self develops. There are multiple reasons for this: The basic integrity of children has not been respected; they have been excessively punished, not had their needs for security and love satisfied, and not been treated with reasonable consistency; and their sexuality as a male or female has not been respected. Not all characterologically disturbed young people have incompetent parents. Some children have a genetic or organic hypersensitivity to stress; the traumatic events in their upbringing may be the result of the child's effect on the mother as well as vice versa. A basic constitutional predisposition to a stress response that arouses conflict in parents explains why one child of a family may suffer from a character distortion when another does not, for example:

A mother was presented by the nurse with her infant to nurse. The baby was slow to respond, the mother became extremely anxious and the helping nurse impatient. The mother became extremely tense, and the baby responded to the change in the musuclar tone with which he was being held by becoming even more balky. At the next feeding, the mother was anxious even before the baby arrived.

This type of interaction holds one genesis of difficulty between mother and child; if these modes of relating continue, an adolescent distrustful of the motives of others and unable to be close to them may be created. Such an individual may become, for example, an infantile personality or a manipulative, chronically fearful liar who, when discovered, feels that contrition is all that is required. Whenever children show recognizable emotional disturbance, parents often accept an unreasonable amount of responsibility but many have devices to avoid this. A call to genetics may avoid a personal sense of guilt. As most families have members who are thought to be black sheep, it is not difficult to appeal to heredity. Sometimes blame is projected solely onto the adolescent, despite the fact that only behavior that is relatively free from unconscious conflicts can be consciously controlled with ease. Parents are often blamed by society for the antisocial actions of their adolescents. But both adults and adolescents are victims when the latter are chronic liars. Adults do not know how to treat such children constructively, and the children continue to try to avoid emotional pain in a sterile and nonproductive way. Distortion in character formation is not only due to parent–child interaction, it may be the result of social system pressures. The emotional involvement of the nuclear family does not necesarily protect children from severe stress applied either by a peer group, extraparental adults, or social organizations. Most obviously, physical or emotional disability inflicted on the child by illness or accident may produce parent–child and character distortions.

Social Systems in the Etiology of Dishonesty

Sometimes, a double standard becomes forced on children by educational systems. Children may be secure at home, honest, and trustful, but this can be spoiled by a bad school experience. It is still possible for children to feel hated by teachers, some schools may have staff who, by their actions, convey that they do not like children and that they dislike teaching even more. In such settings lies of commission are common, lies of omission are ever-present. It is unreasonable to look on children who lie in such settings as disturbed. Their reality testing may be good, and they may lie to avoid unfair and unduly harsh punishment. Peer-group street attachments in underprivileged neighborhoods may force dishonesty on the young. Adolescents, in particular, may have to lie to agemates to remain as in-group members of a gang and to avoid torment. Too often the combination of poor schools with harried teachers in underprivileged neighborhoods where violence and terror rule the streets occurs. Dishonesty and fraud are then incorporated into the personality to make personal survival possible. For example, in parts of the black ghetto adolescents must not show overt signs of anxiety if they are to survive. However loving and fair parents might be, it is difficult if not impossible, to beat the culture of the street; because children, however unconsciously, feel their parents are responsible for whatever happens. Only with adulthood do we accept that our parents are truly not omnipotent. In poor neighborhoods, quite apart from the effect of these on intrafamilial interactions, children and adolescents feel that it is the responsibility of their parents that they live there. They may then lose faith in all adults, including their parents. A lack of confidence in adults makes it impossible to be honest, and distrustfulness becomes pervasive. Parents become involved as part of the bad, unreliable adult world, however good they may be. The behavior of teachers is partially felt by their children to be the parents' fault; they, after all, send their boys and girls to school. Only when children can really see that parents are victims, too, do they begin to forgive them.

Cultural Reinforcement for Lying

The attitudes of society make it likely that adolescents will attempt to use a fantasy solution for difficulties. Politicians have brought both the omission and commission lie to a high art; they are experts at the broken promise and distortion of the truth. Adolescents in conflict about truthfulness are acutely aware of the lies told by the leaders of society. It has been said that an ambassador is a man who lies abroad for the good of his country. Before the days of the mass media this may have been of little significance; today's children and adolescents may be exposed to the lies of the establishment as they appear on television. Lies from national authority figures convey to the listening adolescents a contempt for others. So adolescents justify the dishonesty of the folk heroes of their generation: "Everyone is like that." Their social errors are widely publicized but condoned, since society does not reinforce honesty as a virtue. Like politicians, adolescents are often selective tellers of lies. The truth may be told to members of one's own group, but it may be appropriate to tell outsiders lies. Adolescent drug takers may boast of their purity and honesty but tell lies about who deals in drugs and their source of supply.

In many cultures people find it difficult to be honest about feelings. In some, misery must be hidden, in others, anger. Many parents attempt to hide their differences of opinion and their mutual dislikes from their children. Such transient behavior does not necessarily impinge on children, but pseudopositive feelings produce confusion in them. The justification often given for adult denial of angry feelings toward children is that this type of feeling is hurtful, but children may then not know what actions should convey what feeling. As anger cannot be successfully hidden, a loving remark with an angry look is confusing. Although it is inevitable that most lies will be discovered, the adolescent, preoccupied with his own sense of omnipotence, hopes that magically all will turn out satisfactorily. Furthermore, since only later on in the age period does a sense of the future develop, the present lie is of no significance tomorrow.

Lies may be socially reinforced. Lying is one way of manipulating the environment to create an inaccurate image of the self in minds of others. Some environmental manipulators are considered socially acceptable. To gain entrance to prestigious universities, adolescents go out of their way to involve themselves in extracurricular and responsibility roles in school, because this will look better along with a high grade-point average and SAT scores. The deliberate creation of a false image is, in a sense, a lie. On the other hand, the responsiblity such adolescents choose to exercise in order to be acceptable may ultimately be incorporated into their personalities. An adolescent may behave responsibly in the first place for the wrong reason but may continue this when the reason is no longer present.

In some manipulations truth is distorted to play one person off against another. Adolescents from homes in which parental relationships have broken down, either through lack of communication, separation, divorce, or death, become experts at recreating in all their environments the splits and differences that were so painful to them when they were helpless victims in a nuclear family. Sometimes a parent unwittingly reinforces this technique of relationships by refusing to express an opinion and then passing the child on to the other parent.

Lying as a solitary sympton is usually fairly transient in personality development. A generally secure living environment for most adolescents creates a situation in which lying need only be corrected in a firm, unemotional way. Lying is not, however, the same as a refusal to speak. The latter may indicate a distrust of the motives of others, as does a lie, but it often occurs as part of a sense of loyalty—refusing to tell tales on one's peers in school. A socially acceptable response may, however, become a refusal to name dope pushers and dealers in adolescence. A refusal to talk may be loyal but destructive.

Sleep

Just as fantasy has an economic function in the development of personality, so does sleep. Disturbances of personality growth may show in the exaggerated use of fantasy and its distortions, sleep disturbances similarly appear (Iskower, 1938). At no stage of development is this more clear than with adolescents. On the one hand, adolescents dream less than adults, on the other, an almost typical and stereotyped complaint about adolescents in Western society is the extent to which they lie in bed. It is supposedly impossible to get adolescents up in the morning, their rooms are untidy, they are lazy, they turn day into night, and they are extremely inconsiderate. The external chaos with which adolescents surround themselves is both a measure of their pre-occupation with themselves—they cannot be bothered a great deal with trivia—and an expression of the internal confusion typical of the age period. Common in adolescents is a striking alteration in activity levels; extreme activity, often a flight from the dependent helplessness of sleep, alternates with profound inertia. Morning sleepiness can be caused by late nights, but it is often related to the physiology of adolescence; a maximum growth spurt is a cause of fatigue. Psychologically, a reluctance to wake up can also be a depressive disinclination to face the day. It is an emotional avoidance and withdrawal because the world can feel so tormenting at many stages of adolescence (Schneer and Kay, 1962). Difficulty in awakening, which can begin as a physiological event, can also be a passive way of defying parents and so fighting the struggle of dependence against independence. When an adolescent girl or boy must be awakened by a parent, when no alarm clock will work, then the refusal to get out of bed is both a provocation of mothering and a denial of its need.

Variation in Sleep Needs

Besides the obvious knowledge that human beings need a variable amount of sleep at different maturational stages, the amount an adolescent requires varies from one individual to another. Furthermore, the same individual shows variation in sleep needs through development. Hyperactive children become slothful adolescents. Old people sometimes sleep for hours; at other times they may be very wakeful. By the age of four or five, most children need to sleep about twelve hours a night. This amount gradually reduces until, in adolescence, an average of seven to eight hours at night is required. Young adults may make do with less than this from time to time. Associated with the variation in the amount of sleep people need, appears to be a similar variation in the ease of wakening. Women often take longer to wake than men, although long hours of sleep during the morning seem more common in boys than girls. Irritability is not rare first thing in the morning; family breakfasts that ought to start a happy day are often tense and miserable. Particularly during their growth spurt, many adolescents need much more than eight hours of sleep in any twenty-four-hour period; adolescents may sleep for an hour or so in the early evening. High schools that insist on a rest period after lunch for all their pupils are sensible.

The most usual complaint is about adolescent reluctance to get up; the most important difficulty is insufficient sleep. Insomnia usually implies not being able to get to sleep; some adolescents, however, may fall asleep, then wake up. The general tension of adolescence makes many of them hypervigilant and hyperemotional (Menninger, 1963, p. 167) and, thus, restless sleepers.

Nightmares

A common cause of restless sleep is a nightmare. These last only a short time, are usually remembered when they occur, and adolescents are normally aware of waking up after such an episode. They are, on the one hand, an attempt to relieve tension (Dement, 1960); on the other hand, they create it. A prepubertal child will cry and need comfort from parents. Adolescents will probably comment at breakfast next morning that they had a nightmare, but usually they do not wake their parents. Nightmares are relatively rare in adolescence, although clinically there is evidence of an increase in their frequency at puberty. This is associated with the reawakening of conflicts about a child's relationship to parental sexuality, and nightmares are as common as when a child is four or five. The typical dream of the early age is that of being attacked by a large animal (Blos, 1962, p. 64). In this oedipal period, in which children feel particularly emotionally involved with parents of the opposite sex and are rivals of the parents of the same sex, there is an unconscious wish to get rid of the competitive parent. Early adolescent dreams may be full of extremely aggressive ideas—brains disintegrating, eyes falling out, and so on. These are ways of avoiding panic and concern about the individual being damaged himself. Technically, they are fantasies associated with an earlier anal period of development to avoid castration anxiety. Children and adolescents still function with the talion law: The jealous rage of competitive parent is symbolized by the attack they experience in the dream.

With small children these nightmares are often resolved by the child being told fairy stories before bedtime. In their original form, before they were diluted in the twentieth century, these stories were full of the badness of parent surrogates, the weakness of good parents, and of blood and brutality. However, the stories all end happily ever after; good is triumphant and evil conquered, a subtle way of reassuring children that all will be well.

Similarly, at four to five, children are preoccupied with successful and safe violence; guns and bows and arrows become important for boys. Four-year-old boys may offer to chop off hands, legs and heads of male visitors. Reassurance from the external world and in play is not as easily available to early adolescents. Oedipal fantasies about parents must be actively repressed and, once puberty has arrived can only be played out most indirectly in action. Aggression is controlled by peer-group relationships but often spills out diffusely under stress. Just before tension is relieved by considerable masturbatory activity, prior to the boy's first ejaculation, restless sleep and nightmares are relatively common.

Night Terrors and Sleepwalking

Night terrors occasionally appear in adolescent girls, but they are extremely rare in boys. Even in prepubertal children, however, night terrors are relatively rare. These last much longer than nightmares (usually about twenty minutes) and occur most commonly in early childhood. While obviously asleep, a child is equally terrified and apparently hallucinating. The next day nothing is remembered.

Sleepwalking, a play in action of dreams, is uncommon. Usually it is of no significance, although it may become a persistent symptom that represents a playacting of an unconscious wish or conflict. In spite of a common fantasy, death and damage while sleepwalking, a theme of numerous novels and plays, appears not to have been reported in the scientific literature. If a young adolescent is found sleepwalking he can be led back to bed, and there is no need to awaken him. The concept that it is dangerous to wake an individual in such circumstances presumably protects the youngster from waking up in confusing surroundings. Sleepwalking is most usual after a severe family stress:

Jane, age fourteen, was extremely fond of her grandmother who lived with her and her parents. She had the unhappy experience of taking her grandmother a morning cup of coffee and finding her dead in her bed. She apparently took the situation relatively well, or so it was thought, as she did not appear too disturbed. Jane, however, was referred to a psychiatrist because she continued to sleepwalk to the dead grandmother's room or that of her parents.

Jane was apparently attempting to ensure that more nocturnal tragedies would not happen; it was as if she were trying to reassure herself that the death had not really happened. Since a fear of helplessness or of death is one common cause of sleep difficulties, death in the family makes adolescents fearful of their own vulnerability, particularly when they are helpless and asleep. Menninger (1963, pp. 179–180) reports the case of a young woman who used to sleepwalk to her parents room as part of a retaliation against them.

In many adolescents anxiety precipitated during the day may provoke a situation in which the youngster wakes in the middle of the night and gets up for no apparent reason; this is usually to check that everything is safe in the house. Similarly, some anxious obsessionals need to check that bedroom windows are locked and bedroom doors are open; they will then be safe.

Sleeptalking is quite common, but it is rare for a listener to hear clearly what is said, despite the common idea that secrets are given away because of sleeptalking. The idea behind this fantasy is that the pent-up tensions of the day are released at night.

Most sleep problems are temporary and are usually ignored or handled with reassurance. Persistent sleep difficulties in a tense, worried, unhappy adolescent may be due to situational stress. Specific crises may be occurring, or alternately, adolescents may overreact to day-to-day routine difficulties. Excessive sleep can be an escape from a demanding unpleasant existence. Unlike suffering adults anxious depressed adolescents do not typically

wake up early in the morning feeling terrible, nor do they begin
to feel better at night, as does the depressed older individual.

Insomnia

Insomnia is the most common sleep difficulty of adolescents
and may go back to infancy and childhood. In small children
insomnia often seems associated with general negativism and a
bedtime battle with parents. Children may dilly-dally and be
reluctant to go to bed, or they may find it difficult to sleep, or
both. Parents often feel, angrily, that going to bed has become a
technique of getting attention. So an inability to go to bed or fall
asleep may be associated with patterns of interaction set up
between parents and child over a long period. This is most common with the oldest child in a family. Parents with a first child
are often overanxious. Without child-rearing experience they
may overreact to minor child-rearing difficulties. Many new
parents are not sure that all is well either when their child is
quietly asleep or when it cries. A child may cry and someone
rushes to lift it out of bed. Parents may then show the child off
to friends and relatives. So when the child wakes at night, or even
when it is asleep, it may be brought to be cuddled and admired.
An association of wakefulness at night with parental attention is
thus reinforced. Sleep patterns may similarly be disturbed because
children over three or four months of age are moved while asleep
when babysitters are unavailable. The child may awaken and be
frightened by strange surroundings. A transitional object (Winnicott, 1953), a well-loved teddy bear, or other comforter may
allay this anxiety, but sleep difficulties can be created because
of the ease of modern transportation. A child is moved and
is then expected either to fall—or stay—asleep in new and strange
surroundings.

The inability to sleep satisfactorily in some children may
carry an implicit demand to be reassured and cuddled. Sometimes

parents respond by taking the child to their own bed. Some children may sleep with their mothers for a very long time, but in most societies this type of child rearing continues to make an infant out of a child. A child may wake in order to go to the parental bed. One or the other parent may then be ejected from the marital bed by the sleeplessness of their child. By puberty in Western culture it is inappropriate for children to share their parents' bed at any time. The continued demand of a pubertal boy or girl to do this means that the adolescent cannot abandon a wish to be babied. It also implies an unconscious preoccupation with the sexuality of either or both parents.

In some cultures this is not true. In rural Ireland all the family may still sleep together in one room, the same applies to many poverty-stricken areas of the West. In these circumstances the child may sleep cuddled up to siblings of either sex and parents. Such an individual is obviously exposed to the awareness of parental sexuality, but fantasies about this are obviously corrected by the frequency of the occurrence and the fact that everyone is alive and well the next morning. In primitive cultures at puberty children brought up in this way are moved away to special huts, or they may be given a great deal of sexual freedom with members of both sexes through childhood, so any anxiety or curiosity about sexuality can be worked out through play. Any tensions inside an individual that are created by an awareness of parental sexuality can be played out in action. Cultures such as those of the peasants of southern Ireland, which do not allow any sexual freedom outside of matrimony, cause problems for their children. They are emotionally stimulated with an awareness of sexual activity but given no opportunity to play out tensions in action under a socially acceptable umbrella. This may partially explain the violence, alcoholism, sexual puritanism, and prurience that are common in this culture (Messanger, 1971).

The equation of bed and punishment may also cause difficulty to children and adolescents either in going to bed or in sleeping. If children are felt by their parents to behave in socially

unacceptable ways, it may be appropriate punishment to send
them to a room to isolate them from the rest of the family. If
children are locked in their bedrooms or sent to bed as punishment, such action may produce children who need to have their
door open before they can go to sleep, or going to bed may become associated with parental rejection and guilt.

Sleep difficulties in children may be related to implicit and
explicit family attitudes around resting. Parents may demand
that everyone whisper because a nap is being taken: an association between sleep and quiet is then reinforced. Quiet may be
insisted on because "baby is asleep." Both in the infant and other
siblings hypersensitivity about noise and sleep is created. Parents
may say that, because of some anxiety, they "didn't sleep a wink."
This is rarely accurate, but a family may then relate sleep to
feelings of well-being, and a child may identify with these attitudes. Sleeplessness in word and deed is therefore used both to
get attention and to show anxiety. In adolescents with a long
history of insomnia, the roots of the difficulty sometimes can be
found in those interactive experiences of early childhood. However, there are much more usual causes. If children and adolescents are exposed to a fluctuating bedtime, this can cause insomnia. A failure to offer reasonable security about the time of going
to bed can cause sleep difficulties, and battles about going to bed
are then invited. Whether or not this happens, adolescents almost
inevitably use bedtime as an area of conflict with their parents.
The battle of dependence against autonomy is fought as much at
night as it is in the morning. The child may assess his parents'
giving him more adult status by the demand for just another five
minutes. Because of the implicit meaning of the request, it inevitably and insidiously slips into a demand for more and more.
Particularly in early adolescence, bedtime demands mirror the
problems between parent and child.

The adolescent battle over bedtime is not unlike the mealtime battle of earlier childhood. It is a way in which a child can
successfully defy his parents. A small child can begin to dominate

the household by refusing to go to bed until the father comes upstairs or mother comes up to read to him. The boy or girl may
insist that milk or food be given, that the door be left open, that
the light be left on in bedroom or hallway. In themselves, these
can be quite minor demands to make on parents, and many children need one or the other before they can settle down at night.
If too many bedtime rituals are insisted on, they are an obvious
attempt to exercise control over parents. Similarly, as a child
gets older, it is not unusual to try to delay bedtime because of the
necessity of going to the lavatory at the last minute or the need
for "forgotten" homework to be done. The cry for another ten
minutes is very usual in all children. If they can control parents
by demanding another ten minutes, ultimately they begin to ask
for more and more. Around the issue of sleep, in which control
over the self is abandoned, parents may lose control of their child.
A time extension is a way in which children are shown that
growth is known to be taking place, but the anxious thrust of
early adolescents to take more responsibility than they can handle
often makes firmness necessary. Boys may need their fathers' insistence that they go to bed. A symbolic struggle that may then
take place can be an early adolescent boy's way of having his manhood respected just before the dependence of lying down and
going to sleep is on him.

> Fourteen-year-old Peter was told by his parents that he could
> stay up until 10:30 P.M. as the family had company for dinner.
> At 10:40 P.M. his mother told him to go to bed. He totally
> ignored her request. She told him again and then appealed to
> the boy's father. Peter said, when his father told him to go,
> "Make me." With great good humor and firmness, Peter's
> father wrestled with him on his way to bed.

This typical family interaction conveyed many messages and had
many possible implications. If Peter's mother had forced him to
go to bed with father doing nothing—apart from unconscious
incestuous fantasies that might be aroused by this—the family

attitude that could have been conveyed was that father respected neither the boy nor his mother. Alternately, it could be assumed that father is afraid to support him against mother or vice versa. Peter would be unlikely to see from such a result any feeling that his manhood is valued. When father intervened in the way he did, this control enhanced Peter's feeling that his manhood was valuable and that his father could control his impulsive (and forbidden) wishes and behavior.

A variation in bedtime according to chronological age is significant to adolescents. Older children, particularly in the early and middle stages of adolescence, need to see their younger brothers and sisters go up to bed before they themselves; otherwise, they feel that they are not receiving the increase in status their age justifies.

Merely going to a bedroom does not mean going to bed. Early adolescents may appear to go to bed fairly easily, but then they daydream in their rooms for long periods of time before getting into bed. This is partly a subtle defiance of parental authority, but bedtime is also that time of the day in which adolescent fantasy is likely to be at its most intense. It is partly a flight from the regressive experience of sleep that may also be felt as a threat to personal self-sufficiency.

Sleeplessness in children and adolescents can be associated with severe anxiety. Those who suffer from an obsessional neurosis may experience a turning of thoughts over and over about one or another problem with the approach of a fatigue. Thus, such individuals may find it difficult to fall asleep.

Sexuality and Sleep Difficulties

Only those adolescents who are brought up with religious teaching that masturbation is sinful, or by parents who were overanxious about infantile sexuality, are likely to be anxious about this act. Boys who have trouble about masturbation may find difficulty in falling asleep. This is because self-control is weakened in the half-sleep, half-awake stage that precedes full sleep; anxiety about performing the act may lead a boy to stay awake until he becomes so fatigued that sleep is finally immediate. Masturbation in association with weakened personality controls is then unlikely. This anxiety should always be thought of as a possibility in boys who suffer from sleeplessness. Sometimes it is not the behavior as such but the possible masturbatory fantasy that causes anxiety, particularly in those who have conflicts about homosexuality. Boys may also be concerned about dreams with a sexual and aggressive content, especially those in which they associate sadistic behavior with sexual excitement. Sometimes to avoid the experience of merely lying awake, adolescents may read or listen to the radio until three or four in the morning.

Toward the latter part of midadolescence, often at sixteen or so, when parents have stopped sending their children to bed, transient sleep difficulties may occur. The adolescent is being told in action that he is adult enough to make decisions about sleeping. This threshold of adult responsibility may arouse enough anxiety to make sleep difficult. There are, however, other possible causes of middle-to-late adolescent sleeplessness. The sixteen- or seventeen-year-old adolescent is now likely to be fully mature physically. If family relationships are strained, if the family is isolated from a network of other human beings, adolescents may be lonely. Sleeplessness may then be associated with the problems of sleeping alone.

Lonely adolescents may have an intense need for physical contact. This is evident by the fact that middle-stage adolescents will sit very close to adults of whom they are fond. They do not use physical distance in the same way as adults. When they go to bed, physically mature, middle-stage adolescents and late adolescents, emotionally well balanced, are ready for sexual partners, not just for sexual intercourse and love making but so that a bed may be shared. Children who are lonely and anxious may not be able to fall asleep until they are cuddled, either literally or emotionally, by one or another parent. An adolescent with the body of a young adult needs cuddling from a sexual partner. Today it is very common for young people to be emotionally and sexually lonely. Day-to-day stresses, the association of increased social pressures with early puberty, the attainment of physical maturity by the age of sixteen or seventeen—all these mean that many young people often crave not just sex but a close, loving heterosexual relationship.

Situational Causes for Insomnia

Sleeplessness in adolescents can be caused by a variety of acute anxiety-provoking situations: physical illness, examinations and tests, academic and physical competitiveness, conflicts over money, and sexuality. It may occur after long-distance air travel, which disturbs the built-in time clocks of individuals. A most common cause of disturbed sleep patterns is associated with drug abuse. The alternating use, particularly on weekends, of stimulants and sedatives (speed and downers) by some adolescents disturbs sleep rhythm for two or three days at a time, and is particularly likely with those adolescents who attempt to stay up all night on weekends. Stimulants taken in very high doses may disturb the usual sleep rhythm. A poor appetite on the weekend in a pale, fatigued, irritable adolescent who does not sleep well may be pathognomonic of the use of a stimulant drug.

The proper treatment of sleep difficulties is not by the use of sedatives. These are usually prescribed because it is easier to offer sedatives than to deal with the general conflicts in the personality or life situation of an adolescent. Furthermore, the general drug taking of the adolescent age group is often a type of self medication. If sedatives are then offered by the medical profession as a solution to emotional problems, it is not surprising if adolescents choose to medicate themselves with any of the drugs that illegally circulate.

In younger children and in adolescents daytime hyperactivity may be associated with sleeplessness. Excessive reality demands are a not unusual cause of sleeplessness in children and young adolescents: Unkind teachers who give excessive homework and are overcritical, parental conflict and physical deprivation, and peer-group tensions should be considered first as a reason for adolescent stress. Only if these are not present should more specific assistance be necessary.

Many of the transient upsets of adolescents occur as the result of day-to-day pressures that play on the individual. If these can be understood, and the young person offered emotional support or the stress removed, most upsets will subside, especially in a stable, loving family. The problem, if the etiology of sleep difficulties is not known, is whether a policy of masterly inactivity should be pursued or whether more active intervention is required. Sleep difficulties lasting more than a few days are almost always an indication to seek behavioral help.

References

Bateson, G., and Mead, M. (1942), *Balinese Character*. New York: New York Academy of Sciences.

Blos, P. (1962), *On Adolescence*. Glencoe, Ill.: Free Press.

Bradley, N. C. (1947), The growth of the knowledge of time in children of school age. *Br. J. Psychol.,* 65: 197–217.

Dement, W. C. (1960), The effect of dream deprivation. *Science,* 131: 1705–1707.

Friedman, K. C. (1944a), Time concepts of elementary school children. *Elem. Sch. J.,* 44: 337–342.

———— (1944b), Time concepts of junior and senior high school pupils and of adults. *Sch. Rev.,* 52: 233–238.

Greenson, R. (1949), The psychology of apathy. *Psychoanal. Q.,* 18: 290–302.

Iskower, O. (1938), A contribution to the psychopathology of phenomena associated with falling asleep. *Int. J. Psycho-Anal.,* 19: 331–345.

Menninger, K. A. (1963), *The Vital Balance*. New York: Viking.

Messanger, J. C. (1971), Sex and repression in an Irish community. In *Human Sexual Behavior*, ed. D. S. Marshall and R. C. Suggs, 3–38. New York: Basic Books.

Murphy, G. (1947), *Personality: A Biosocial Approach to Origin and Structure*. New York: Harper and Brothers.

Schneer, H. I., and Kay, P. (1962), The suicidal adolescent. In *Adolescents, Psychoanalytic Approach to Problems and Therapy*, ed. S. Lorand and H. I. Schneer, 180–201, New York: Paul Hoeber.

Winnicott, D. W. (1953), Transitional objects and transitional phenomena. *Int. J. Psycho-Anal.*, 31: 89–97.

13

Psychological Disturbances of Adolescence and Their Treatment

In adolescence adult demands begin to be made on the personality, so existing emotional difficulties may come to the fore apparently for the first time. But most labels applied to adolescent maladjustments are crude and inadequate (Masterson, 1967, pp. 17–21). They do not really indicate separate personality problems: Effectively, they pick out symptom clusters. They do not represent specific illnesses as do medical labels, nor do they generally indicate the kind of help an adolescent might need. Some personality problems that appear in adolescence, because of a combination of social stress and physiological turbulence, indicate that development into psychological adolescence has not yet taken place. Other syndromes are typical of the age period and represent a partial failure of emotional development at this stage. The former are typically personality problems; the latter failures of identity development with, or without neurotic difficulties.

Most typically the disturbances of adolescence appear in a defiance of social norms. Society is preoccupied with a triad of socially defined antisocial behavior: sex, drugs, and delinquency. Although disturbed adolescents inflict pain on their environment, this does not mean that they themselves do not experience psychic pain. Nevertheless, particularly in early adolescence, it is almost always the pain precipitated upon others that produces the request for help. Most usually, preexisting personality disturbance emerges during adolescence because of an imbalance between the stresses and supports in the physical and personality growth of the adolescent, the family, and the total environment.

Appearance of Disturbance

The adolescent who suffers emotional collapse does so either at the height of the pubertal period, just after the period of maximum growth; at the beginning of the middle period of adolescence, the start of the period of identity differentiation; or at the beginning of late adolescence, a time of coping and identity consolidation. These three peaks are in the middle of the junior high school years, at the beginning of the senior high school years, and in academic individuals in their first year of university. It is common for disturbed adolescents to show symptoms just as they are about to change from one school to another or have just done so or, alternatively, as they leave high school. At a time of internal stress the anxiety of having to face a new situation arises, and breakdown is likely to occur. Among those who are likely to take part in antisocial behavior, usually nonacademic adolescents, a peak of delinquent behavior occurs in the six months before the possible school-leaving age of sixteen. Young people who leave school at sixteen, live in large cities, and have insufficient strength inside their personalities and inadequate support from without, have an unduly high job-turnover rate in those societies with full employment; in others they fail to find work. There is an increase in referral for psychological help in the six months before adolescents leave school to seek higher education or in the first six months of a college career. Students are often so pressurized to attain academic success that their emotional growth is retarded. They may break down in their first year at the university or during their last two semesters, when they are threatened by real life, with no further external supports able to offer a socially acceptable outlet for dependent needs.

The Effect of Psychological Disturbance on Maturation

In trying to be helpful to adolescents in distress, the causes of disturbance within society, the family, and the individual have to be understood if damage is to be repaired. Some believe that help for the child who behaves in a delinquent or antisocial way need not be different from that needed for the nondelinquent and that symptoms have no significance; in adolescence this is a fallacy. Antisocial behavior is often exciting and gratifying. Further, the distortions that such delinquent adolescents inflict on the world change their perception of it. One boy will insist that everyone smokes pot, another that the whole world is crooked, a third that he only knows homosexuals. Since the way the world is perceived is partly what influences the development of personality, a symptom that began as an attempt either to avoid the experience of frustration or to solve an internal conflict, can become an end in itself. Adolescents need to feel that the world is consistent if they are to use it to develop their identity; thus they always attempt to keep this state. Disturbed youngsters surround themselves with people similar to themselves and thus misperceive the nature of the environment. Further, adolescent maladjustment tends to produce a world that is felt as highly persecutory; the negative reactions aroused by disturbed adolescent behavior are painful to the youngster and ultimately a personality perceiving the world as tormenting is produced.

Thus, adolescent psychological disturbances affect the development of identity, that conscious sense of individual uniqueness that is meaningful in terms of past experience and is consonant with how one appears to others (Erikson, 1968, pp. 155–165). Those adolescents who cannot establish this sense of being in a way that they feel is satisfactory have no sense of solidarity with their world. They often see themselves only as part of an out-group of society. Of necessity, the attachment to this is quite tenuous. In all symptom clusters in adolescence there is, to some extent, a failure of identity formation, and often the symptoms are an attempt to solve the feeling of empty desolation associated with role diffusion.

The concept of identity is particularly useful because it gives helping adults a goal in their work with adolescents who suffer from a failure of identity formation. The young person only knows that he is seeking a relief from chronic tension in ways that may be more or less destructive, the tension must be avoided almost at any cost.

Identity Crises

Adolescents suffering from an identity crisis may show their difficulties in impulsive behavioral ways. They are often filled with diffuse rage against their parents whom they may perceive as highly invasive of their personalities: Impulsive acts of destruction may be directed at family property, often that belonging to their mothers. They may steal with little obvious gain, and they are usually caught. They may make suicidal gestures (Lewin, 1950) or enter willingly into sexual promiscuity or drug abuse. An identity crisis does not necessarily imply a pervasive failure of personality development; it may be a function of developmental disturbance at adolescence. As is so often the case, the severity of the disturbed behavior does not necessarily imply an equally disturbed personality, at any rate in depth. On the other hand, the first evidences of a seriously disturbed personality may appear as an identity crisis, because the adolescent has been unable to make meaningful emotional attachments in individuals outside the nuclear family. Most usually the more immature personality shows itself in a diffuse inability to make decisions.

Identity Diffusion

Some adolescents suffer from *chronic identity diffusion.* They are unable to settle on a vocational choice, or on whether to be generally academic or not. They cannot commit themselves to a sexual role, and, even if others seem to be involved, their sexual activity is both masturbatory and self-centered.

Adolescents who suffer in this way most easily abandon any sense of self they might have. They are particularly vulnerable to group contagion (Redl, 1942, p. 580) and rapidly seem prepared to abandon anything that conveys an awareness of their own special individual uniqueness. The drug scene particularly appeals to such young people, but even without this they fail to fulfill their potentiality either academically or vocationally. Often they feel unable to make meaningful emotional contracts with anyone: They may have intercourse, but they do not make love. The most common cry of such young people is "Who am I?", "What am I?", "What do I want?" Sometimes they complain of a desperate feeling of complete emptiness.

Adolescents who suffer from chronic identity diffusion are likely to experience acute confusional states that are often misdiagnosed as a schizophrenic reaction. If this happens, and the youngster is placed in a typical psychiatric hospital, which has a socially aberrant way of life, the adolescent may then affectively withdraw and appear sicker than he really is. Some may appear as heroin addicts and may be improperly placed on methadone, thus being given the false identity of a drug addict. Or they may commit delinquent acts, attacking the authority structure of the society in which they live; the label of juvenile delinquent is applied, and the adolescent adopts this as a pseudosolution to explain what he is.

Therapeutic Assistance for Identity Problems

In social systems that allow meaningful emotional contact with other human beings, both peers and extraparental adults, most adolescents with a problem of identity formation can be significantly helped by an understanding adult who does not have formal training in psychotherapy. However, if the identity difficulties are caused by early damage to the personality, important emotional attachments are difficult, if not impossible, and specially trained therapists and therepeutic settings may be necessary. Adolescents who suffer from identity diffusion have major problems of trusting the other person. In social systems, specially therapeutic or not, such adolescents often test out the value of other people by antisocial behavior designed to assess whether they are really cared about. The problem is that the adolescent suffering in this way is over involved with his own tenuous sense of self, but he does not like or love himself. In order to be able to do this, he first has to introject and then incorporate the image of a loving other. To establish the value of this individual, he has to behave in antisocial ways both to ensure that the other person is powerful enough to control aggression, and that aggressive behavior will not lead to rejection; only then can love be felt and be relied upon. The distrust is not the distrust of paranoia; it is based on an assumption that one cannot possibly be cared about. Thus, the motives of others become highly suspect and must be tested and retested.

These difficulties are present in the therapy of adolescents. In one-to-one situations their anxious hostility has to be understood and interpreted. In social therapy similar distrust is likely to be present initially.

In psychotherapy there are particular problems around its termination. On the one hand, a therapist should not fight adolescents' wishes to try out a new kind of identity for themselves when they wish to leave therapy; on the other, if therapy is abandoned too quickly, the identity problems recur. The issue is whether a desire to leave therapy is real because the adolescent wishes to test out the strength of a new personality, or whether it implies the attitude "if you loved me you would not let me go."

Neurotic Problems of Adolescence

Some adolescents suffer from neurotic difficulties (Josselyn, 1954). They show specific symptoms that are an attempt to resolve an inner conflict of contradictory desires. For example, the child who does not want to leave home because he is afraid of what might happen to his parents when he is away, but who wishes to go to school at the same time, may develop an irrational fear of attending school, a school phobia. The concept of neurotic symptoms in an otherwise healthy personality does not apply in adolescence. Neurosis always implies a general personality impairment in young people. At the very least the neurotic adolescent also has an identity problem. Identity formation is affected because the way the world relates to the adolescent changes, because of his sickness the youngster's own perception of the world is further falsified by his anxiety; so his concept of a way of life and image of people to be incorporated into the personality is distorted. It is a medical convenience to talk about neurotic illness as if it were unrelated to general personality difficulties.

Typical neurotic symptoms in adolescents are phobias, depression, and pains without organic cause, particularly head- and stomachaches and obsessional symptoms. The adolescent may be preoccupied with a thought he cannot get out of his head. Sometimes the individual has to repeat the same action to an extent that may seriously inconvenience his life; going back to see whether the light has been turned off, making sure doors are closed, arranging clothes in a specially meticulous way, and being generally overmeticulous.

Most neurotic difficulties will not be resolved without expert psychotherapy, although youth workers and teachers can certainly help such young sufferers by accepting that they have difficulties but expecting the maximum performance of which they are capable.

Physical Illness and Personality Development

Longstanding physical problems in adolescence affect the adolescent's perception of himself, his relationship to the world-at-large, and intrafamilial relationships. The latter is demonstrated by the problems of diabetics. In childhood they are forced to be overdependent on their parents because insulin has to be administered by father or mother. When puberty is reached, the battle of autonomy may be fought by a refusal to take insulin. Thus, diabetic adolescents have a self-destructive weapon easily available that can be used to provoke parental anxiety, make them feel impotent, and be death-defying.

Similar conflicts appear in epileptic children, with additional problems produced by the process of physical growth. Epileptics who have usually been given their medication by their parents have particular difficulties. Control is a crucial issue during adolescence, so medication may be refused as part of the adolescent's wish to test out his own controls: Can life be managed without medication? This is felt as particularly important since adolescents with epilepsy have the hidden anxiety that they may have a seizure during sexual intercourse. Just as with diabetics, the adolescent who is liable to seizures, may also refuse medication as part of an autonomy struggle with parents, or pediatricians, who may have come to be felt as parental.

Chronic physical symptoms without organic cause are the most common indications of emotional upset in adolescents. Fatigue or vague physical ill health with no known etiology are indications that adolescents are not coping successfully with psychological stress. Chronic tics, including nail biting, indicate an anxious youngster who may become easily tense under minimal stress. Bedwetting is not uncommon in adolescent boys and is always a symptom of emotional disturbance even in the rare event that an organic cause is also present. Asthma and chronic skin diseases are specific medical conditions that also indicate psychological distrubance.

A very common skin disease of adolescence used to be acne. It would appear that the incidence of this may be decreasing as nonendocrinological factors seem to be attenuating. Many adolescents nowadays, for example, boys with longer hair, are generally

cleaner and wash more frequently than their short-haired prede-
cessors. Or they may be more secure about masculine identity as
a result of the currently more sensible attitude toward sexuality.
So issues such as cleanliness and personal security that are relevant in the etiology of acne became less significant.

It is regrettably common for many adolescents to become permanently physically deformed following accidents. These young
people may appear to deny the significance of the deformity, by
engaging in physical activities, for example. However, anxiety
symptoms commonly appear in late adolescence, when many of
these young people seem impelled to avoid sexuality, because they
feel they will appear unlovely to a sexual partner—a problem for
boys as much as for girls.

> Kenneth was a seventeen-year-old boy who was severely burned
> by an accident involving a high-tension electrical cable. The ac-
> cident occurred when he was with two friends: one was killed;
> one had a bilateral leg amputation; and Kenneth was severely
> burned around his buttocks. He also had a below-the-knee am-
> putation of one leg.
>
> From being an outgoing boy with an active social life,
> Kenneth became quiet and withdrawn. His parents persuaded
> him to see a psychiatrist as they became concerned about his
> bitterness and what they felt was the excessive use of marijuana.
> In the course of therapy Kenneth said, "I can't stand to look at
> myself in a mirror. What do you think a girl would think if she
> saw my leg and ass?"

Once-weekly therapy, in which Kenneth talked freely of his un-
desirability to girls and was helped to see it as a projection of his
own feelings about himself, led to a reduction in marijuana smoking and an improvement in his schoolwork. He found a girlfriend;
the first time he had intercourse he kept his prosthesis on; he was
then, on other occasions, able to remove it.

Techniques of Therapeutic Intervention

The intervention of the sensitive adult, when young people are exposed to acute trauma, is rewarding for him and it can dramatically rescue the adolescent. When adolescents are the victims of accidents, caring adults available to young people need to be able to be perceptive about the underlying conflicts of their lives, which the injury will reinforce, to work with them in an emotional atmosphere that respects individual integrity, and to try appropriately to meet their needs. Adolescents may suffer today, but they can become part of the mature adult population of tomorrow, if efforts are made to assist them through those acute conflict situations they cannot handle alone. If these conditions exist, many can resiliently cope with severe stress. On the other hand, when an adolescent exposed to trauma is isolated from caring adults who can intuitively offer help and emotional support, the best that can be hoped for is adequate, formally organized psychological intervention. A failure to obtain this may produce a crippled, damaged, and damaging personality—both are too expensive for most societies. Surgeons and their staffs involved with adolescents who are injured need to be knowledgeable about adolescent psychology and techniques of psychological help.

Adolescence as it affects the behavior of the child with a chronic illness needs to be discussed by a pediatrician or family practitioner, prior to puberty, with parents. As soon as feasible, children need to be given responsibility for their own medication, which becomes something the doctor discusses with the child. Anxiety about sexuality needs to be appropriately considered. Reassurance should not be facile, but neither should an iatrogenic anxiety be produced by telling the youngsters of things he might worry about that would never occur to him. If physicians or others have a good general relationship with adolescents this is the backcloth against which concerns about chronic illness can be discussed. Dermatologists, for example, who indicate willingness to discuss the life of adolescents with them, rather than only look at their pimples, are enormously appreciated.

Sexual Difficulties

Sexual difficulties commonly appear during adolescence. For example, some boys still worry about masturbation or the fantasies that go with it. They may fear that they will not be potent or that there is something wrong with them physically, but they are often reluctant to mention these fears to anyone. Sometimes they feel that the persistence of this act means that they are immature. A similar situation occurs when boys in midadolescence become anxious about homosexual feelings. Usually such boys are not sexually excited by the presence of the other boy's genitalia; the real issue is one of identity, with the implicit question as to whether one is sufficiently manly.

Promiscuity is a typical symptom of identity diffusion in a girl. It usually appears at fourteen or fifteen and is the girl's attempt to establish a feeling of wholeness. This symptom is also typical of a very severe failure in maturation, however, that might be seen in hysterical or infantile personalities. The relationship is not with the boy as a person, but with a part of his body. A girl takes the boy's penis into her vagina as the infant sucks its thumb. Such individuals are often very demanding with their boyfriends—as clinging as an infant to its mother. And just as a mother may feel that her infant tries to control her, the boyfriends of promiscuous girls may feel that their girls try to control them. The girl is then liable to be rejected because the boy begins to feel that even the act of intercourse does not justify the demanding way she treats him. The girl's fear of rejection promotes her rejection: To reassure herself that she is worthwhile as a woman she may then get pregnant.

There are particular problems for adults who wish to help adolescents with sexual difficulties. Sexually disturbed young people often find talk about their sexual activities gratifying and sexually stimulating, as can be seen from their appearance. Youngsters assume a rather glazed expression or they may start to shift uncomfortably in their chair. Sometimes adolescents are brought to doctors by their parents, or they come themselves. Since sexuality is used developmentally as a way of asserting privacy and separateness, therapists in such situations cannot tell parents why their children seek help. The young people themselves have to decide what their parents should be told, although in action therapists cannot take sides against parents by colluding in silence.

Whether or not adolescent girls should be given contraceptives may be an issue. Early adolescents who behave promiscuously are always seriously psychologically disturbed, as are those who form intense sexual attachments with older males. This disturbance may be due to serious social or personal pathology. In the event that no treatment for either of these is possible, it may be that collusion with society's failure to be helpful is ethically justified. However, protecting the individual adolescent from the miseries of illegitimate pregnancy allows society to continue to offer inadequate treatment resources for the psychologically disturbed or do anything about social pathology.

For more mature middle-stage adolescents and onwards the situation is a little easier. Doctors do well, however, to point out to girls for whom they prescribe the pill, or the intrauterine device, that their expectations of a sexual relationship are likely to be different from those of boys; the latter have less need for a feeling of permanence and may find the natural feminine request for this frightening; they may then be rejecting.

It is important when trying to help boys with their anxieties about masturbation and homosexuality not to be facile and reassuring. They may be told by an adult who is interested in their welfare that the anxiety is common; they also need to be told that if it does not abate they should come back. If an adolescent is told not to worry and his anxiety continues, he may find it difficult to admit this. The intended reassurance fails to help, and the adolescent is made to feel even more odd because the problem is still present.

Obesity and Anorexia Nervosa

Because they result from interrelated factors in the physiological, psychological, and environmental experiences of the individual (Bruche, 1973, p. 6), obesity (Wallace, 1964) and anorexia (Sperling, 1967) are common problems in adolescence.

All adolescents show a variation in weight and the distribution of body fat, but manipulation of body size by overeating or starvation are indications of personality maldevelopment. The issue is whether or not these conditions are progressive. Sometimes these adolescents have been fat children; often their problems are related to family attitudes towards food and love. Sometimes such adolescents, particularly girls, may be identifying directly with their mothers.

Gross obesity distorts adolescents' relationships with peers and adults. They are related to not as individuals but as fat. This, in the middle stages of adolescence particularly effects the development of sexual identity. Fat adolescents may either be heterosexually ignored, or behave in a highly promiscuous way. Sometimes obesity may be a flight from heterosexuality; sometimes it represents an angry dependent rebellion within the family. In this, dependence on food is very similar to dependence on drugs and alcohol. It is a regressive attempt to solve the problems of anxiety, whatever its cause.

There are two possible approaches to the treatment of obesity in adolescence. Generally intensive psychotherapy is difficult and there are few reports of success in the literature (Bruche, 1973). Group therapy is probably contraindicated in adolescent obesity as the acceptability of fatness is socially reinforced. One approach that has been successful is to admit obese adolescents to general wards, preferably for adolescents, and put them on a 200- to 400-calorie diet, which ensures that they will lose one pound a day. While on the medical wards these adolescents are given educational, recreational, and vocational activities; they also see a psychiatrist regularly, whose goal is to help the reinforcement of an acceptable sense of masculine or feminine identity. When the adolescents have reached an acceptable shape, they move, keeping the same therapist, to an adolescent psychiatric ward. The young people there do not relate to them as fat and thus a new body image is societally reinforced. After some three months in this environment the young people are returned to the community.

This type of treatment can be highly successful, but it is inordinately expensive. Complications are that many obese adolescents became very aggressive as they lose weight, thus they are very difficult to handle on medical wards. Furthermore, it is not unusual for their mothers to smuggle food into the hospital for them.

Obese adolescents should never be given appetite suppressors. Amphetamines in such youngsters may offer the replacement of dependence on food with dependence on drugs.

Anorexia nervosa commonly appears for the first time in adolescence. It is commonly associated with severe depression that hides behind a facade of bland denial and it can be suicidal in its intensity. Some adolescents appear to gain positive satisfaction from the helpessness their starvation produces around them. Food becomes a battleground in which parental figures are gleefully attacked.

John was a fifteen-year-old boy whose father was a master chef. At puberty he was sent away to school, but only at the end of the pubertal period did he begin to lose weight. This loss occurred at the time when other boys were beginning to be heterosexually interested, and ultimately John was sent home in a state of severe starvation.

John's starvation had multiple roots. He consciously felt sexuality to be bad and was trying to starve himself so that he no longer got erections; he had never masturbated. He also got enormous satisfaction from driving his father to a fury because he would not eat his good food. When he was hospitalized he would force himself to vomit and would hide food if he possibly could. This boy fits a well-known psychological picture (King, 1963). Typically, he was highly preoccupied with food but determined not to have it. He also had an omnipotent denial that he could be hurt by abstinence.

In many adolescent girls it is hard to find conscious sexual and autonomy conflicts; for them it is as if thinness and an afeminine shape has become an end in itself. This has been called a weight phobia (Crisp, 1970).

Therapy for anorexia nervosa involves either the whole family, or the adolescent requires long-term hospitalization. Mere weight gain is often not enough and a behavior-modification approach that does not treat underlying pathology may cause a suicidal risk in those who are basically depressed (Blinder *et al.*, 1970).

Pregnancy and Abortion

When unmarried girls become pregnant, adults try to be helpful in a variety of ways. An abortion is more and more seen as the acceptable solution. Although this may be socially convenient, it often carries the implication to a girl that the important adults in her life do not see her as fit to be a woman. If lack of security about her feminine role is the emotional conflict that has led her to getting pregnant in the first place, abortion increases one problem as it solves another. Other girls become pregnant, not because they want a baby but because they need to be pregnant. A baby is seen as a doll to be cuddled. If a child is born, insecure girls are not able to cope with the demanding greed of a new infant without considerable emotional difficulties.

After an abortion an adolescent girl often appears to show no psychological effects other than relief. However, usually about six months later, when the baby would have been born, girls who are coincidentally in psychotherapy report episodes of severe depression. The clinical evidence is that many insecure girls attempt to become pregnant again at this time; partly this is to reassure themselves that they have not been damaged, partly to replace the murdered infant. If abortions take place after an adolescent girl has felt the baby move, she then seems to feel herself to be murderous immediately thereafter. If the parents have helped arrange the abortion, she projects that feeling onto them, as well as onto the doctor who performed the operation. This occurs especially in adolescents whose thinking is still concrete. Girls who have this experience are irrevocably hurt by it, and abortions at this stage are more damaging psychologically than having the baby.

There are no psychological indications for abortion; there are only psychosocial justifications. Adolescents who have abortions should receive counseling help thereafter, because a pregnancy—like any other adolescent action with antisocial connotations—is likely to be a request for personal help. An abortion, however, is a magical solution, and, if magic is offered, talking is often felt as useless and tedious. If counseling help is offered to illegitimately pregnant girls who are to have an abortion, a relationship with a therapist needs to be established prior to the abortion, so it can be continued thereafter. Social and educational help is obviously necessary. To process adolescent girls through abortion clinics is a medically effective, but psychologically inadequate way that incites further emotional difficulties. Ideally, a clinic for pregnant adolescent girls offers counseling and reality assistance, as well as the possibility of termination of the pregnancy.

Pregnant girls who are to have their babies are often sent away from school partly because of society's anxiety that others will be tempted to follow in their footsteps, partly because of concern about the attitudes of other children's parents. But girls almost always know when one of them is being sexually active. There is thus, little justification for removing a girl from school because she becomes pregnant. If the pregnancy of a girl were felt as shameful, there would appear to be no alternative but to hide her; the attitude of the young in these cases, however, can be more mature than the attitudes of the older generation.

When girls are unmarried and having a child, they need emotional support and help from adults who care about them. Unfortunately, they are often the victims of society's unconscious punitive attitudes. Homes for unmarried mothers may be emotionally frigid and cold places.

Adoption poses special psychological problems for unmarried adolescent mothers. If they do not nurse and hold the baby during the lying-in period, it is very difficult for them to mourn the loss of their child, as it has never been real to them. For them to do this, and then hand over the baby with no personal counseling to help them mourn the loss, does not seem humane. Nurses, however, often project themselves into the situation and insist that unmarried mothers who are not going to keep the baby not see and hold it. Mothers who give up babies for adoption need therapy both to understand the etiology of their need to become pregnant and to mourn the loss. Only then is repetition likely to be avoided.

Society makes it particularly difficult for unmarried mothers to keep their babies, even if a satisfactory father substitute can be found. Children brought up by one-parent families without an adequate parent substitute of the opposite sex are very likely to be emotionally crippled. If unmarried girls bring their babies home to the nuclear family, they are often in competition with their mothers for the care of the child; the girl loses.

Mental Illness in Adolescence

Mental illness proper is comparatively rare among adolescents, but the lack of adequate or effective treatment facilities makes it a major social problem. Mental illness, schizophrenia, and manic depressive psychosis are unfortunate diagnostic labels applied to adolescent illness. These labels have all tended to become pejorative and often provoke fantasies of inevitable personality deterioration. The classical descriptions of schizophrenic syndromes as inevitably deteriorating are inaccurate and a result of illness plus inadequate treatment. As a result of these descriptions, these diagnoses still make adults feel that they cannot help at all and that only the technically trained can be of use. But schizophrenic illnesses do not lead to inevitable deterioration and are treatable (Miller and Clancy, 1952). The less young people are labeled and the less the environment rejects them, the more quickly can those who suffer in these ways be helped.

The idea that these illnesses lead to personality disintegration has grown up because their natural history in adolescence is almost unknown. Most of the clinical descriptions are based on observations in mental hospitals. If adolescents are placed in disturbed, socially aberrant environments, such as those in many mental hospitals, their personalities almost inevitably deteriorate (Miller, 1954). Most hospital routines involve a timetable in which there are hours of enforced idleness that hardly assist adolescence development. Those young people who desperately need competent psychiatric hospital help already have difficulties in making satisfactory identifications. They are likely to deteriorate if they are subjected to the social lunacies of a typical hospital environment for more than a very short space of time.

Schizophrenic adolescents can be kept away from long-term hospitalization if they obtain skilled help from an outpatient clinic and if they have adults and other adolescents in their lives who relate to them as people. The ideal treatment is to hospitalize such youngsters only during the very acute phase of the illness.

Since intensive psychotherapeutic help in adolescent schizo-phrenia is rarely available, schizophrenic symptoms should be looked upon as a stress response, and efforts should be made to either reduce the patient's sensitivity to stress or reduce its inten-sity. Tranquilizers tend to have this effect in adults, but they do not appear to work satisfactorily in pubertal adolescents who have a high level of circulatory growth hormone. The optimum ther-apy for them includes supportive therapy and work with the family to reduce the intensity of their aberrant responses to their child's illness.

The problem associated with the diagnosis of schizophrenia is that the label makes others feel that these are impulsive and dangerous individuals. This is not necessarily true at all and may be related to the fear all human beings have of madness inside their own personalities.

Schizophrenia may rarely result in antisocial or aggressive behavior. When this happens, there can be no guarantee that schizophrenia will be diagnosed. Unless society routinely takes the trouble to listen to its adolescents, an illness underlying sur-face behavior may be ignored.

Tim, age sixteen, was in a juvenile detention home for making a violent assault first on his mother, then on other women. No one had spent sufficient time with the boy to allow him to say that the devil was instructing him to kill people. The world had reacted as if he were a bad aggressive boy, rather than a severely disturbed, disorganized mad boy.

Bill was sent to a school for delinquents in need of care and protection because he was constantly running away from home. He had not told anyone in his environment that he heard voices telling him to do this. Ultimately, Bill was found to be suffering from a brain tumor that explained his delusion.

Manic depressive psychosis is difficult to diagnose in adoles-cents but it responds dramatically to treatment with lithium.

Adolescent Suicide

Depression in adolescents is a common symptom that may be associated with transient maladjustment, personality difficulties, madness, or severe stress. It causes particular concern to adults who have charge of such youngsters, particularly because they make suicidal threats.

The frequency and type of suicide attempts by adolescents are socioculturally determined. Suicide is rarer in Britain and the United States than in some parts of Eastern Europe. Suicidal gestures, as distinct from attempts, are quite common in the West, and there is some suggestive clinical evidence that suicidal attempts among adolescents in the United States are currently increasing in frequency, apparently associated with a decline in the incidence of syringe hepatitis and toxicity due to drug abuse. It is usually the isolated, rather withdrawn adolescent who kills himself (Schneer and Kay, 1967), and often there appears to be little or nothing adults could have done to prevent it.

> Tom was an eighteen-year-old boy who was admitted to the adolescent medical wards of a university hospital with multiple physical complaints. No organic cause was found for these and he was seen by the psychiatrist attached to the ward. The boy had not been able to make a satisfactory adjustment away from his parents, and it seemed reasonable to work with him in brief therapy over the issue of his being able to separate himself from his family.
>
> Initially Tom appeared to do very well. He discussed some of his sexual anxieties thoughtfully, his somatic symptoms disappeared and plans were made to discharge him from the hospital to continue therapy at home. The day before his discharge he went to the hospital chapel, covered his face with a plastic bag, and after a three-hour search he was found dead.

He had given no clue to his competent therapist of his suicidal intent; the only evidence that could be retrospectively found was that two days earlier he said to an adolescent girl patient, with whom he was out walking, that he did not think suicide was always wrong. With this boy, as with similar episodes with others, great guilt is almost always aroused in those individuals who have been emotionally involved with an adolescent who successfully commits suicide. Of all the aggressive acts of which people are capable, suicide is one of the most aggressive; it is a hostile act directed at loved ones, at society, as well as at the self. The survivors are always left wondering how they failed.

An additional problem is that since they are always unconsciously angry with the suicide the mourning process for survivors, particularly brothers and sisters, is more complicated and difficult than is the case in a natural death.

Those disturbed personalities who make suicidal gestures to call the attention of the world to their emotional difficulties can never be relied upon if they promise not to hurt themselves, not because these adolescents are bad but because their need for help is so desperate that they will say anything to get immediate approval from adults. This need to be gratified here and now is so great that they cannot predict anything of their own behavior. They are not deliberately lying; their truth constantly changes.

Meaning of Antisocial Behavior in Adolescence

Adolescence is such a turbulent age that it may be particularly difficult to assess the significance of difficult behavior. As with all individuals adolescents need to balance within themselves the wish to behave impulsively, and thus relieve tension, and the need to control this behavior. The more uncomfortable an individual becomes within his environment, the stronger may be the wish to behave impulsively. The weaker the personality controls, the more likely it is that impulsive behavior will occur.

Adolescents have one particular additional problem. They have to exercise the controls that are required by civilization, yet they are living in a time of rapidly changing standards. Differing and increasing demands are made on them as they grow up. They have to try to free themselves from childish feelings of dependence on their parents; otherwise they will never feel adult. They have to cope with physiological changes within themselves that cause psychic turbulence, if not turbulence in outward behavior. So it is almost inevitable from time to time that most adolescents will appear to be behaving in a highly unreasonable way. Most of this behavior settles down; the problem is to decide when it will do so and when adults, whether parents, teachers, youth workers, or family practitioners, should try to offer something more specific than usual day-to-day care.

People do not always see disturbance for what it is, and they sometimes tend to approach the surface behavior of children without real consideration of underlying causes. The disturbances of adolescence usually show in some form of difficult or antisocial behavior. Just to react to this repressively is not helpful, as the problem may go underground only to reappear a year or two later. Equally, to be overpermissive will increase the adolescent's anxiety; there is a need to provide external control.

If the stresses from which the adolescent suffers lead to antisocial behavior, there should be no conflict between the needs of society for protection and the treatment of the individual; it is impossible to help a disturbed adolescent if, in the process, hurtful attacks on others are condoned. When authority figures act as if antisocial behavior has no social implications, they will not be able to aid the individual concerned. It is not possible to assist an adolescent in difficulty if his hurtful actions are sanctioned by whomever is trying to be helpful. If the causes of difficult behavior are not understood, any response is likely to be appropriately useful only as a matter of pure luck. Bad behavior may merely be the object of rebuke; this may be enough only if it occurs as part of a transient emotional upset.

Appropriate control by a loved, admired, and respected adult may be highly meaningful to the adolescent in his care. In trying to help adolescents to handle their own destructive and aggressive impulses, grown-ups often do not understand that the most effective control of disturbed behavior can occur only when an adolescent trusts and likes them. This becomes a particular problem in the average high school where the pupils do not have sufficient contact over a sufficient period of time to respect the adult as a person. Teachers are not seen as people, only as occupiers of roles. This forces schools to use tariffs of punishment. The carrot and the stick are inadequate ways of impressing the young. Often minor upsets that are noticed by teachers are ignored by counselors because "no one else has complained." Thus, the meaning of unusual behavior is lost. Nevertheless, aggressive behavior must be controlled, accepted, and understood; if it is not, the stress produced by such behavior may make the situation worse both for the adolescent and his enviroment.

All adolescents have a need for privacy from authority adults. This means that there should be hesitation before any more than a routine response to misbehavior is considered necessary. Otherwise adolescents are likely to feel that their private world is constantly being invaded. Before investigating some of the more private motivations of adolescents, concerned adults should consider how antisocial an action is and whether or not the adolescent will respond to a relatively superficial response. When routine attempts to be helpful to young people in this way fail, it is then that there is an indication to look for causes. Usually this does not happen; people in the environment tend to give up on difficult adolescents and wait for them to go elsewhere. Particularly in some high schools the staff appear to feel that they have no alternative but to wait for the difficult adolescent to reach the age when they may legally leave or be ejected from school.

All too often, when delinquents are seen in a juvenile court, thev have a long history of persistent bullying, or other types of aggressively disturbed behavior, to which previous adult responses appear to have been stereotyped. Sometimes the disturbance in the individual is so great that nothing could have been done, but previously inadequate reactions may be due to the inadequacy of a school's social setting, its teacher's lack of training for the task they have been called upon to perform, or anxiety about confronting the child's parents with the idea that psychological help may be needed.

Effect of Antisocial Behavior on the Environment

The behavior of the adolescent must affect his environment and his family. Thus disturbances can become cyclic: More stress can be fed back into the individual from his environment, which is then put under greater stress, producing more individual disturbances. The severity of the disturbed behavior may thus be a measure of the disturbance within the social situation, not merely of that within the individual. The following episode comes from a school in England:

> David, a particularly small fifteen-year-old, became more and more upset at school. He engaged in whatever antisocial behavior seemed to be occurring. He was known to be a troublemaker, and on one occasion he and a group of his friends involved themselves in a bout of marijuana smoking. He ran away from school frequently and was abusive to the staff, who felt that despite his academic progress they could no longer tolerate him, and he was expelled.
>
> David's father had been divorced by his mother when he was seven. His stepfather was extremely fond of him, but David was still suffering from the separation. Within himself he was struggling to establish a firm sense of masculine identity. His school still used physical punishment, and David felt that if he were beaten it would be a humiliation. He was afraid that he would cry—an intolerable threat to his sense of manhood—and he was consciously afraid of the homosexual threat in having to bend over to be beaten on the buttocks. In spite of his many fantasies about the brutality of beating, David was provoking by

his behavior a situation in which he was likely to be beaten. He asserted himself by refusing to allow this to happen and created a head-on collision with the authorities. He and they maneuvered themselves into a situation in which there was no going back; neither would give in to the other. The school felt that it must have control, have him conform to the rules; he in his turn became more defiant and difficult.

Ultimately, the school and the boy were feeding disturbed behavior into each other. The only solution that the school could see was to send the boy away, and as soon as this happened he settled down. This led his parents to believe that all was now well—regrettably far from the truth. After having moved from school to school, thus repeating the loss of significant adults in his environment that began with the loss of his father, he became dependent on the use of marijuana.

This whole episode was also a result of a failure to understand the significance of emotional stress in the early lives of difficult adolescents.

One problem of working with difficult and disturbed adolescents is that many adults are quite unsure as to what level of optimum performance to expect from an emotionally disturbed adolescent. Many of those who work with young people do not understand that disturbances are unlikely to be helped unless adults expect the maximum performance of which the individual is capable. When adults are not guided by experts on this issue, or if they are not highly experienced, they may expect either too much or too little from their pupils:

James, an asthmatic sixteen-year-old boy, with a father who was a highly successful alcoholic businessman and a mother who was a depressed, anxious woman, reacted to family stress by failing to turn in his homework. In addition, he cut some of his classes. The principal of his school reacted to this by suspending him at once and threatening to expel him if he broke the rules once more. He also took the opportunity of ordering James to cut his extremely long hair. This handed the boy a weapon that he angrily could and did use against himself and his parents. He immediately acted up again and stayed out of school.

A woman teacher who rightly perceived a thirteen-year-old boy in her class to be severely disturbed, spent so much time in containing his upsets and made so few demands upon him, that the morale of the whole class suffered. She oversympathized with the underprivilege she sensed in her pupil and began to take his side against the rest of the class. It was as if he became the good boy and the others became bad. The rest of the class became more and more difficult to handle as they felt, reasonably, that their teacher was not as interested in them as she should have been.

Assessment of Symptomatic Behavior

Adolescents typically show disturbance by inflicting pain on the environment, rather than by experiencing pain themselves. By hurting the environment an adolescent indicates to the adult world that something is wrong, so adults need to understand the specific ways in which youngsters convey distress.

The extent of the adolescent's destructiveness, either directed towards the self or others, needs to be assessed. In doing this, the age, social situation, and general stress under which an adolescent might find himself have to be understood. For exemple, temper in an early adolescent with minimum provocation is less significant than a similar outburst in the late teens. A refusal on the part of a boy or girl to make reparation for a destructive action, often symbolized by a refusal to apologize, is often an indication of psychological troubles. The constant repetition of irritating behavior, despite action taken to stop it, can mean that the adolescent is in difficulty.

Adolescents in psychological distress often look it. More unkempt than their peers, they seem pale, listless, and fidgety; they look as if they need a good night's sleep. The daydreaming of early adolescence may persist for years, rather than months, and an inability to concentrate may go on for longer than experience would lead one to expect.

Persistent behavior that deviates from the norm of the group may indicate disturbance, if the values of the system meet the developmental needs of the young. The difference between patently unusual behavior and acceptable nonconformity is the key issue. That adolescents do not conform to what they see as an unreasonable rule does not mean that they are psychologically upset. Social change is often created by the pressure put on society by young people. Conformity is not necessarily a sign of mental health; sometimes it indicates passive aberration.

Disturbed behavior may be a reaction against the imposition of what the adolescent perceives as alien values. This is an issue in ethnic conflicts in the school system, but more often it is related to social-class values or academic preoccupations about nonacademic adolescents. Some people define behavior as disturbed because they do not like it.

> The principal of a high school became extremely upset because a large number of adolescents were milling around in the halls. After berating them, he discovered that they were a group of nonacademic youngsters on a scavenger hunt arranged by their class teacher, who was delighted by their capacity to work together.

If schools impose middle-class values on black or white working-class adolescents, they are attempting to make them desert the standards of the social group from which they come. In any school that has a social mix and that does this, persistently difficult behavior will likely occur in one or the other group. This will not necessarily indicate permanent psychological disturbance, nor will it indicate how the adolescents will behave when they leave school. This conflict is a particular issue in high schools, rather than the primary school. Until children reach adolescence, they are more involved in the emotional life of the family than they are in the world outside. Home is the important emotional base, and it is unlikely that grade schools will create a severe conflict of values in children; when vital decisions have to be made, the child will follow the values of home. After puberty the child's need for emotional independence from his parents makes him more susceptible to the influence of the school; if this influence is too pervasive, the adolescent then has a severe value conflict, which may lead to overdependence on peers or intense conflict with either parental values or those of the school.

If in any one school there is a social mix it may be hard, for teachers to decide whether any particular pattern of behavior is abnormal. The local norms and culture have to be taken into account in assessing its possible meaning. For example, in some schools it is not unusual for early adolescent boys to be playing covertly with their genitals at the back of the room, but a sixteen-year-old who does this is likely to be upset. Mutual masturbation up until midadolescence should not cause undue alarm in an all-male, closed environment, but this depends on the general stress the boys are exposed to at the time. In any overrestrictive setting homosexual behavior almost certainly indicates transient emotional disturbance; the nature and quality of the behavior may indicate whether or not a disorder of character formation is also present.

Sometimes adolescents may ask for help by prolonged disturbed behavior or by actions that are highly unusual:

> As part of an assignment to write on any subject he liked, Kevin, a fourteen-year-old boy, gave his teacher a long, highly pornographic essay. A day or two earlier he had accidentally dropped a lurid paperback on the floor of his class. His teacher recognized that the boy was in need of some sort of aid and felt that merely to punish the boy would not be appropriate. He thought that Kevin was expressing contempt or hostility for the school, and Kevin was sent to the school social worker, who talked to him in a firm but kindly way about the unacceptability of his behavior,

which did not recur. There was no punishment, and the teachers reacted to the behavior helpfully on an explicit level.

Kevin perhaps was trying to show how worried he was about his sexual feelings. It might have been helpful if he had been asked about this, but the fact that the behavior did not recur could have meant that Kevin took the school's non-rejection of him as an acceptance of his sexuality. This would certainly have helped him.

Frequently adults who try to help do not know whether a problem has been solved, or merely driven underground. Those people who take on the job of trying to aid the young have to bear the uncertainty of never being quite sure whether they have been useful or not.

Dishonesty

The adolescent who lies does so either to avoid trouble or to bolster up a feeling of personal inadequacy. Early adolescents may still produce childish fantasies and behave as if they were true. It is the persistence of the behavior that should cause alarm, but its significance partly depends on whether lying is part of the social norm of the adolescent's group and the general environment in which the youngster lives and works. The same applies to cheating, which some groups take more seriously than others.

Temper Outbursts

Another disturbed group consists of those who can relate to others yet have major tantrums whenever they are frustrated. Sometimes they feel they have to gratify themselves at any cost; today drugs are extensively used for this purpose. Promiscuous girls, for example, may seek a purely physical relationship with a boy to avoid feeling any immediate psychological pain or anxiety. Boys who become involved in wantonly destructive behavior may also be unable to tolerate frustration. However, it is always important in assessing the significance of such behavior to find out to which conflicts and pressures the young have been exposed.

Underachievement

Underachievement is the typical antisocial act of academic youth. They do not normally behave antisocially in the community-at-large; their technique of showing anger toward the family and the school is to fail to perform adequately at an academic level. The characteristic qualities of delinquent behavior are present in underachievement: It attacks the individual himself, the social system as a whole, and carries with it a perverse gratification. It may not be noticed because little has come to be expected of an individual adolescent or because it is part of a syndrome that has come to include withdrawal. In the latter case, quite seriously withdrawn behavior through a significant part of a school career, even if the young person appears to be functioning at a moderate level, may indicate quite severe psychological disturbance. This is missed as a manifestation of difficulty because conformity is so highly valued. Social systems that require passive acceptance from adolescents may not be aware that compliance which is seen as indicating a good child can be problem behavior. A combination of the obedient withdrawn adolescent who never does quite as well as expected, and a highly rigid school, may result in a failure to perceive severe emotional difficulties. In many situations the adolescent who never disturbs anyone is naturally thought of as being in good psychological shape. Those adolescents who never bother parents or other adults in their life are usually troubled. Such withdrawn young people are extraordinarily difficult to help, and there are very few centers in the psychiatric world equipped for them. They may suffer in that they cannot involve themselves emotionally with other people, either adolescents or adults. It is very difficult for adults to become anchor points for adolescent development if the young cannot relate to them.

Not all disturbed behavior, however, is impulsive or unconsciously motivated. It may be quite conscious, and it may be a direct plea for help.

> Martin, a boy at a fairly rigid conformist British school, wanted to change some of his courses at an advanced level. He could not see a way in which the school would agree to this (although the school would, in fact, have agreed to a change). Martin, therefore, decided quite consciously that the only solution was not to work. Ultimately, he would be removed because he was not working; he would then be sent somewhere else where he would be able to do the courses he wished. This highly disturbed piece of behavior arose because the boy had assumed that the world of his school would be hostile to him, just as he felt his parents were. It is easy to see how he could assume this degree of hostility in a school where the boys felt extreme conformity was demanded.

Many university students appear to get poor grades out of choice. Often these are people who begin to resent the academic treadmill. For a medical student, continuous education under considerable pressure may have been going on for eight or nine years since entering high school. Some medical schools quite properly do not drop individuals permanently who make poor grades; rather, they send them on leave of absence for academic, medical, or psychiatric reasons. A student who wants a year off from academic studies may deliberately do poorly to get it. A not unreasonable goal is achieved by a deliberate piece of disturbed and somewhat antisocial behavior.

Underachievement (Kimball, 1953), the persistent failure on the part of an adolescent to achieve his known academic potential, often remains unrecognized as an indication of disturbance, yet it probably is a most common symptom of emotional disturbance in the academic young. This can be highly destructive to the individual, particularly in those educational systems where progress depends on age, even when underachievement lasts only a few months.

Schools in which teachers have sufficient contact with young people so they can recognize the situation often report that adolescents "could do better" over a long period of time; it usually does not occur to them that this may be a symptom of emotional maladjustment. In most high schools, where teacher contact with pupils is minimal because teachers remain with students only one semester or two and have too many to whom they must relate, it is often not even recognized that a pupil can do more if he enters in the stage of underachievement.

Schools that are sensitive about underachievement as a possible symptom of upset, may well wait for pupils to pass through the turbulence of early adolescence, before coming to a decision as to whether there is any call for specific psychiatric help. The recognition of this disturbed symptom exposes the involved adult to a particular stress: Since society fails to provide adequate resources to help these adolescents, it is usually impossible for the individual to obtain psychiatric assistance. If underachievement is not generally seen to indicate disturbance, this assistance will never be made available.

If underachievement persists after the end of early adolescence and if help is not then sought, the young person may remain inadequate for the rest of his life. When he leaves school this inadequacy may be more apparent: Bright individuals find it difficult to perform jobs they find boring. Yet someone without formal qualifications may have to take such a job. The phrase "could do better" from a school may, during early adolescence, indicate developmental difficulties only. In midadolescence it may indicate psychological disturbance, chronic depression, an unresolved conflict, or a failure to develop a firm sense of self.

Underachievement may also occur in adolescents who reach puberty at sixteen to seventeen, since a late developer is preoccupied with his failure to develop physically as well as his contemporaries. Late maturation is a worry for boys because they significantly assess manhood by comparison with their agemates. Late development in girls is fortunately quite rare. Those who experience it feel intensely that they are not sufficiently feminine and that they will never be attractive to the opposite sex. A boy is reassured by a late growth spurt because this makes him a big man: A girl feels that to be very tall will make her even more sexually undesirable; she may think boys do not like to go out with taller girls.

Adolescents who develop late may appear to be quite bright but to lack the capacity to tolerate frustration as equably as others. They ofen underachieve because of anxiety during the usual years of early adolescence and pubertal turmoil during part of what for others are midadolescent years.

Today underachievement is commonly associated with a dependence on a marijuana high. Smoking marijuana appears to reduce the ability to retain knowledge in some adolescents, particularly if joints are smoked after doing homework and before going to bed. Furthermore, when the drug is used during the schoolday the dreamy depersonalization it creates makes effective learning difficult. This is often an etiological reason for underachievement; in chronic marijuana smoking users often report feeling "pretty stoned" until noon or later after they have smoked.

A seventeen-year-old boy was referred to a psychiatrist because of a sudden falloff in academic achievement. Following a loss of a girlfriend he had begun to smoke five to six joints daily. He found himself disinclined to work and unable to concentrate. The frequency of his marijuana use was reduced with intensive therapy, and, as he smoked then only on Saturday night, his grades returned to their usual level.

All workers with young people need to understand ways in which boys and girls show emotional disturbance. Sometimes being a good listener is enough; the patient recognition that there is a difficulty over which the youngster has little control may make it possible for a self-righting mechanism to appear. An upset adolescent benefits from becoming aware of the positive loving qualities of people in his environment. Therapy is often directed towards reducing the feeling of persecution experienced from the world, so that positive qualities can be felt and incorporated into the personality.

The disturbances of adolescents mostly show us symptom clusters that are now associated with sex, drugs, and delinquency. Each of these topics merits separate consideration, but in each cluster the underlying difficulties are often the same.

References

Aichorn, A. (1935), *Wayward Youth*. New York: Viking.

Bruche, H. (1973), *Eating Disorders*. New York: Basic Books.

Blinder, B. J., Freeman, D. M. A., and Stunkard, A. J. (1970), Behavior therapy of anorexia nervosa and effectiveness of activity as a reinforcer of weight gain. *Am. J. Psychiatr.*, 126: 77–82.

Crisp, A. H. (1970), Premorbid factors in adult disorders of weight with particular reference to primary anorexia nervosa (weight phobia). A literature review. *J. Psychosom. Dis.*, 14: 1–22.

Erikson, E. H. (1968), *Identity, Youth and Crisis*. New York: Norton.

Josselyn, I. (1954), The ego in adolescence. *Am. J. Orthopsychiatr.*, 24: 223–237.

Kimball, B. (1953), Case studies in educational failure during adolescence. *Am. J. Orthopsychiatr.*, 23: 405–415.

King, A. (1963), Primary and secondary anorexia nervosa syndromes. *Br. J. Psychiatr.*, 109: 470–479.

Lewin, B. (1950), *The Psychoanalysis of Elation*. New York: Norton.

Masterson, J. F. (1967), *The Psychiatric Dilemma of Adolescence*. Boston: Little, Brown.

Miller, D. (1954), An approach to the social rehabilitation of chronic psychotic patients. *Psychiatry,* 17: 347–358.

———, and Clancy, J. (1952), The rehabilitation of chronic schizophrenic patients. *Psychiatry,* 15: 435–443.

Redl, F. (1942), Group emotion and leadership. *Psychiatry,* 5: 580.

Schneer, H. I., and Kay, P. (1962), The suicidal adolescent. In *Adolescents, Psychoanalytic Approach to Problems and Therapy,* ed. S. Lorand and H. I. Schneer, 180–201. New York: Paul Hoeber.

Sperling, M. (1962), Psychosomatic disorder. In *Adolescents, Psychoanalytic Approach to Problems and Therapy,* ed. S. Lorand and H. I. Schneer, 202–216. New York: Paul Hoeber.

Wallace, M. W. (1964), Why and how children are fat. *Pediatrics,* 34: 303.

14

Social Organizations and the Treatment of Disturbed Adolescents

Principles of Care

Any recommendation that is made to help disturbed youth needs to take note of the available community resources. Psychiatric services, child care, group homes, probation services, student health centers, and a variety of free clinics all have to try to cope with an overwhelming demand, and their resources are bound to be inadequate. Nevertheless, there is a difference between an insufficient quality of well-delivered care and of poorly delivered service. Although the quality of care varies from place to place, generally the many formal agencies should work on certain principles (American Psychiatric Association, 1971). The presence or absence of these is informative as to the quality of care provided;

1. Each individual within the organization should be helped to achieve an optimal level of growth.

2. The integrity of each adolescent and his family should be respected.

3. Respect for the maturational level of the individual should be at least equal to that of his chronological age.

4. The program should respect the striving for autonomy of each adolescent, and the needs of the child should not be sacrificed to the orientation, personal or theoretical, of the staff.

Just because staff are expert in one field, they should not auto-matically assume that this will meet the needs of young people in their care.

5. The significance of parents, peer groups, extraparental adults, and social norms in the personality development of individual adolescents should be respected. Adolescents in residential care should not be "institutionalized" by being exposed to an "emotional deficiency disease" (Bettelheim and Sylvester, 1948) or being asked to identify with a way of life that is so aberrant that it produces a variety of pathological psychological reactions (Miller, 1965, pp. 63–77). In particular, the capacity of young people to be creative in the community should be enhanced, not destroyed.

6. Imagination, creativity, and intellectual ability should be equally respected. The physiological and psychological needs for space, activity, and community contacts of each adolescent in care are as important as an attempt to resolve an adolescent's intrapsychic conflicts.

7. Each adolescent is a total person, the physical state of the adolescent should be considered as important as his emotional well-being, and vice versa.

8. The dependent needs of adolescents should be respected, which means that adult staff have the responsibility not to abandon young people in their care. The physical environment in which youngsters are cared for should be warm, safe and non-institutional and respect the tactile and perceptual sensitivities of the young, as well as their need for privacy.

9. Since adolescents live in a drug-taking environment, therapeutic agencies should prescribe these with great care.

10. There is no place for punishment in the residential and nonresidential care of adolescents.

Few institutions in which adolescents are cared for meet these requirements; along with the specific provisions of delivery systems to cope with both personal and social maladjustment, ways of preventing adolescent personality distortions are needed. Not only will society never provide all the treatment services that are required, the generally unsatisfactory facilities by which society often demonstrates its unconscious hatred for its young are unlikely to be improved in the near future.

Educational Settings as Treatment Agencies

It has already been stressed that the school is vital to the development of healthy young people. This is equally true of the disturbed adolescent. A good school can be particularly helpful to those young people who have been recognized as having specific emotional needs. And just as a good family practitioner is interested in treatment and prevention, a good school is involved with positive growth as well as helping the transient disturbances of its pupils. A family doctor refers for further help those few of his patients whom he cannot diagnose and, thus, cannot treat or those for whom he does not have adequate treatment facilities. There is an analogy with the school system. Most disturbed adolescents will be automatically helped by a good school; those that are not will be recognized and either specifically aided in the school by the use of school social workers, specifically trained teachers, counselors, or appropriate curriculum adjustments. Alternately, they will be referred to specialized agencies. Grammar schools may be able to recognize disturbed behavior because the children stay in the same group; junior high schools and beyond more often fail to do this.

Special Educational Settings

There is a general recognition in the educational system that special facilities are needed, either in the general school system or separately, for the mentally retarded. There is far less awareness of the needs of the emotionally disturbed. However, in recognition of the importance of the school setting many countries provide special schools that they hope will resolve the particular difficulties of emotionally disturbed children. Children may be sent to these by legal authorities or child-care services; sometimes, if special educational facilities are provided within the general school system, they may be placed by the school authorities themselves. In America the preference seems to be to place emotionally disturbed youth in special classes in the ordinary high school. This method is probably not as helpful as the special day schools for maladjusted children that are common in Britain. Boarding schools for emotionally disturbed children and for those labeled as delinquent are common. These are often single sex, and, since a co-educational environment is certainly emotionally healthier, it is striking that disturbed children from broken homes, often with only one parent, go to a school that is staffed and filled with only one sex.

Educational Philosophy on the Treatment of Disturbance

Both in special schools and experimental schools for ordinary children certain interesting ideas have been put forward; some do not make for a growing environment. One advocates that disturbed children will be helped by being loved, which is usually taken to mean that they should live in a permissive society in which their expressed wishes should be gratified (Berg, 1968). Alternately, such children are felt to need only external control of their aggression. The film *Warrendale* illustrates an approach that children will be helped by a type of emotional catharsis in a controlled environment. A further concept is to design an environment that is run only with behavior-modification techniques. There is something of value in all these ideas, but a good setting fits the treatment technique used to the needs of the individual child rather than the reverse. Certain principles apply in the treatment of disturbed children. The children need to feel cared about (Shields, 1962). Their aggression should be controlled so that they find it difficult to inflict pain on themselves or others. The opportunity must be given to play out safely their most dis- turbing conflicts in an understanding environment. Apart from these principles, such environments need to help their adolescents grow as people, which means that they should provide oppor- tunities for the development of imagination, creativity, and phys- ical, academic, and vocational ability. Finally, loving adults are needed who, apart from child-caring roles, should preferably have another vocational identity the children can recognize.

Causes of Institutional Failure

Experiments sometimes have failed because society has found it difficult to tolerate change or because the schools have not been able to meet the needs of their pupils. Failure can be subtle and disguised by the fact that difficult children are re- peatedly placed elsewhere. On other occasions a setting dete- riorates very rapidly or is closed because of some scandal. Finally, many poor institutions continue, particularly in the field of de- linquency, because of a variety of emotional and economic needs of society-at-large. The protagonists of the idea that love is enough do not appear to understand that it is not sufficient to offer love and patient understanding to a deprived, aggressive adolescent. The designers of such experiments appear to have an oversimplified world of good and bad and tend to see critics of their approach as bad, themselves as good. This concept is identi- fied with by children is such settings who acquire the idea that some staff are bad and some good.

With disturbed children this splitting of the world is in- evitable, particularly if they cannot be offered formal psychother- apeutic help. What is then important is that they see the people nearest to them as good, those farthest away as bad. In a school setting this means that if anyone has to become a bad authority figure it should be the principal. If he ensures, either consciously or not, that he is seen as the good member of the community, other staff will be likely to be seen as bad, leading to inevitable manipulation of the staff by the children and increasingly disturbed behavior. Staff become angry with each other, and this, in turn, feeds more disturbance into the community of children. It is no use to imply that all staff should be expert and to blame some for being overauthoritarian. Good administrators have to create good schools with a proportion of inadequate staff and a turnover of some of their best teachers.

If techniques of emotional catharsis are used staff sometimes unconsciously provoke disturbed outbursts in their charges, perhaps in the unwitting service of their own, rather than the children's, needs. In World War II an effective technique of treatment for battle neurosis was to enable the psychologically wounded soldiers to reexperience a traumatic experience under hypnotic drugs. The success of this has apparently led to the false belief that catharsis of painful emotional experiences was a solution to the more chronic ills of civilian life.

Successes have been reported with well-planned group homes for young people and in skillfully organized settings for delinquents. These organizations always report better results with boys than girls for a good many reasons: Boys who show disturbance call the attention of society more dramatically to themselves; they act up in the community early in their difficulties. Girls first retreat into the family, which is often acceptable to parents. They are not seen generally as emotionally sick until they are in a worse state than the equivalent boy.

Careful studies of failure have also shown areas in which confusion can arise. The common denominator for success appears to be the capacity of adolescents to recognize the value of a human relationship and accept controls within it, the recognition of the integrity of each individual being, the use of implicit social expectation, the provision of resources to make the development of identity possible, adequate vocational and educational training, and adults who are seen as valuable, who are not frightened by the aggression or the seduction of the young. Adults particularly need to be able to understand and help dissipate the persecutory anxiety of the disturbed adolescent.

Role of Adults in Helping the Emotionally Disturbed

There are two main problem areas in the care of difficult young people. If staff, particularly men, have only child-caring roles, they are likely to threaten the tenuous sense of autonomy of the disturbed adolescent, even when they appropriately meet dependent needs. This arises because they do not offer themselves as models occupying socially recognizable roles. If they do, such individuals can be identified with by boys and can offer girls the interest that is needed to support their developing sense of femininity. The absence of this supportive aspect of child and adolescent care means that adolescents in institutions are more likely to regress or become overtly destructive. The problem is not dissimilar to that in penal settings, where a most highly valued member of the institutional community is the prison guard. A man or woman doing a job that is a model of nonproductivity is not an appropriate identification figure for a delinquent adolescent who, unsure of his own sense of self, looks to adults for models.

Sometimes adolescents threaten young staff, often because the latter are so like the former. In such situations, if staff are not offered adequate emotional support, they become so anxious about getting close to adolescents that they are physically neglectful: Health needs of the young are not met; the surroundings demonstrate a lack of care; and adolescents are treated in environments that may appear clean, sterile, and cold or drab, neglected, and deteriorating.

Family relationships affect the treatment of adolescents. An important determinant of upset behavior in the young is disturbed family interaction. Yet there is a confused belief in some quarters that if disturbed children in special boarding schools return home frequently their poor relationship with their parents will necessarily improve. This has led to a system in Britain where delinquent children are put in schools as close to their homes as possible. Intense therapeutic effort may be made with adolescents whose personality is hopefully still quite elastic. Highly intermittent visits from social workers with excessive case loads are thought to be enough to assist a family in which there are difficulties with individuals, and pathological interactions must be helped as well.

There is some evidence that separation of some disturbed children from their disturbed parents is helpful if placement is in a social setting that really meets the child's needs with great skill and sensitivity. Insofar as a parental help is concerned, in the adolescent age range there are two relevant approaches: young adolescents who return to their homes, particularly those in early adolescence, need to have parents who are helped. Otherwise, the youngster is likely to return to the same pathological environment from which he came and that will still influence him. Older adolescents from the middle stage onwards have to learn to cope with their parents as they are. It is less generally necessary to expect parental change, and social work help should be designed to help parents maintain their child in a therapeutic setting for as long as necessary. With either older or younger adolescents in treatment settings, the return for long visits without skilled help offered to parent and child is almost certainly not helpful. If institutions designed to treat emotionally disturbed children and adolescents close for vacations, the action is usually designed to meet the institution's needs rather than those of the children.

Most emotionally disturbed adolescents should be able to receive help in a good school that is not specially designed for the sick but does meet general adolescent needs. Some schools are reluctant to admit disturbed adolescents because it is thought that they will be upsetting to otherwise well-adjusted boys and girls. Although this anxiety often occurs in an ordinary school, well-balanced adolescents can tolerate upset behavior in their contemporaries, although adolescents who are themselves under stress are likely to be made anxious by a boy or girl whom they perceive as disturbed. Early adolescents are more threatened by disturbance in others than are those from the middle stage onwards; they are so anxious about their own controls and their own physical integrity that crippling of any sort in others tends to be frightening. As a result, early adolescents scapegoat the weak and incompetent. This only happens with middle-stage adolescents when they are in environments in which their developmental needs are not met. Regrettably, the sixteen-year-old who is known to have been in a psychiatric hospital will almost certainly be tormented by his peers in a typical impersonally structured American high school. In such settings the madness of disturbed adolescents is felt as an emotional threat; it produces situations in which the threatened group may reject such individuals by bullying or teasing disturbed youngsters to provoke more disturbed behavior. The rejection is an attempt on the part of the members of the group to deny that they have the potential for such disturbance inside themselves. Bullying is part of this denial. The teasing means that the members of the group are proving to themselves that they can control disturbed behavior in others. Thus, they believe they can control it inside themselves. This behavior does not occur with healthy middle-stage adolescents when they go to schools in which their emotional needs for significant interpersonal contact are met.

Psychologically, good schools that are willing to try to help the maladjusted can admit a certain number of disturbed adolescents without disturbing the environment. Adolescents respond to implicit expectation and peer-group pressure. If too high a population of emotionally disturbed young are placed in the average good school, with their greater needs for both nurture and control than an equivalent-age individual, they may shift the way the whole school structure functions. There is then a regressive pull on the normal adolescent who may still be strug-gling with childlike needs. It is impossible for an outsider to specify how many disturbed children a school can take. Each school must decide for itself. It is probable that most schools are too anxious about this and could handle more children who are known to be troubled than they actually accept. The average school has about 10 percent of its population suffering from some degree of emotional disturbance at any one time; 2 percent are probably severely disturbed. The latter tend to be a fairly fixed group of individuals; since most disturbance is transient, the former are different individuals at different times.

In the private sector of education, and to some extent even in the public school system, each school has special qualities that make it able to help some youngsters and not others. Schools are, however, often uncertain as to the type of adolescent they are best able to help. When they are in doubt, technical assistance, usually from a psychiatrist, should be made available. Unnecessary rejection of young people can cause guilt to teachers and suffering to disturbed adolescents and their parents. On the other hand, to take young people whom schools cannot help may be even more unfortunate:

A small private co-educational Quaker boarding school, which was extremely anxious to be helpful, agreed to take Debbie, a girl from an unhappy and divided home who behaved in a provocative way towards authority. But the school had not faced the fact that its staff were having difficulties among themselves. The women staff were more rigid and conformist in their social attitudes than the men. This led to tension between the girls and boys, and further anxiety made Debbie liken life at school to life in her divided home. She did her best to drown her anxiety by becoming as provocatively difficult to the women as she had previously been to her mother; for example, she accidentally left cigarette butts on a table by her bed. The women began to tell the headmaster how wrong he had been to take her. The examples of her provocation became numerous.

Debbie managed, even when she was wearing a school uniform, to make it appear seductive; inevitably the teachers were annoyed. When they became repressive, she gave them a lecture on liberal morality. Although she was doing better academically than ever before, and for the first time made real friends among her own age group, the tension in the staff concentrated on Debbie to such an extent that she became a scapegoat. The principal felt that he had no alternative but to send her home.

A major problem that any one faces in handling the seriously disturbed adolescent is knowing when to ask for expert help. Ideally, referral to a psychiatric clinic should be made when pediatricians, family practitioners, teachers, youth workers, or parents have satisfied themselves that they are not being helpful. This, of course, requires that helping adults both get to know children and also know how to recognize disturbed behavior. Alternately, they may know from experience that a particular adolescent's difficulties are likely to be too great for them to handle. If possible, help should be sought *before* things have reached such a pass that the presence of an adolescent within a social setting can no longer be tolerated.

Self-Righting Mechanisms in Adolescence

To a certain degree the idea that, insofar as emotional disturbance is concerned, one can snap out of it, or, alternately, grow out of it, continues to exist, not only in the United States but also in many other countries of the Western world. Like so many of the concepts of society, this has a kernel of truth. Because of it, necessary attempts to get help may be prevented or delayed, but it is fair to say that it may also allow young people the chance to try to solve their difficulties by themselves. To be able to conquer difficulties obviously enhances an adolescent's self-esteem; this is clearly desirable. The important thing is that the price should not be too high. For example, drug dependence, especially on such substances as marijuana is probably colluded in by nonactivity on the part of many adults, schools, and youth centers.

The psychic turbulence of some young people's adolescence may lead to an automatic correction of childhood upsets. The change in the attitudes of the adolescent towards the self and the resulting attitude changes on the part of parents, teachers, and others may create a self-righting mechanism during adolescence. The possibility of relating on an emotional level to adults who are new in the young person's life may give a second chance for mature development. This is particularly true in a social environment in which people are sensitive to adolescent needs.

On the other hand, a change for the better may be more apparent than real; the adolescent may repress his internal conflicts and appear to function as if nothing is wrong. In this situation, there is frequently little emotional energy left to meet the challenges of the real world. The adolescent may pay the price for his superficial improvement by failing to develop his full potential.

The self-labeling propensity of adolescents may also discourage adults from referring them for help. Many are fearful that young people sent to a psychiatrist may then describe themselves and explain away their actions in terms of being emotionally disturbed: "I'm sick, I will act accordingly." The propensity of adolescents to acquire a fake identity may make it very difficult to motivate some to seek help. Adolescents with homosexual difficulties may announce themselves to another person with "I am homosexual." Conflicted young adolescents may use such organizations as the Gay Liberation Movement to reinforce their false identity. Those who are emotionally distressed may find it difficult to say: "I am me, I am a person." Instead they are all too ready to wear the label that is available, or that society gives them, to obtain a false sense of security. So young people may call themselves freaks, straight, greasers, and jocks. Potentially helpful adults are likely to worry when adolescents flaunt an eccentric label: Are they really disturbed? Or are they exaggerating a minor difficulty for effect? Can anything be done anyway?

Any labeling of adolescents is liable to create difficulties. Many are all too often prepared to adopt the identity they are given by their immediate world. When they are tagged by schools as failures by being put in low academic tracks, they tend to respond and see themselves accordingly as failures. When the young are saddled with formal diagnostic terms that imply a poor chance of recovery, the people around them tend to be so influenced by these that recovery is made more difficult.

Fear of Psychiatry

A further reason why adolescents are not referred for help when they need it is that many people are both ignorant about, and suspicious of, psychiatry. Some believe that all patients lie on a couch, others that psychiatrists deal only with those who are mad:

> In one European country a psychiatrist telephoned a boy's teacher and said that he would like to discuss a boy's difficulties with her. Later that evening the psychiatrist was telephoned at his home by the teacher's husband. He was highly suspicious and demanded to know why the psychiatrist wanted to interview his wife.

This fear of psychiatrists still exists in many societies, and represents a dread of the unknown forces inside each human being. Many teachers, for example, often believe that for their pupil to see a psychiatrist implies that they have failed to perform their job adequately, or they are afraid that moral weakness and grave mental illness will be detected in the adolescent. These attitudes rub off on adolescent patients who may say that they think the job of a psychiatrist is to see whether or not they are crazy.

If teachers do not consciously hold these attitudes themselves, they often assume that parents will feel ashamed of their child's need for help.

A teacher at an excellent school wanted a girl who had been stealing to see a psychiatrist. The letter she wrote to the girl's mother about this was so vague, talking of a "psychologist friend of the school," that the mother had no idea what the teacher was trying to say. When the mother found out what was happening, after giving permission for a psychologist to talk to her daughter, she was shocked and angry.

Quality of Psychiatric Care for Adolescents

The concept of peer-group counseling is often used so adults can avoid the responsibility of facing emotional disturbance in their charges. It is much easier to get an adolescent of fifteen who is smoking pot two or three times daily to talk to marijuana-smoking young adults in their early twenties and imagine something constructive is being done to face the real distress of the youngster.

In one high school a drug-help group was set up in a room in the school to talk to the students who so wished about drugs. Apparently very successful rap sessions were held. Obviously no formal follow up was possible but a group of students said at a drug-education discussion that all the students who took part in the sessions were more heavily into drugs after the sessions than before.

Peer counseling is offered in particular to institutionalized delinquents and minority-group students; alternately the latter may be given a poorly trained social worker or counselor of the same ethnic group because, supposedly, the children will more likely be understood, irrespective of the quality or the training of the offered helper. This is racism at its worst. What matters is the quality of help offered: The more deprived the youngster, the better it should be: Regrettably, this often is not the arbiter that is used.

If an adolescent does reach a clinic, the chances of his being adequately helped are at present extremely small. The training of psychiatrists, social workers, and teachers in understanding the problems of children and adolescents is often defective.

> An adolescent psychiatrist gave the last lecture of the whole course to a group of graduating social workers at a well-known school of social work. In the question period one student said, "How do you talk to adolescents?" Nowhere in the course had any significant discussion about techniques of relating to adolescents been given.

Too many clinics have given in to the overwhelming need for help from young people and process them as if they were on a moving staircase, spending insufficient time with them or their families. Psychiatrists who are trained to work only with children often may find it difficult to relate to adolescents. Theirs is much the same problem as that of an infant schoolteacher who feels out of his depth with boys or girls of fifteen.

Traditionally, adolescents have been considered difficult to help in psychiatric clinics. Adolescents are often reluctant to see themselves as needing help of any kind from adults. They particularly resent being sent to a child-guidance clinic. To wait in a room in which parents and children are also waiting and to be seen in a playroom for small children—all this makes the adolescent feel that he is being treated as a small child. Service delivery for adolescents is unsatisfactory. Many clinics tend to have very long waiting lists, and adolescents are usually referred for help at a time of crisis. By the time the clinic is ready to see him, he is often unwilling to turn up, or in some way or another the problem seems to have faded. The need for help is then no longer considered necessary by anyone; doctors, teachers, parents, or the youngsters themselves. This is particularly likely because parents, if not schools, are always hopeful that matters will right themselves. Sometimes staff from referring agencies may become so resentful of what they see as the cavalier attitude of psychiatric clinics to their needs, implied by long waiting lists, that they give up requests for help in despair.

Expectations of Psychological Help

Too much may be expected from psychological assistance. Disturbed adolescents, parents, and youth workers generally feel that there should be an immediate and dramatic improvement. Teachers, parents, and adolescents may find it difficult to accept that psychological progress is not likely to take the form of a straight line upward but rather a wave motion on an upward curve. Psychiatrists should make it clear to involved adults and their patients that there can be no magical change. If they fail to do this, both the adolescent and those involved with him may prematurely withdraw in disappointment. Of course, on occasions change is rapid, and this contributes to the unreal picture of the omnipotent psychiatrist:

> One sixteen-year-old boy was referred for help after having been troublesome for about three years. Andrew was depressed and felt that the teachers were expecting him to be troublesome. He felt that little was to be gained by staying in school. Whenever he found work difficult, he walked out. His teachers responded repressively; Andrew became more outrageously provocative. A late developer, he behaved as if he were really adolescent. He was argumentative, difficult, exhibitionistic, easily upset, and in constant trouble. By the time Andrew came for help, puberty had started. The fact of referral changed the teachers' attitude towards him; they decided that he must be disturbed and, therefore, became less critical. Andrew experienced with immense relief the physical changes that he had thought would never occur. He

was able in three or four sessions to discuss his feelings about his teachers and his late development. His behavior changed dramatically. He became a successful member of the school where it had been thought that he could never have a responsible position. As a result the staff began to expect equally dramatic changes in many of their more disturbed pupils. There was a flood of referrals for help, which rapidly dried up when the equivalent magic was not produced.

Not all adolescents can be helped in outpatient psychiatric clinics; formal psychiatric treatment, in particular individual or group psychotherapy, may have little to offer to adolescents who cannot make relationships. In psychotherapy the understanding a patient develops with a therapist makes possible the control of disturbed and antisocial behavior. The patient then needs to develop those relationships that alone can enable him to grow.

The stormy course of some adolescents' treatment tends to become intolerably difficult for the world and people around them (Miller, 1957). This sometimes has inevitable, if unfortunate, consequences. Because it is difficult to predict when change will occur, a social setting may reject an adolescent just at the point of improvement. Frequently, if adolescents feel a change in themselves, they resist the process automatically. The individual may engage in a burst of disturbed behavior as if to prove that nothing has changed. One is as one has always felt oneself to be; nothing is different. At this point interested adults are likely to feel that the situation is now intolerable: We have done all we can and there is no point in trying any further.

It is essential that psychiatrists and other workers with young people should understand one another. For example, psychiatrists often feel bitterly that they get no cooperation from schools. The teacher and the psychiatrist then create a distance between themselves. Each has no real idea of what it is that the other expects, and they make few attempts to find out.

It is also important that school social workers be supported by psychiatrists. Without adequate psychiatric help expectations may be aroused that cannot be fulfilled. The better the worker, the more likely is it that he or she will discover and release disturbed behavior. Adolescents who sense difficulties within themselves usually cannot go directly to a person they know to be helpful; they have to act out a request for assistance. Once moderately upset children are helped within a school, the more disturbed adolescents will surface. A school social worker will not have the personal resources to help severely disturbed adolescents, who will attempt to get help by behaving in a disturbed way. The school social workers are then in the same impossible position as psychiatrists who work in poor penal institutions. By their assistance to some, they may encourage young people to believe that they will get help for their difficulties; when adequate aid is not forthcoming, such individuals may feel acutely disappointed and teased.

Teachers and other adults should use the psychiatrist in a sensible way. Some are so anxious to help adolescents whom they perceive as disturbed, or whom they have referred to a psychiatrist, that they make help very difficult. Unwittingly, they may put themselves and the psychiatrist in a ludicrous position:

> Lewis was sent for help at the age of fifteen because he had stolen $2.00 from a changing room. Despite the fact that he was warned that further bad behavior might mean supervision, he followed this with a series of minor infringements of school rules. Between his first and second appointment with the psychiatrist, he was caught by a teacher with a packet of cigarettes. He was told that he would be suspended, unless your doctor specifies otherwise.
>
> The boy felt the school was saying: "We will reject you unless we are told not to do so." Meaning to be helpful, the school authorities effectively told Lewis that they did not trust their own judgment and they gave the psychiatrist a power over his life that could not be helpful. Lewis felt obliged to be overpolite to the doctor and found it difficult to talk freely about how he felt about himself, his parents, and the school. He now

had to be on his best behavior because the psychiatrist had such power over him.

Often, children are suspended until a psychiatrist is ready to say that they are fit to return to school. This is futile; behavior is also a function of the quality of the environment. A similar pattern is created when children who steal in school are sent home with the statement that they can return if a specialist recommends this. It is not surprising that in most parts of the Western world referral to a psychiatrist is still seen as a last desperate resort. The psychiatrist may become the policeman for disturbed young people. It is not uncommon for them to be warned that they will be referred to a psychiatrist unless they pull their socks up.

Need for Nonpsychiatric Help

The deficiencies in the psychiatric services and the difficulties involved in using them means that skilled assistance is needed even more from the staff of schools. Even with a good psychiatric service, there are some adolescents who can probably only be helped in educational settings; schools and youth clubs can be very helpful to some adolescents who find it difficult to make one to one human relationships and who thus find it very hard to use psychotherapy. The general atmosphere of a school may help such young people make tenuous and not very emotionally meaningful relationships, yet get satisfaction from performing useful and worthwhile tasks. Too many demands are not then made upon such adolescents and they may find satisfaction in the numerous activities, physical, imaginative, or academic, that may be available.

To understand the disturbances of adolescents and how to treat them, it is necessary to sort out three factors: the type of symptoms, the capacity of the individual to make meaningful emotional relationships with others, and the etiology of the upset.

It is important to consider built-in stress and supports that impinge on the individual in three areas: the family, the environment, and the personality of the individual as it affects the perception of the world. The maximum helpful effort can then be placed where it will carry the most weight. Sometimes the main thrust will be in the control of behavior, some types of drug taking, for example; a change of environment or help with the family or personality difficulties may be indicated at other times. Any one individual may need different kinds of help at different times, but, whatever is done, young people need a continuity in their relationships with helpful adults. If continuity of care with the same group of adults is not provided, much effort is wasted, as adolescents are highly sensitive to the loss of meaningful adults. The assumption is sometimes made that if an adolescent is in formal psychotherapy, other relationships do not matter. For example, court social workers commonly abandon their relationships with clients when a decision for outpatient therapy is made. Quite apart from the fact that external controls may be needed in an adolescent's life, psychotherapy, when the therapist provides the only meaningful relationship in an individual's world, is almost bound to fail.

Prevention of Maladjustment

The networks of society should be preserved and strengthened if prevention of maladjustment that offers the most hope for the development of healthy young people is to be possible. Individual dedicated teachers and youth workers can perform remarkable tasks in poor school systems and neighborhoods, but society cannot rely on the lifeblood of very special human beings. Many social organizations are necessary, but the stability that society lacks—and without which many adolescents find it difficult to develop—can be recreated in the world of school with the skill of many people. The resilience, charm, creativity, and loving qualities of humanity can be seen in sharp focus during the ad-

olescent age period. The destructive anger and hatred of mankind can also be most vividly present at that time.

The psychological mettle of the young is tested and retested
by present day society. In some ways we are now permissive;
this is probably desirable if it allows young people to make emotional contact with each other and the world. Permissiveness becomes destructive licence when it makes possible the exposure
of individuals to intolerable stress and conflict. The issue for our
society is how to allow for the creativity of mankind while containing its aggression. We can do this only if we learn from our
own history; people can direct their energies outward in a constructive way only when they have a safe and secure emotional
base from which they can grow.

With sufficient resources we can repair the damage we have
already caused; with the use of human skills we can create environments that help people to grow up. Some schools protect the
children of underprivileged neighborhoods from needing to take
part in destructive antisocial acts; some communities have already
been created in which human families easily relate to each other;
some societies care for their aged and their young. A dedicated
individual can rescue a nearly destroyed adolescent. We have the
capacities; society cannot rely on the provision of more and more
technical help.

Before remedial action to help adolescents grow is possible,
the way in which social systems fail to meet their developmental
needs must be understood. When, for example, community mental
health organizations deal only with the symptomatic manifestations of social-system malaise, they may help the preservation of
an inadequate social organization. If, for example, distressed and
disturbed youth are removed from schools, helped, and then
returned, little may be done to look at the fundamental maladjustment within the organization as a whole.

A decision may be made by helping people not to work intensively with a disturbed family because an individual child may
grow up, and grow away from it. The same decision made about

a social organization that significantly affects the lives of generations of young people, should be made only after the most thoughtful deliberation.

References

American Psychiatric Association (1971), *Standards for Psychiatric Facilities Serving Children and Adolescents.* Washington, D.C.

Berg, L. (1968), *Risinghill.* Harmondsworth: Penguin.

Bettelheim, B., and Sylvester, E. (1948), A therapeutic milieu. *Am. J. Orthopsychiatr.*, 18: 191–206.

Miller, D. (1957), The treatment of adolescents in an adult hospital. *Bull. Menninger Clin.*, 21: 189–198.

———— (1965), *Growth to Freedom, The Psycho-Social Treatment of Delinquent Youth.* Bloomington: Indiana University Press.

Shields, R. W. (1962), *A Cure of Delinquents.* London: Heinemann.

15

Principles of Adolescent Therapy

Just as in general medicine it is self-evident in helping young people that the etiology of any disturbance has to be understood before any appropriately helpful recommendations can be made. Unfortunately, in psychological medicine, whether therapy is given by nonphysicians or MD's, this concept is not generally applied. Often, the type of assistance depends on the discipline of the helping person. Sociologists think in sociological terms, psychologists in individual psychological ways, psychiatrists may have psychological or sociological orientation, but add the use of medication. Within any one discipline, there are numerous orientations: the psychotherapies—group, family, individual; behavior-modification techniques; milieu therapy and therapeutic communities; the use of somatic treatments. Even within these orientations, the individual may be offered assistance that is related to such factors as the time a therapist may have available. A psychotherapist with one free session a week offers this; a group therapist with a vacancy in a group makes the place available.

In medicine the discovery of certain drugs and surgical techniques has made it possible to improve, at any rate potentially, service delivery. In helping adolescents, the equivalent may well be in assisting those social organizations that impinge on adolescents to understand their role in helping or hindering personality development. Just as the individual diagnosed as suffering from a pneumococcal pneumonia may now be treated with the appropriate antibiotic, so may schools, youth centers, extraparental adults be asked to respond in appropriate ways, if the etiology of adolescent maladjustment is understood. To date, attempts to help disturbed adolescents are often hindered by the rigidities and unawareness of social systems and people working with distressed young people often do not know what type of help should be sought.

Insofar as schools are concerned, they will be of little use to those of their population who are in emotional difficulty unless they have become more sensitive to the needs of all individuals and are able to be responsive to them. The behaviorists' concepts of mass conditioning are currently widely, if inadequately, applied; there is little evidence that more of the same will significantly reduce alienation and emotional disturbance. Furthermore, there is evidence that respect for individual needs pays dividends.

Social Organizations as Therapeutic Agents

The necessity for schools to provide for continuity of human relationships has been repeatedly stressed. With this in mind, schools could further help their pupils, particularly late developers, by becoming more sensitive about the use of maturational norms in academic placement (Jones, 1969). After the age of eighteen or so, when adolescents begin a university education, they usually enter an educational system that does not normally consider the individual student's age, at any rate prior to age twenty-five, as a criterion of likely academic progress. In community colleges, high school subjects are taken irrespective of age.

This approach could be applied to all high school education. If children could stay together for certain nonacademic courses for a considerable part of their day; specific academic subjects would be followed by students of different ages without any dis-

crimination against the late developer. Such a student could begin a course later than the majority of pupils, but there would
be no pressure on him to catch up to those chronologically older
than himself. If American teachers could accept the European
concept that it is not necessary to teach each subject every day,
and if the concept of a half-day off twice a week were adopted,
schools could have a viable house system, establish small-group
continuity, and allow children of different maturation levels to
use specialized central facilities for certain academic and vocational activities. What would then be needed would be more adequate training for teachers in human development and techniques
of interpersonal relationships.

Within a school, one aim of a teacher should be to provide
emotional support and care, while adolescents learn along with
academic or vocational knowledge, that impulsive needs for gratification cannot be met. A baby is harmed if it has a mother who
rushes to give it a bottle before it cries: To meet needs before they
are expressed imprints on the human personality the image of an
unreal world. An environment that does not allow an adolescent
to experience frustration does not help him mature. There is,
then, no evidence that it is desirable to abandon in academic and
nonacademic subjects the need for a high standard of achievement and pride in productivity. This does not mean that a community should attempt to create frustration by being rigid and
depriving. Equally frustrating environments can be unwittingly
created by people determined to banish them; it is a mistake to
imagine that to be totally loving is to be nonfrustrating: too
much love can produce intolerable frustration since it makes people feel helpless and impotent (Bettelheim, 1950).

Relief of Tension and Anxiety

During growth the young may not be strong enough to with-
stand tension and anxiety. Their wishes for the immediate relief

of frustration may be greater than their capacity to delay an action that they may know to be unwise. Internal conflicts are then acted out on the community or directed against the self (Freud, 1920). For example, if an adolescent wants to pass an examination, but because of a general depression finds the subject boring, he is likely to forget to do his work, fall asleep, and lie to himself. Teachers are disappointed and often irritated, and the youngster suffers with an unnecessary failure. If adolescents are not aware of what troubles them, or if they feel hopelessly misunderstood and ill-treated, antisocial behavior is more likely. An adolescent who appreciates his surroundings will do his best in them. A common fantasy of the large high school, which has abandoned meaningful emotional relations as the norm, is that adolescents can be controlled by a tariff of rewards and punishments. Well-adjusted adolescents who feel positive about adults will accept control and will not see controls as punitive and arbitrary. A young person who feels loved and cared for by an adult can often abstain from self-destructive impulsive behavior for the other person, if not for himself.

It is not unusual for children who have done well academically and socially in high schools up to grade ten to fail in grade eleven and start to behave in a socially aberrant way. This change may occur because it is no longer possible at age fifteen or sixteen for the average adolescent to contain impulsive behavior for the sake of parents; to do so sacrifices autonomy strivings. A poorly developed sense of the future, particularly in boys, is no deterrent to the gratification that may be obtained from impulsive behavior. An intellectual understanding, without emotional awareness, that present behavior affects future activities is likely to increase a potential level of anxiety and so enhance the probability of impulsive behavior, which becomes an attempted escape from frustration.

John, a boy of sixteen who had made straight A's in grade ten and D's and E's in grade eleven was referred to a psychiatrist because he missed 120 class periods in one semester. He said, "I know my parents want me to do well and last year that was enough, but now I hassle with them all the time; particularly my mother. I want to go into a profession, but this worries me; and I can't get my head together enough to do any work."

At the start of grade eleven, John got all new teachers, two he had liked in grade ten no longer taught him. He neither knew, liked, or valued any of the staff presently teaching him. In schools the most liked teachers tend to get the best results; they are the ones who find it easy to keep a class interested and involved. It is in contact with individuals such as these that adolescents are likely to suspend difficult behavior. One year of such people is not enough. There is no reason, however, why one teacher should not be able to teach the same group of children a subject over two to three years.

Problems of Good Teaching

All adolescents dislike and resent losing people who are important to them. A good adult leaving an adolescent arouses at least irritation, at most despair. The anger of separation has to be worked out with the individual who is leaving. If it is not, the next adult will have a doubly hard time in forming a new relationship.

The teaching situation may, however, be more complex: It is often not enough to say that the teacher should be liked. Those teachers who wish to respect the integrity of individuals and not repress them will probably try to provide a liberal education setting. Unfortunately, disturbed adolescents who are likely to become aggressive will tend to see such teachers as weaklings. In a generally rigid school the frustrations forced on them in class will be acted out in the classroom with the more understanding teacher. In such an authoritarian school, the new teacher with the attitude that rigid external control need not be a suitable teaching mechanism may be forced to be as repressive as others. The more a school fails to help its difficult adolescents, the harder it is for a teacher who has an authority role in such a setting to have a good relationship with pupils. All authority adults tend to be tarred with the brush of the environment in which they work. Very remarkable personalities may be able to hold out against this pressure; others have no alternative but to conform or leave.

Environmental Norms and Helpful Adults

It is desirable that adolescents feel a consistency from people who wish to influence them; thus, the environment should fit the message that the individual adult within it wishes to convey to the young. With society-at-large, this is not possible. In smaller settings that more directly impinge on the individual—schools, youth clubs, colleges and universities—where reasonable consistency between environmental and individual attitudes is lacking, attempts at human relationships on the part of individual adults with the young are likely to be difficult. If a teacher talks about mutually helpful human relationships in an environment in which these do not generally occur, he is felt to be insincere or helpless. This is important in schools but especially in institutions for those who are labeled delinquents. Some staff in an unsatisfactory environment may make a particular effort to care for the individuals within it. Although they may give real help to individuals, they are unlikely to be used as models by the adolescents in their charge. Inevitably, such people are insufficiently valued by the environment and what they say is inconsistent with what their presence implies. Although such teachers may appear to have good relationships with their charges, these probably never have the depth they would have in a more constructive setting. The provision of good psychological treatment and general emotional care depends on the ability of an environment to meet the developmental, intellectual, emotional, and vocational needs of its charges. A good teacher or counselor working in such settings should be able to make relationships with adolescents that will help them incorporate into their personalities the positive values of the world in which they live. In a setting that fails to meet appropriate human needs, the young are very suspicious of all authority adults. If their doubt abates, and they begin to use counseling help, they will expose to their counselor the corruption of their own relationships and those with other adults in the system. This exposure is an implicit demand that something be done. Usually the counselor has no power to reform and the adolescent feels cheated. Any faith in authority adults that may have been developing is also dissipated. If an attempt at reform is made the institution may, with many rationalizations, try to get rid of the person who is perceived as attempting to discredit it.

When adolescents develop good relationships with teachers, in environments that meet their needs, they can discuss their feelings and become freer to cope with themselves and the demands of the world outside. The capacity to communicate feelings in words is not as developed in early adolescence as it is later on. Nevertheless, direct interest from teachers is as important to this age group as it is to others, because they need to feel that someone cares about them. Teachers who can convince pupils that the latter are significant as people are then in a much better position to help in a crisis.

Teachers have an important role in helping young people understand something of what is going on in the world around them, particularly now when adolescents are faced with problems of general and political morality, sexual behavior, and distracting temptations in society. Issues such as drug addiction and the use of alcohol and cigarettes are recurring worries. In their habitual behavior adolescents identify with what adults do rather than say. If teachers or parents use cigarettes, any exhortation from them not to do this is likely to be valueless. When adults smoke secretly in their common room, adolescents are likely to do the same in the

washroom. If teachers feel forced to go on strike or refuse to perform extracurricular duties, their message to their pupils is that
direct action is the appropriate response to grievances. It is impossible for adults who are responsible for the care of adolescents
to be beyond reproach, but if adults are aware of their own inevitable inconsistencies they will allow for their effect.

Individual and Group Relationships

It is sometimes believed that group approaches to the young
are simpler than one-to-one relationships. Such group approaches
depend on a good working relationship between adults and young
people. Adults should be able to listen to adolescents and help
them with their individual difficulties—whether help is explicitly
requested or not—before they can help a group with its conflicts. The teacher who is valued by pupils because of a skill at
sport, in a classroom, or in the arts should be able to establish an
individual working relationship with each of them. It is then
possible for adolescents to have someone to whom they can turn
as individuals. They can also discuss conflicts that trouble them
as a group.

Adolescents, because of their fear of dependence, often
find it difficult to express gratitude. Even if an adult has been
helpful in an individual relationship, an adolescent may complain
that "he tried to talk to me but he was a phony." He may feel
the adult was not sufficiently understanding or did not care
enough. The lack of appreciation that is sometimes shown by the
young often leaves adults, who are made to feel inadequate, reluctant to try to help. Teachers who relate to their adolescent
pupils are often unreasonably put in the position of amateur
psychiatrists, yet the need is so great that they really have no
choice but to try to be useful. Probably no other organized group
in society has the same opportunities to aid adolescents as the

well-trained teacher; only after the pupil has left school may they be offered deserved appreciation.

Changes within the school system routine, apart from helping all adolescents mature, would make it possible for schools to respond very specifically to the needs of individuals. It might then be possible for any one child to specify the type of group placement that ought to be made, the type of subject to be taught and its technique, and the nature and quality of adult relationships.

More out-of-school activities should be available. Although formal classes of various sorts, usually adult education, take place in high school buildings at night, these only skim the resources. If a school has facilities for recreation and the creative arts, they should be available to the public, including adolescents, outside school hours. It is absurd to leave them unused in the evening and during school vacations. The arguments that it is too difficult to clean the buildings or that destruction will occur are unconvincing.

Use of Youth Centers

In addition to whatever is provided by home and school, adolescents need various youth centers in their neighborhood. At the present time, these tend to be organized by churches in smaller communities; in many large cities boy's clubs are run in association with the Boys Club of America. In many places there is remarkably little cooperation between youth clubs that may jealously guard their membership. Often the most affluent neighborhoods have the best facilities, although the situation in most cities and suburbs, where youth facilities are notably lacking, is deplorable. In the inner cities the facilities for youth are as deprived as the rest of the neighborhood.

Adolescents do not usually move very far in cities; most of their activities occur within about a square mile of their homes. Therefore, adolescents should have neighborhood centers with organized recreation; the same or other centers should provide outlets for creativity. Also needed are unstructured settings equipped with a food bar, a record player, and a TV set, and grown-ups ready, if asked, to provide an opportunity for interpersonal relationships across age groups with no formally organized activity. Such youth centers can be housed in different kinds of buildings, which (with the provision that poverty is no help) should generally fit the character of the neighborhood. The interior of the youth club should be designed to meet its particular function. In smaller cities and towns, the club should be centrally placed, rather than at the periphery of the community. The hours of such centers should meet adolescent needs; a drop-in unstructured center, for example, should be open every day of the year, if it is to be genuinely useful.

Techniques of Relating to Adolescents

All workers with young people—teachers, school counselors, probation officers, physicians and social workers—generally feel the need for more adequate training in interpersonal relationships and personal counseling techniques with adolescents. They should know of the effect of environment on human behavior, particularly as this applies to the setting in which they work. Professional staff may also need training in using and understanding the problems of voluntary helpers, who are essential if a youth center is to convince the adolescent that the community-at-large cares for him.

Besides specific psychotherapeutic techniques there are some general guidelines that might be of value to those who wish to relate in a useful way to adolescents in distress. It is common for specific contact to occur with adolescents at a time of crisis. Although an adolescent may ask for help in words, he more often implicitly demands help through an antisocial act. The helpful adult needs to understand what is behind the adolescent's difficult behavior, and it is tempting, in looking for the answer, to ask the youngster why he behaved in such a way. This is usually a sterile question. If the adolescent knows the answer, he may choose to lie; if he does not, he may feel obliged to produce a specious reason. Although he thinks he knows, his answer may be inaccurate. Asking such a question is likely to make a young person feel persecuted, discussing his general life suitation is much better. If the adult covers the adolescent's general social situation, work, and family relationships in an interview, the explantation for the difficulty often becomes clear.

Adults who are out of touch with their own inner experience of feeling and imagination, who are unaware of their own conflicts and who are preoccupied with their own status find it difficult to help the young. All grown-ups interviewing adolescents should ask themselves at least three questions: What is the youngster likely to be feeling now? How has this feeling been modified by interviews with me and other authority figures in the past (Gill, *et al.*, 1954, pp. 106–107)? What are the adolescent's expectations of the situation, how has he been told about it, what is his perception of the interviewer's role?

Authority Role of Adults

The adolescent's reaction to the adult as an authority figure is an important indication of his state of mind. In all human beings experiences of the past condition responses in the present. The reaction to authority in the here and now is based partly on a previous perception of authority. So if a doctor or a personal or academic counselor or teacher in a school or university attempts to relate to an adolescent, the latter's reaction will be determined by many factors: It will be based partly on childhood experiences of authority from father or mother, partly on the experience of authority in hospitals and clinics, schools and colleges, partly on the general feeling of personal security of the young person concerned. In educational settings the response also will depend on the reputation among the student body of the staff member who is acting as a personal counselor: how has he treated the student in the past? What is his reputation in society-at-large? The issue of reputation in an institution needs to be particularly understood by personal counselors. Minority students are likely to feel that only members of their own ethnic group can understand them. The prejudiced individual of any race is hardly likely to be a good personal or vocational counselor, but the issue is really the competence of an individual, not his skin color or ethnic group. Also important is the depth of a counselor's education and its breadth. All people do not live in the same way, and the specific identity of different ethnic groups needs to be understood.

Freedom of expression with adults who have authority is impossible, if it is not promoted in the whole life of the community. In schools where nobody expects children to ask questions in the classroom, it is quite unreal to expect them to talk freely to adults in an interview.

Some adults working with adolescents are clearly agents of authority; others may feel that this is not their role, that it is their responsibility to help young people choose whether to conform to the wishes of society or not. Rebellious young people may believe that their actions are based on an experience of inner freedom, but the rebellion may be an attempt to break out of an internal strait-jacket.

Whether the adult is an agent of authority or not, it is desirable that adolescents feel that adults are on their side but not against parents or society. Since antisocial behavior is usually self-destructive, the adult should try to convey, without being pompous, that he wants to help stop it. His attitude should be: let us see how you and I together can be of use to you.

Reduction of Stress in the Interview

The basic principle for successful human relationships is to
help the other person feel at ease. Even a confrontation about
antisocial behavior will be more effective if the adolescent has a
good relationship with the adult who is involved. But good will is
not always enough.

Adults may know that condescension is unsatisfactory in
interviews; however, what influences the client is not necessarily
the intent of the interviewer but what is perceived and received
emotionally. Those young people with whom stressful situations
are being discussed are particularly sensitive to what they think
the interviewer thinks of them:

> A boy with a rich, powerful alcoholic father was sent to see a
> professor of psychiatry because the staff of his prep school was
> alarmed about his frequent outbursts of temper. Harry was
> fifteen and a late developer; there were as yet no signs of puberty.
> In his first interview he was seen by the professor in the presence
> of his staff and students. Harry replied to all questions in mono-
> syllables. The professor thought that the boy might be suffering
> from an acute personality disintegration, possibly schizophrenia,
> because of his withdrawal.
>
> In a subsequent interview with a psychiatrist who was not a
> professor Harry said that he thought the professor was much too
> important to talk to him about his troubles. Harry then spoke of
> his feeling of inferiority because he was small; other boys teased
> him and called him queer. It was more difficult for him at school
> because his father always collected him at vacation times in a big
> expensive car; other boys were critical about this. Unwittingly,
> the professor was repeating for Harry the painful experience that
> he had with his powerful, successful father.

In this case the boy misperceived the intention and feelings
of the professor, who cared about the welfare of young people.
In other situations attempts to help by those who do not like

adolescents—or the particular youngster concerned—are seldom effective.

Adolescents are sensitive to their treatment prior to an interview as well as to what happens within it. An offhand secretary can greatly disturb the young; rigid registration procedures in hospitals, in which individuals are kept interminably waiting, form letters, and lateness for appointments imply a lack of caring to which the youngster is likely to respond negatively. What the interviewer actually does is as important as what he or she says. Taking notes in order to remember what is said at the time may arouse a whole gamut of feelings in the other person, varying from worry as to what is being written to a feeling that it must be critical. Sometimes an adolescent may feel that the interviewer is more interested in the quality of the notes than in his own feelings and ideas. If notes must be taken, it is important to recognize how anxious this might make young people and to tell them why notes are important. Much the same sort of concern can be aroused when a report is read in front of an adolescent with no comment about its content or where it came from. Inevitably, the individual must wonder what is being read and why. If an interview bears a possibility of criticism or chastisement, the adolescent's anxiety can prevent the adult's comments from having any long-term effect or value.

For an adolescent being interviewed for the first time two issues need resolution: the perception and understanding of the situation held by the youngster, and the interviewer's frank statement as to his or her understanding. Adults who value words as significant communication tend to underestimate the importance of action (Sullivan, 1951). Adolescence is an action-oriented age; adolescents interpret—and sometimes misinterpret—the behavior of adults, and they themselves often communicate by their actions. Anxiety is most commonly shown by behavior: the way an adolescent sits, the obvious tension of fingers, agitated movements—all these may show that he is experiencing tension. If these signs of tension do not disappear during an interview, it means that the adolescent is not able to respond and become more comfortable. When the attempt to help the youngster feel at ease obviously does not succeed, it is reasonable to comment on this in a noncritical manner. Adolescents have conflicts about exhibitionism and can easily feel they are being observed; their automatic inclination may be to feel embarrassed and criticized when a comment is made about appearance, particularly because adults often pick on this. Adolescent hypersensitivity may turn a helpful comment into a persecutory one.

An adolescent who does not respond to an understanding remark about his apparent tension may often be helped by a more oblique technique: "Sometimes people are so often criticized about the way they look that they get hurt by anyone noticing it." This type of comment leaves the adolescent able to reject an idea if he wishes.

Personal Relationships, Control, and Punishment

All interviews should have a goal: Adults should have in mind what they want to learn or convey. In schools personal interviews between a staff member and a pupil may be concerned with the problem of controlling the latter's disturbed behavior. Some feel that the way to exercise control in such situations is to apply a conscience pressure, to be an external agent for the adolescent. They imply to the youngster that he is not really aware that what he has done is wrong and that the only way to show this is by punishment. It is arguable that punishment, as distinct from control, is ever justified. But even if it is, it becomes valueless as a regular or reflex response to behavior. Punishment is particularly futile if applied by an adult whom the adolescent considers worthless and who he knows does not love him. For late adolescents a necessity to punish represents a failure in development or inadequacy in the interpersonal relationships of the social system to which they belong.

It is naive to assume that the person who is put in a helping role will necessarily feel comfortable. Many teachers, for example, understand that there are complex motives behind the behavior and words of their pupils. Because such teachers are concerned about the adequacy of their own response, they prefer to react by avoiding the issue; they act as if there were no problem at all. All adults who have signicant emotional attachments with young people have to face problems of inadequacy and guilt. The person who wishes to feel important—or omnipotent—should not work with adolescents.

In their relationships with their children parents can always find situations in which they wish they had behaved better or been more understanding or less permissive. Similarly significant extraparental adults, with a formally assigned helping role or not, may be defensive about what they have done in the past. One way to handle this discomfort is to hide behind the concept of role: Certain actions were not performed, for example, by teachers as people but because they had to play the role of teacher. It is then assumed that the pupil, or society, will find the unacceptable act more tolerable.

Corporal punishment is a typical example. In those states that continue to tolerate corporal punishment in their educational institutions, some adults feel defensive about it; most feel uncomfortable about having to inflict pain, although they may find unconscious satisfaction in doing so. The conflict is eased by the conviction that beating is part of the role of a teacher or, in residential institutions, care worker, and has nothing personal about it. This is not how the young see it. The boy who gets beaten in a Boys' Town or some such organization is likely to be a less mature member of the society; he is quite unlikely to appreciate a distinction between what is done personally and what is done as part of a role. If such a boy does not value the adult who beats him as an individual, and does not feel that he is cared about, he will react either by an emotional withdrawal ("I don't care") or with fear, according to the severity of the beating. Another possible reaction is contempt. If the boy does feel valued and cared for he will probably react to the beating with a feeling of slavish dependence, particularly if it has been painful. Advocates of "spare the rod and spoil the child" rationalize that adolescents agree with them. A pupil treated with excessive harshness may react by identifying with what has been done, so adults who may be criticized by an outside authority for such punitive behavior can usually show that adolescents support them. Teachers who beat their pupils have the gratification of being told by them that the action was right.

No one authority adult can effectively dissociate himself from corporal punishment used in a social setting. Within any social organization staff appear to support each other: Adolescents feel that if staff work in an organization where beating occurs, they implicitly agree with this type of behavior. Thus there is a mutual responsibility when a beating takes place. Staff may attempt to deny this, but their denial will not be accepted by pupils.

Calling upon adolescent victims to support some particular aberration within a system is widespread:

> In a meeting of adults and adolescents to discuss a "disciplinary policy" for a local school system, a school administrator asked a fourteen-year-old girl if she thought peer group stability was necessary. Her reply was "Oh no, I think it's so nice to have to get a new set of people every semester." The administrator beamed at this confirmation of a statement previously used by him to justify a no-change policy.

Some adults feel that talking to children should be tried but they have no real expectation that it will be helpful. They will warn a boy about unacceptable behavior and then use violence to repress it. The following story was reported in the English magazine *Where* (Miller, 1969):

> George was eleven. Big for his age and very strong, he hadn't been in the school for more than a week before a little boy in his

grade was brought to the assistant principal with a bruised mouth. George had hit him, "because he hassled me."

The principal tried to talk to him in a humane, reasonable, and persuasive way, but the same kind of incident was repeated three times in the next month. He decided George should be handed over to the school social worker who had time to go into his background thoroughly and establish a good relationship with him.

The social worker reported fair progress: he thought he was getting somewhere. Alas, no, for the next victim was a girl. It was established that she called George "four-eyes" (he wore glasses) and he retaliated by striking her very hard on the breast. The assistant principal reported as follows: "I had a chat with George. I found him likeable and frank, but he had, so he said, a terrible temper. I decided that he needed to be taught a sharp lesson, but held my hand until the social worker had seen the parents." He went on to say that the father, a long-distance truck driver, had taught George to use his fists, "but only to look after himself." The mother said George did as he liked when her husband was away, that he was an easy boy to be with at home but was very rough with other boys. The social worker thought, as I did, that George was out of hand and needed checking now.

"I had George in and told him that the next time he hit anybody without being hit first I would beat the stuffing out of him. Within a fortnight George was brought to me for giving a smaller boy a black eye. I thrashed him and said that next time I would double the dose, I did.

"Since then, over a year ago now, there has been to our knowledge no more bullying."

The more violence an adolescent or adult has within himself, the more he will see violence as appropriate for the control of others. The violent adolescent who is beaten for his violence applies exactly this same technique to try and control other people, usually with less discretion and control than the violence that was applied to his person. Such an adolescent is likely to become an adult who approves of violent techniques of control.

Counseling Roles in Schools

Personal counseling roles have been given in some schools to social workers. If this is done, more than one social worker for two thousand or more children is needed. Furthermore, the isolation of this role from others is unrealistic; for most children personal help is most easily accepted from someone who has another role, one that is understandable in the social context in which the adolescents and adults work. Some adults may have administrative authority within the school, but this should not isolate them from offering personal help to the children. Ideally, any adult should be able to help any pupil who makes the approach. In practice, certain individuals not necessarily designated for a care role are the ones who are approached. Some feel quite inadequate to deal with the emotional problems that are brought to them. This difficulty in personally counseling adolescents, and the fact that most school staff have not been adequately trained for it, have led to the idea that the responsibility for the emotional care of school boys and girls should be given to specially created school counselors who would no longer have an educational role.

The specially trained school counselor should have sufficient skills to help adolescents in distress, and he should have a special role in relating to parents. But the presence of such school counselors may encourage other teaching staff to opt out even further from occupying a significantly personal role in the lives of the pupils. The concept shows a good deal of confusion. Middle-stage adolescents are most reluctant to confide in an adult whom they may perceive as an agent of their parents. In any case, all too often the adult consciously or not takes sides in a child–parent struggle. Furthermore, to ensure good relationships between adolescent and adult in schools all teachers need both counseling skills and a sensitivity about the effects of social environment on human behavior. Rather than having specially trained school counselors, it would seem better to change the quality of courses in schools of education and to offer all present-day teachers a chance to learn more of human relationships and of the difficulties that adolescents may experience.

If human relationships in a school are well developed, teachers may then be said to "teach" human relationships: first by setting an example in the living social environment of the school, and next by meaningfully imparting facts and attitudes verbally. But loving attitudes can only be imparted to adolescents in an atmosphere where human beings care for each other. Sex education demonstrates the issue. If pupils are not treated with consideration by teachers, they tend not to respect each other. It is reasonable if sexual behavior is discussed to indicate that intercourse should only take place as an act of love. This concept is not very meaningful if it is offered by someone who is felt as uncaring. Similarly, there can be no very perceptive discussion of the disadvantages of sterile autocracy, if the teacher leading it behaves like an autocrat.

Human Relationships and Service to Others

All communities have a need for service that can be met only by voluntary effort: the care of the aged, the crippled, and the helpless. All adolescents need to feel needed by the world in which they live. Service to the community should be in the school curriculum of all adolescents as soon as the turmoil of puberty is over. However, it is impossible for a school to direct its pupils towards community service, unless the pupils feel the school is helping them. Schools that appear not to care will not get their pupils to help others. When teachers are considered distant and uncaring, real cooperation from adolescents will not be forthcoming. They may appear to go along politely with the demands made upon them, but jobs are poorly performed; more aggressive youth merely refuse. Service to the community cannot be like a school football game in which the attendance of spectators is insisted upon by a roll call with punishment for absentees. Community service offers adolescents the chance to make contact with all ages and to feel valued, but they must first feel respected by the adults who lead them towards this service.

The discussion of human relationships between adult and adolescent in this chapter has primarily been applied to schools and their staff. The principles apply equally to pediatricians and their adolescent patients, youth clubs and youth workers, the staffs of penal institutions and psychiatric hospitals, and young people in the community who are helped by many types of social workers.

Problems of Training

Apart from understanding the psychosocial implications of human development, special training in understanding human relations and in counseling techniques—whether by regular training groups (Miller, 1967) and seminars, special vacation courses, or for the few, the sabbatical year—is a necessity for adults who have responsibility for the care of the young. In an ideal society this training would also be an integral part of the course for youth workers and teachers at college. The national shortage of trained people to help those who work directly with adolescents makes the planning of training difficult, and it is likely that the present shortage of such experts will last indefinitely. To deal with this problem a self-help technique, with only occasional technical input, in which people working with the young pool their experiences and learn from each other would seem to be a realistic solution.

If the breakdown of communication between the adult and the adolescent is to be repaired, care should be continuous from the individual adult and the environment. The essence of successful human relationships with the young is common sense and sensitivity. Though these cannot be *taught,* extra skills can be learned. The so-called gap between the generations need not exist if adults treat young people with consistency and understanding.

Psychotherapy

Attitudes toward psychotherapy are ambivalent: either it is thought to require no special skills or it is considered to be a highly esoteric art. Some of the principles and techniques of psychotherapy are highly relevant for those who would be of use to the adolescent in personal distress.

Because adolescence is midway between child- and adulthood a number of the techniques of relating to the world that belong to childhood remain during the period of adolescence, and this produces special treatment parameters. Specifically, action communication is highly significant. Verbal communication may still be much less indicative of how the youngster perceives his world, and this has implications in psychotherapy, both family, group, and individual, expressive or supportive. In adult psychotherapy verbal communication is most meaningful with middle-class adults, much less so with working-class groups. It is, however, even less meaningful for pubertal adolescents than for adults from all social classes.

Adolescents may have to be sent to see a psychiatrist by their parents; it is not necessary for early adolescents to wish consciously to come for help. Only very disturbed or very manipulative early adolescents are likely to express this wish. Parental pressure is still needed in midadolescence, but it is the responsibility of parents to have their child seen by a potential therapist, who, after the first interviews has to mobilize the adolescent's motivation so that a general willingness to attend without parental pressure becomes evident. In late adolescence parental pressure may be applied, but the motivation to attend, in situations other than acute personality disintegration, generally must be the patients.

Initial Approach to the Adolescent as a Psychiatric Patient

The attitude of an adolescent to any treatment process is bviously multidetermined. Apart from attitudes that may previously have been created by his environment, treatment begins at the moment of refcrral to a psychiatrist. Most adolescents up to the maturational age of fifteen or sixteen do not come willingly. An adolescent under this age who seeks psychiatric help is usually in very serious psychic difficulty. Most will have been sent to a therapist. They will not have said in words, "I want help," but will have arranged, usually by antisocial behavior, to get into a position in which help will be offered. Repetitious disturbed behavior in an adolescent usually represents a shout for assistance.

The adolescent's acting out a request for help puts a peculiar responsibility on the psychiatrist. Prior to the referral the adolescent has shown the ticket of admission for assistance to school teachers, parents, pediatricians or others. These authorities may then ask for a psychiatric consultation. An affirmative reply but a delayed initial appointment may imply that the psychiatrist does not really think the youngster or his behavior is important. Adolescents usually request help by creating a crisis; apart from the implications of a delayed response, a long wait may mean that the opportunity to assist is gone. Adolescents act out their request for assistance when the structural supports in their environment are failing; the relationship with their parents or their environment has become overstressful. At the crisis point a new personal environmental homeostasis has not yet been established, and this is the point of optimal intervention.

The success or failure of an attempt to help an adolescent may depend on the initial approach to the individual. Parents should not be called or written to and asked to bring the adolescent. That perhaps intolerable message implies that the adolescent is a dependent member of the nuclear family. The potential helping adult preferably should write, rather than telephone, offering the adolescent an appointment. A telephone call may be felt to be seductive or overcontrolling. The therapist should mention that he has been told of some of the difficulties leading to the request for a consultation; the adolescent is also protected from being told of the interview on the morning of the appointment.

Communication with an adolescent is most significant in a waiting room. In disturbed adolescents, in particular, conflicts about dependence pose as a threat to autonomy. The interviewer's actions in a waiting room may indicate to the adolescent how he is seen. Shaking hands with the parents first and then with the adolescent has a different meaning from greeting the adolescent first and then acknowledging the presence of the parents. Either way, a message is given to the adolescent about who in the family is seen as most significant.

Crisis Referrals

Acute crisis referral may occur when young people appear at a hospital emergency room, acutely confused from drugs or otherwise, or following a suicidal attempt. Communications from professionals are highly meaningful at such a time. If adolescents are talked down from a bad trip and then sent home, they may understand that assistance will be offered to help drugs be safely used. The message in the drug toxicity may not have been well recognized.

Suicidal attempts or gestures require special care. If adolescents are sent home after a suicidal attempt—once it has been established that there is no danger to life—and told to contact a psychiatrist the next day, the implication may be that neither the individual nor the action is taken too seriously. Admission to a hospital after a suicidal attempt is always indicated until it has been established that there is no further risk of self-destruction.

Even though it may be clear that this is not the case, the attempt needs to be felt to have been taken very seriously by authority adults. If adolescents are seen in an emergency room after such behavior the emergency room physician, or psychiatrist, should make a specific appointment for the patient on the next day. Preferably the same person will see the patient, although this may not be possible. Parents often need to deny that their children are suicidal so to leave it to them to make an appointment may be as unsatisfactory as leaving it to the adolescent.

The Role of Therapy in the Prevention of Disturbed Behavior

Adolescents have a perception of themselves as all powerful. When they relate to an adult whom they see as personally helpful, they project their own feeling of omnipotence and assume the potential therapist has this capacity. Adolescents in the initial stages of a therapeutic contact thus see the therapist as an extension of themselves, and this explains the importance of the contact an adolescent might have with a potential therapist or secretary or receptionist. If a psychiatrist has a secretary who is felt by young patients to be unpleasant, the psychiatrist is blamed for he is supposed to know about this behavior. To an extent adolescents who are taking adult steps to autonomy may be like the two-year-olds who are first trying to be independent. When they fall and hurt themselves, they may blame their mothers, who were supposed to know of such an eventuality. When an adolescent trusts an adult enough to allow him to be helpful, such a therapist is supposed to be prescient; he is felt as responsible for the behavior of all his staff. There is some truth in this assumption. Psychiatrists who do nothing when they hear of such episodes show disrespect to the patient.

A particular problem in the outpatient treatment of adolescents is that they will act out their tensions unless this process can be interrupted by therapeutic intervention. In early adolescents conflict and psychic pain are projected onto the environment; others rather than the adolescent experience the pain. In the first stages of therapy a major task is to help young people not act out their conflicts in such a way that chances of assistance will be destroyed. An adolescent who continues to hurt society will not have such behavior tolerated, and the initial wish to be helpful on the part of adults disappears, replaced by a punitive response. To allow therapy to take place, outpatient adolescents must begin to feel positive about their therapists. With prepubertal children therapists have more time, because the disturbed behavior of a child is usually contained within the family. A nine-year-old may tell his parents that he hates his therapist, but he is unlikely to rob the neighborhood store or become a drug toxic to demonstrate how futile are attempts to help. If adolescents do not begin to like and value adults who try to help them, they continue to act in self-destructive and aggressive ways. Thus, for adolescents to contain the self-destructive behavior that has brought them to treatment, therapists must be seen as omnipotent, interesting, and involved. Therapists are, however, not omnipotent, they are often devalued by society, they may not be sufficiently interesting, and the adolescent may demand an impossible level of involvement.

Some who work with adolescents seem to be successful with them while they are seeing the youngsters. As soon as such a therapist goes on vacation, however, or the apparently successful therapy ends, the adolescent is exactly where he was before, because the issue of omnipotence has never been resolved. The therapist, too gratified by the positive feelings of his patient, is willing to accept the omnipotent role; he never deals with the angry, anxious experiences that spilled over into the self-destructive behavior that had brought a boy or girl to treatment.

Communication Between Therapist and Adolescent

In all circumstances, crisis or not, action communications from therapists to adolescent patients must fit those in words.

Sitting behind a desk implies a wish to keep a distance; note taking may lead the patient to assume that the primary interest of the interviewer is in his data collection. The adolescent's initial intent is to try to assess the personality of the interviewer.

The usual formal method of taking a psychiatric history implicitly demands that the adolescent meet the needs of a psychiatrist, rather than the reverse. Collecting information from an adolescent about his life, asking him to perform simple psychological tests or to name the President may only show that the adolescent can be maneuvered into a situation of obedience and passivity, if it does not imply that he is merely an object to be studied. In order to understand the adolescent, knowledge of upbringing is important, but a formal history cannot be taken as with some adults. Formal history taking distorts the adolescent's communication technique with adults, and it is crucial to understand the adolescent's natural ways of interacting with others: The physical distance an adolescent puts between himself and the interviewer is as significant as evidences of anxiety that do not dissipate in the course of an interview. In an inital interview tension and anxiety are inevitable. Learned superficial techniques of verbal communication may produce apparent interaction, but unchanged tension is highly significant nonverbal communication. There are two levels of communication in an adolescent interview: What is said, and what is done. Useful understanding can be gained by consideration of what might be communicated if the adolescent could only be seen and not heard.

Because adolescents communicate partly by play—although the play is unlike that of children—it is technically difficult to handle such communication. The adolescent in therapy, or in a meaningful emotional relationship with an adult, may play out his difficulties in action, just as small children resolve maturational conflicts by direct play activity.

In Britain train watching is a common habit of early adolescent boys. They go to train stations and check the numbers and types of trains entering a main-line terminal. A discussion by a boy about a train coming in and out of a station may carry meanings similar to the play with trains of a smaller child in play therapy.

Adolescents may also play at being in therapy or may even play the role of being a young person in relationship to adults. Adolescents will talk of their play and, thus communicate. Formal play probably has little place in adolescent psychotherapy. Some therapists have the special ability to use "squiggles" (Winnicott, 1971); others play checkers with their young adolescent patients. However, the latter is probably of value only in these early adolescents who cannot yet significantly involve themselves in verbal communication because of their stage of puberty. This is the stage of development at which one silent boy said in psychotherapy: "It is not that I do not want to talk to you, nothing comes into my head and I cannot." Adolescents must try out roles—subidentities —as patients, young people, sick people, delinquents, hippies, freaks, even, on occasion, being straight. All these may be seen by the same psychotherapist with the same patient over a period of time. Adolescents may use themselves in a psychotherapeutic session as if they were the toy with whom they were actually playing.

An adolescent was being interviewed in a one-way vision room, and the session was being observed by a group of medical students. Although he knew about the student's presence and had agreed to be seen, the patient was uncomfortable, had many anxieties about what the students thought, wondered who they were, and felt that he had really little chance.

The boy, who was highly delinquent, arrived in the interviewing room before the therapist. When the latter arrived, the patient was standing by the mirror with a chair as if to break it. This threat was both a test of the therapist and a communication about the situation.

The boy had not been seen before; the therapist knew little about him. Nevertheless, a highly significant interaction from the start of the interview was inevitable. The therapist had to decide whether he would try to interpret to the boy what he thought the action might mean or whether he would try to therapeutically counteract. The therapist sat down calmly and seemed to be cool about the behavior. He said that he understood that the boy had strong feelings about the interview. He could always break the mirror if he wished, and the interviewer indicated that he would make no effort at physical restraint. The interviewer went on to say that the roots of his situation needed to be understood. He was implicitly telling the boy that he recognized his anxiety. In this way reassurance for the boy was counteracted; the comfort of the therapist acted as a control for the patient.

Motivation and Relationships with Parents, Therapists, and Other Adults

Conscious motivation is usually present only in those early adolescents suffering from severe psychic pain, very depressed, or psychologically disintegrating individuals. It is not, however, unusual for family psychopathology to show itself under the guise of adolescent maladjustment. The adolescent is the family's way of obtaining help, although in these situations the motivation is not usually that of the young person.

The pubertal adolescent is narcissistically involved with the self, and feelings and conflicts are inevitably projected into the adult world. Hence, the youngster feels the problems are not really his, they are the world's or his family's. There are always special difficulties in the therapy of early adolescents who experience a psychic dissolution. Many such adolescents are particularly preoccupied with the need to gain control over themselves because of the physiological changes of puberty. They have hardly any capacity for self-observation, and it is hard for them to join in a therapeutic alliance with a therapist. They are more likely to see the therapist as a valuable adult with whom they might identify. Furthermore, any anxiety that may be produced by referral for psychiatric help is a further threat to a tenuously developing ego. The implied dependence and incompetence are threats to adolescent self-esteem.

The important technical problem in initial interviews is to note the marginal, often nonverbal, communications of the adolescent that convey that magic is wanted. The recognition of this unstated wish is, of course, therapeutic omniscience. If a therapist does not make clear that he knows that the adolescent wants a magic solution, and that this is unattainable, the adolescent feels cheated. Either he does not return, or he plays a pseudo-therapeutic game to appease these authority figures who sent him for help in the first place. In initial interviews one must be sufficiently omnipotent that acting-out behavior will be suspended and the adolescent will return voluntarily; at the same time, however, the knowledge must be conveyed that the therapist cannot be omnipotent. If adults temporarily feel that their therapist is disappointing and useless conscious motivation may be relied on to keep them coming for therapy. With children, parental motivation has a similar effect. However, for many adolescents who see psychiatrists communication with parents has broken down. The reason for referral may be loss of parental control; parental wishes are not carried out because they are too threatening or are no longer valued. The therapist must then keep a sufficiently positive transference so that the adolescents will continue to attend, while at the same time trying to help them cope with their angry feelings about themselves and their world. Parents may still be needed to prevent an abrupt withdrawal from therapy, particularly when the patient feels disenchanted with the therapist and the value of therapy. Since insight is valueless unless it is felt to be true, patients will not understand their anger unless they feel it with the therapist. At the same time, they must care enough about the therapist to continue. This need to sustain ambivalence is one reason for the storminess of adolescent psychotherapy. Parents, moreover, are often highly mixed in their attitudes to therapy. A sick adolescent is also a dependent child and may be gratifying for parents. Often parents cease to pay their child's treatment bills on time as improvement begins to take place.

Success in treatment is related to an accurate diagnostic appraisal of where the weight of therapy should be placed and to the setting of realistic goals. Group therapy, individual or family work, or environmental changes all require an assessment of a predicted outcome in any individual.

Aims of Therapy

Changing the personality structure of an adolescent is generally not a realistic therapeutic goal. An appropriate direction is to aid the normal growth process, to assist adolescents to gain autonomy from the dependent infantile ties to the nuclear family, and to help them make final firm identifications as men or women. The therapist should aim to assist young people obtain that inner freedom from conflict that will allow them to live fuller lives in today's disturbed world. Help for parents is usually pointed at assisting them in the resolution of their personal conflicts and not using their child as part of a family conflict. Since there is, in a sense, a conflict of interest between parent and child, family therapy has little place as the only treatment for adolescent maladjustment.

Adolescent conflicts may so weaken ego functions that an impaired capacity to use human relationships is produced. Instead of receiving a positive feeling of love, affection, and value from their world, even when it is offered, disturbed adolescents feel highly persecuted by their environment and the people in it. The people to whom they relate are felt as unloving. The parents of conflict-ridden adolescents are well aware of this; other adults sometimes accept adolescent alienation as age appropriate. Although disturbed adolescents may allege that they are only understood by their own generation, this often is more of a wish than a fact. Many do not feel understood by anyone. They cling to their peers as a drowning man to a lifeline, but they may feel as persecuted by their agemates as by adults. Adolescents may say they want no contact with adults; they really wonder whether adults are prepared to care for them. Perhaps the most that all but highly intensive therapy does, is reduce the amount of persecution that the adolescent feels from his world. Angry feelings have to be worked through and understood in the therapeutic relationship; catharsis is not enough. In the course of therapy the patient becomes aware that his angry feelings do not necessarily destroy good relationships. The negative feelings that become focused in the therapeutic situation may contribute to the adolescent's not wishing to attend therapy. Moreover, people in the adolescent's world, particularly parents, may be feeling that the adolescent is doing extremely well and they are less likely to support the idea of continuing therapy. For this reason many young people leave therapy permanently, but the feeling that all is going well, and that only the therapeutic situation is tormenting is not an indication for termination. On the other hand, if the therapist is seen as the only benign figure, therapy is rarely going satisfactorily.

Successful adolescent psychotherapy requires, apart from a therapist, the availability of other people to whom the adolescent can relate. If these are not present and if the patient does work through some of his angry feelings, the only available positive relationship is with a therapist. Adolescents then have no way of freeing themselves from dependence on therapy.

Need for Social Networks

Adolescents recommended for psychotherapy need people in their world, in the past, present, and potential future, who care about them. Social isolation may be a contraindication to outpatient therapy. An adolescent with a history of very tenuous or very negative relationships with parents or others is in a difficult psychotherapeutic position. When such an adolescent has just moved to a community, a typical junior high school, for example, it may be almost impossible for many months to make relationships with peers or teachers. Such distressed adolescents may not progress in psychotherapy because they cannot find people in their world to whom they can relate. Teachers are too distant, and a potential peer group is overinvolved with itself.

Again, therapy for the adolescent requires a diagnostic assessment of the stresses and supports in the adolescent's world. The potential for growth of church groups, youth organizations, and so on, may have to be considered, if a school system cannot provide adequate human relationships. Sometimes, if these are absent, psychiatric day care may be necessary. Placing a disturbed adolescent in a meaningful social network does not in itself lead to emotional growth and conflict resolution. Without such relationships, the chances of successful psychotherapy are slim.

Need for Relief of Symptoms

An important aspect of therapeutic work with adolescents is to enable them to make firm positive identifications. Because symptoms may produce persecutory responses from the environment—for example, underachievement arouses rejection and anger; drug taking arouses intense concern over external controls; bedwetting leads to hostility from those concerned with the adolescent's cleanliness, even if some vicarious satisfaction is gained from the activity—symptomatic relief is a necessary prerequisite to further emotional growth. Without it, it is unlikely that an environment that has been made hostile by disturbed behavior can become supportive.

Some therapists used to believe that relief of one symptom without resolution of the underlying conflict would automatically lead to the production of another symptom. This is only rarely true. That theory presupposes that environmental support and the perception of love have little effect in the development of a healthier personality. Symptom relief is justified in those patients who have a capacity to make positive attachments to people in their environment; more emotional growth can then be expected than might otherwise occur. The technique by which the symptom relief is a particular issue especially insofar as medication is concerned.

Medication in Adolescent Treatment

In adolescent treatment medication should be used sparingly. Antidepressants, perhaps because of their chemical relationship to growth hormones, seem only to have a placebo effect in adolescents. Early adolescent schizophrenics do much less well with the tranquilizers than those whose growth phase of development is over, or then adults. Apart from these biochemical reasons tranquilizers also cause psychological stress. Most ataractics affect muscular tone, and physical activity is an extremely important way of relieving emotional tension in adolescence.

Giving medication also teaches adolescents that this is an appropriate way of handling anxiety and further presupposes that therapists are able to be magicians. Except in specific organic diseases sedatives are particularly contraindicated in adolescents; they do not help general states of tension, and adolescent sleeplessness can usually be resolved by a combination of psychotherapy and environmental management. Therapy implies that it is difficult to work out emotional problems; a pill contraindicates this concept and reinforces the common message of society-at-large that escape through drugs is acceptable.

A major treatment problem today is the illicit use of drugs. As part of a test of a therapist's value, adolescents may arrive at a therapy session stoned. They may want the therapist to be aware that they are toxic (that is aware of them as individuals), or they may want something to be done about their behavior. The hostility of drug taking to the therapeutic process needs to be recognized. Depending on the substance, drug-toxic adolescents suffer from greater or lesser depersonalization; in this psychological state they are not able to have a satisfactory observing ego. Although the capacity to reinvolve oneself with a reality situation under external pressure is greater with marijuana than with alcohol, the effects of drug toxicity cannot be interpreted away. Whatever else may be done in such a therapeutic session, counteraction is forced on a therapist; some types of psychotherapy may then cease to be possible.

Termination of Treatment

The termination of therapy with adolescents poses many problems. Often an adolescent will express the idea that he wishes to try himself out in life without continuing therapy. This attempt at autonomy should generally be respected, although it is a temptation to persuade an adolescent to stay in therapy, particularly if psychopathology is still evident. The real question the adolescent is raising is whether the therapist sees him as capable of autonomy. It is probably better to risk the adolescent's having to return for more therapy—though he may be angry because he was allowed to go too soon—than to crush an attempt at independent growth. It is important that this concept be understood, if only intellectually, by an adolescent's parents.

Although in the psychotherapy of the middle and late adolescent a therapist may have little direct contact with parents, he should see them at the end of the assessment phase of work with the adolescent before therapy formally begins. He should ensure that parents have someone with whom to communicate their anxieties, if this role is contraindicated for the therapist. At the termination of therapy, the offer should be made to see parents again, although they rarely accept this.

References

Bettelheim, B. (1950), *Love Is Not Enough*. Glencoe, Ill.: Free Press.

Freud, S. (1920), Beyond the pleasure principle. In *Standard Edition*, 18: 7–66. London: Hogarth Press, 1955.

Gill, M., Newman, R., Redlich, F. C. (1954), *The Initial Interview in Psychiatric Practice*. New York: International Universities Press.

Jones, H. E. (1969), Adolescence in our society. In *The Family in a Democratic Society*, Comp. Community Services Society of New York, 70–82. New York: Columbia University Press.

Miller, D. (1967), Staff training in the penal system. In *The Use of Small Groups in Training*, ed. R. Gosling, D. Miller, P. M. Turquet, and D. Woodhouse, 98–112. Herts, Eng.: Caldicote Press.

—————— (1969), Aggression in adolescents. *Where*, January 4.

Sullivan, H. S. (1951), The psychiatric interview. *Psychiatry*, 14: 361–373.

Winnicott, D. W. (1971), *Therapeutic Consultations in Child Psychiatry*. New York: Basic Books.

16

The Treatment of Disturbances Produced by Death and Divorce

Some adolescent maladjustments occur principally because of a disturbance of the balance of stress and support that exists in the immediate environment of the individual, commonly death or separation of a parent. It is difficult to know which is the more painful: death, final and irrevocable, or separation, perceived as bewildering and teasing (Robertson and Bowlby, 1952). It is probably impossible for any child to deal adequately with either experience unless he is helped by adults other than his surviving parent. As the family networks of Western civilization are broken up, this throws a particular responsibility on pediatricians, family practitioners and a whole variety of youth workers.

Problems of Mourning

It is necessary to mourn to get over the death of a loved one. The traditional mourning is subtle and complex: the dead person is buried in the ground beneath a headstone (which perhaps reassured our ancestors that he would not return to haunt them); he is talked about, wept over, laughed about; his faults are reviewed and his abilities are discussed (Draper, 1965, p. 126).

He is even blamed: "How could he possibly leave me?" The grave is visited quite frequently. Often, after the burial, a party is held to celebrate his departure. These processes allow the adult to play out feelings of guilt, anger, grief, despair, and loss; paradoxically, they may also show relief that the death has occurred at last.

All the mixed feelings in the adult who loses a loved one are present in the adolescent who loses a parent. The mourning processes of adulthood, however, are not so easily available to the young. At one time the very obvious rituals of adult mourning allowed the young to experience these at second hand. Not being mature enough to deal with death themselves, they could experience grief reactions in a way with which they could cope, through adults. Today these formalized gestures of adult society are going; it is no longer commonplace in the Western world for people to mourn in a way that meets their psychological needs. The ritual of the funeral home with the synthetic-looking corpse and the family isolated with their grief is no substitute for the adequate mourning experience of some more primitive societies. Particularly in American culture, where the outward expression of sorrow is not particularly acceptable, the loss of a loved one causes an additional stress even for adults, because they are no longer allowed satisfactory social outlets for grief. Mourning rites are as old as man: it can only harm people when they are abandoned. The lack of these rites hinders adults from helping the bereaved adolescent by their example, because *they* no longer show how to cope with death. Some adults isolated with their grief have been known to die prematurely. Adolescents in this plight may lose their zest for life and are likely to become cold, unloving people whose capacity for loving and caring is prematurely withered.

Death in the Hospital

Because most hospitals forbid children under the age of twelve to visit adults, the death of a parent in the hospital means not only that the dying parent may be denied the opportunity to make peace with children but that children feel that their parents abruptly and mysteriously left them. Children cannot be shown by parents that they are not responsible for their death; they cannot apologize for leaving. The behavior of hospitals, intended to be helpful, ends by being emotionally painful to all.

Before the age of puberty children do not really understand that death means a permanent separation, and even after puberty this is probably not really appreciated. The current fashion of not allowing children to go to funerals increases this difficulty. Death is not emotionally comprehensible, even to adults, until they become emotionally aware that they will die themselves. It is possible that this awareness only reaches many adults in the early thirties. Up to then the healthy know they will die but they do not really feel it to be possible. It is therefore hardly surprising that children and adolescents have difficulty with death.

Effects of Parental Loss

A child or adolescent may cope with loss by an immediate denial (Bonnard, 1962, p. 160) of feeling. If, as is likely, the survivors in the family fail to recognize that this is happening and believe that the death has been taken well, the young have an even greater need for outside help, a need of which they are often not consciously aware.

> The mother of a daughter, age ten, whose husband had just died, was unsure whether she should let the child go to the funeral. She therefore asked her daughter what she wanted to do. "Go to the funeral and then to the movies" was the reply. With relief she accepted the child's partial denial of feeling as a solution: The child's grief was apparently slight. It did not occur to the mother that more than this would be necessary to help the child over the loss.

If children cannot be helped to mourn the effect of parental death or separation they are left as they grow up with an unresolved traumatic experience within their personalities. The damage this causes depends to some extent on the age at which it occurs and whether it is the mother or the father who is lost.

Children who have never known their mothers because they were abandoned through death or desertion are likely to suffer gross damage to their capacities to be loving human beings, unless they obtain a permanent mother substitute. An infant must have mothering or it cannot survive at all (Greenacre, 1952). Sometimes the child who has no real mother is looked after by a series of women: This multiple handling can cause severe personality damage. Sometimes a consistent mother substitute is available for the first months or years of such a child's life, and then there is a change. Such children suffer like those whose real mother has just died. It becomes difficult to provide them with an adequate mother substitute because they may initially rebuff adult attempts to help them. They cannot trust the new adult not to go away, and they project their anger against the lost parent onto the new parent substitute. Often these children become adults who appear unable to make close and warm relationships with others; they may be helped to make a good adaptation, rarely are they able to be truly loving.

Children who have never known their fathers and who are brought up by women alone with no father substitutes are also likely to have severely damaged personalities (Deutsch, 1944). How great the damage is depends on other factors in the environment; the degree of physical and emotional deprivation, the presence of possible father substitutes, and the inborn sensitivity of the child. Without an available father figure, such children have no inner image of fatherhood; when boys become fathers themselves, they do not know how to behave in this role.

This particular problem is demonstrated by the generation who as children hardly saw their fathers until they were five or six—if at all—because of World War II. As men today, they find it very difficult to provide their sons with a model of fatherhood. The girls suffered quite differently: They have a strong image of mothering but no experience of fathers as consistent, loving, and supporting figures. Thus, as mothers themselves, they have no expectation as to how their husbands should behave. Such women relate to their husbands as their mothers' did to them, often in a controlling, mothering fashion, rather than as a mistress, lover, and wife. Similarly, in the present decade, the underprivileged matriarchal societies that may exist among some poverty stricken groups, present a continuing problem. If the young men are not helped to be adequate fathers, they abandon their new family when they feel their children are competitors for their mate's affection, usually when the infant is about three months old (Miller, 1965). So the process is repeated, and a succession of children from disturbed, one-parent families is created.

Age and the Loss of a Parent

Children who have lost a parent before the age of five or six pose special problems for adults who wish to help them when they reach adolescence. A lack of satisfactory mothering is likely to create someone with a damaged, isolated personality who finds it difficult to make a meaningful emotional relationship with adults (Miller, 1965). Those children who lack satisfactory fathering have difficulty in making relationships with adults, but they have suffered less: If such a consistent relationship is available to them they can use it after much preliminary testing.

Parental loss when a child has had the solid emotional experience of a loving parent through the first five or six years of life has a different effect. The child has an image of an apparently loving parent who has chosen to go away. This feeling that the action was deliberate is inevitable, because a child cannot conceive that his parents can be helpless, and the fact of death cannot yet be understood. The parent is felt to have been a deserter, and the only explanation possible is that this has been done because the child is bad. An older child may also feel that the parent is bad to have left, but the conscious concept of parents as other than good is difficult for those who are younger.

Effects of Divorce and Separation

The same feeling is aroused by divorce and the withdrawal of one parent, usually the father, from the scene. That the parent is still alive makes the situation less irrevocable; however, the child cannot later alter the feeling of having been deliberately abandoned because the parent did choose to go.

A parent of the opposite sex leaving home is felt in a sense as a sexual rejection. Often the children of such a separation yearn after the departed parent until a remarriage takes place. The behavior of the child may then have the flavor of "hell hath no fury." The same may occur when a widowed parent remarries:

> Jane, age eleven, reacted to her mother's death by looking after her two younger brothers, keeping house for her father, and being a model child at school. Her father remarried when she was thirteen. The same week she ran away from home with a seventeen-year-old boy whom she had just met. Two years later she was seen in a juvenile detention home with a long history of promiscuity and absconding. No one had discussed with her the feelings of loss she felt for her mother or her anger at her father for then deserting her for another woman.

Those adolescents who lose their parents by divorce or separation are in some ways in a more difficult position than those who lose a parent through death. Healthy emotional growth requires that children feel loved by their parents. Divorce or separation may imply that the child is secondary in their life; children must come to terms with such a notion. Young people find it difficult to express to other adults their feelings about this, sometimes because they are trapped by a feeling of family loyalty and do not wish to take sides against one or the other parent, always because there are few built-in social supports for the children of divorced parents. Occasionally adolescents will simplify the issues and make one parent bad and the other good, treating the parents' separation with a facade of extreme cynicism. Inside themselves they are often as grief-stricken, bereft, angry, and despairing as the adolescent who has lost a parent through death. In trying to help such young people, it is important that therapists do not allow themselves to be maneuvered into taking the side of one parent or the other. It is, however, farcical and alienating to tell an adolescent who does complain about his father or mother that he "really loves" his parents; he won't feel it to be true and will consider the adult to be talking nonsense. The adolescent does not want agreement that the parent is bad; he'll want recognition of the fact that he feels this. Divorce arouses intense mixed feelings if one parent deserts the other. If a father leaves home for example, adolescent children particularly feel that their mother should have been able to stop father from going off with another woman. She is blamed as a failure. If, however, the mother successfully dates men, her sexuality becomes even more anxiety provoking. Adolescent daughters may become anxious when they get boy friends, in case they should be as much a failure as they felt mother to have been. This may be sexually acted out. Boys partly identify with what they feel as the sexually predatory behavior of their father; they also get gratification from protecting their mothers. Yet they also have a profound contempt for women who cannot keep their men. Boys and girls may both identify with a parent whom they see as a sexual failure.

John's father had left his mother when he was twelve. She told

him about the new wife with scorn and loathing, and John refused
to have any communication with his father. Consciously, he had
no feelings at that time of anger or contempt for his mother.

John worked extremely hard at school, was a straight "A"
student, and at the age of eighteen was admitted to a prestigious
university. He had never had a girlfriend. Shortly after entering
as a freshman, John met a girl and after about three months had
intercourse with her. He knew she was seeing another boy all
the time but preferred to think this was of no significance. Four
weeks after they had intercourse, John was told by the girl that
she might be pregnant. This was confirmed, and two weeks later
John paid $250 toward her abortion. The obstetrician told John
that his girl was ten weeks pregnant, but the youth felt that must
be a mistake. John came to see a psychiatrist after the girl left
him for the original boy because of acute feelings of failure, and
the unshakable idea that if he had been more sexually able his
girl might have stayed with him.

Identifying with his mother, John put himself at the losing end
of a triangular sexual situation.

Effect of Parental Death

From the age of five to the end of early adolescence, the
feeling that is aroused by the death of parent is the same; the
intensity of the experience is more easily handled as the individual's capacity to understand reality matures. For the adolescent who has lost a parent through death, father or mother may
have been buried in reality but cannot be buried by the self
without outside help. The image of the dead parent stays alive
inside the child and adolescent. Feelings about this are likely to
torment the individual, either consciously or unconsciously,
through adult life, if they are not resolved. Many years after the
death of a parent, when mourning processes ought to be finished,

the adolescent may still weep about a dead father or mother, or feel a pervasive sadness when the loss is recalled.

It is difficult for an adolscent boy to accept control from his mother; the absence of a father in the house makes it hard for the boy to obtain a satisfactory feeling of self. A girl brought up without a father finds it equally hard to value herself as a woman. One way of dealing with the loss is to identify with the dead parent. A dramatic change in older adolescents may occur following parental death: A boy or girl may suddenly seem to everyone to have become exactly like the dead father.

> Judy was a fifteen-year-old girl who was placed in a juvenile detention home because she repeatedly ran away from home, became extremely drug toxic, and was then picked up ill in cafes, side streets, or in the summer on the sidewalk. The behavior had been going on for two years.
>
> In an interview, Judy told a psychiatrist that she hated her mother, but she said, with tears in her eyes, that she had loved her father who had died when she was twelve. She was asked what he was like. "He was a chronic alcoholic, he did not get on with mother. They would have a row and he would leave home and we would not see him for two or three days. Then someone would bring him home; he had passed out. He would dry out for a day or two then they would be at it again."

Apart from these internal difficulties, the fatherless child or adolescent has particular social problems. The friend with two parents is envied, and often the individual who has lost a parent when a child has the unconscious conviction that the world now owes him a living—having experienced such a loss, he feels entitled to things. Similarly, many children who feel starved for affection frequently steal from the person who they feel is depriving them (Bonnard, 1962, pp. 162–163). The adolescent who has lost either parent commonly responds with an expectation that society will provide. When he grows up, he is often unreliable, particularly in handling money and at work.

One-Parent Adolescent in School

The adolescents who are most likely to suffer in the school system are those from one-parent families. Fatherless boys and girls, particularly, need a male teacher who is prepared to be interested and involved with them over the years. Such a teacher can enable such children to live rather than to exist, if he can tolerate their inevitable preliminary testing of his personality. It is easier for an adolescent to accept substitute fathering than substitute mothering, because mothers are expected to involve themselves in their child's life more intimately than fathers. Substitute mothering is, therefore, that much more difficult.

Unfortunately, the school does not automatically respond to a child's loss of a father by ensuring that male figures are available. Even if they did, the loss would be rapidly reexperienced because adult–pupil relationships rarely last more than a year. This means that significant males for such a child may have to be sought outside the school. This need is met more often for boys than girls. The girl who loses a father may be forced into early heterosexual relationships as the only way of finding a significant male figure. Often such girls seek contacts with older men in this way; when they are abandoned, they feel the bereavement again. Often they themselves precipitate this behavior but it is still a teasing and tormenting experience. An adult who wishes to help fatherless children should be aware that they may feel teased by gestures that seem appropriate. An invitation home to dinner or an offer of a visit to the lake may be felt as an invitation to be a child of the family.

Feelings Associated with Loss

Of all the feelings that are aroused by loss the one most socially acceptable is grief. Children are allowed to cry; adoles-

cents are also allowed to show their misery to an extent, even
though in many cultures boys are thought to be unmasculine if
they weep (Jersild, 1963, pp. 193–194). But other emotional
experiences surrounding death make it difficult to handle inside
the self.

The idea that the dead parent has deliberately chosen to
go away leads children and adolescents to feel angry, both with
the dead parent and with the surviving parent for letting the
event happen. Adolescents also tend to make all experiences
their own, perhaps because the most unacceptable experience
for them is helplessness. To avoid this helpless feeling adolescents
—even though they may also appear to disclaim responsibility
for relatively trivial difficulties—will accept responsibility within themselves for the profoundly disturbing incidents that
befall them. The young person feels that he has sent the
dead parent away. His guilt may be increased by the realization
that competition for the affection of the surviving parent is
over.

The effects of anger, personal responsibility, and grief exist
irrespective of ethnic groups or social class. A vocational guidance counselor working in a Scandinavian youth employment
office was concerned about a boy who had difficulties at work
since leaving school at sixteen:

> Gary's father had died when he was nine; his mother had married
> for a second time when he was twelve. When he was fourteen,
> one of his half-sisters had drowned. According to school reports
> he had been very good in subjects such as arithmetic, physics, and
> chemistry, but he had no interest in social studies and had found
> religious instruction particularly irksome. He was very intelligent
> but restless.
>
> At the youth employment office Gary had been given a large
> battery of psychological tests. These showed that he was capable
> of leadership but incapable of making friends. His level of
> achievement was high; he was thought to be fluent and imag-
> inative. It was deduced that he was unstable and sensitive and

suffered from a good deal of anxiety. He was said to be restless, unsettled, and lonely, and to have a need for reassurance.

Gary had only five interviews with the counselor over eighteen months, although he visited the employment bureau looking for jobs at least twenty times. At first he had wanted a job in a distant town with an uncle, and there had been some attempt to send him to the training school of a paper mill. The principal, after interviewing Gary, felt that he was unable to accept him. He then worked for six different employers, staying in one job for one and a half months at the most. Whenever he had a job in which promotion prospects were likely to be excellent he quarrelled with the foreman and was fired. The counselor felt that there was no chance of this boy ever working successfully because of his quarrels with authority. Gary's story was bewildering; he appeared to have been given every chance and it was suggested that he was really a psychopath and nothing could be done. Routine efforts at systematic help having failed, the response was to apply a label.

The story could be understood in the following way. The school had not understood the reason for his restlessness and while he was there, no one had helped him with the underlying conflicts that helped create it. Nevertheless, the structure of the school had offered him a good deal of emotional support. When this was withdrawn the painful experiences of his early life, the death of a father and a sister, were recalled. The unresolved feelings of anxiety and guilt led to self-destructive behavior. Feeling himself to be dangerous in relationships with others, Gary constantly put himself in a situation in which he could not be close to people, because those he loved might die. In addition, he was so angry with authority figures, because his father had "left" him, that he had constantly to quarrel with them; hence, the difficulty with his foreman.

The youth employment officer was unaware that there could be any cause of Gary's behavior other than work shyness; he had tried to help by seeking changes and by criticizing Gary whenever he lost a job. The officer had not been able to consider changes that might have met Gary's particular needs, for example, a job in which the foreman would not be disturbed by his rudeness. It could have been explained to a potential employer that Gary needed to keep himself somewhat isolated from supervisors; the employment officer might have insisted that Gary show he could keep just one job before making further attempts to find him a position to suit his talents. This would have given him some opportunity to expiate his feelings of guilt by doing menial tasks. If his school had been helpful to him when his father and sister died, by giving him the opportunity to talk about his feelings to a sympathetic adult with some sensitivity to the effects of loss, he might not have been left as a late adolescent with an intolerable self-destructive burden of guilt.

Whenever people suffer anguish, they need to share the experience. It may appear that adolescents do not want to do this; they say, leave me alone, because sharing may seem like a return to childlike dependence. Although the adult may accept this stated desire for isolation, the need to share remains. Sooner or later the bereaved child or adolescent has to be able to express in actions or words his feelings about his loss. The child facing the emotional confusion aroused by parental death may not feel anything: the experience of loss may have to be denied because it is too overwhelming. The adolescent, possibly more aware of his feelings, may not be able to share them because he is afraid that he might break down and weep or in some other way show that he feels desperately unsure of himself.

An adolescent who is aware of the grief of the parent who survives will wish to be helpful, not hurtful. It may, for instance, be impossible for him to show his angry feelings. If the adolescent were to allow his mixed feelings about a dead parent to become conscious, these would probably be considered as bewildering, idiosyncratic, or mad. Furthermore, the adolescent may also blame the surviving parent. He may angrily feel that a caring mother could not possibly let her husband die.

In pushing aside confused feelings about the loss of a parent, the adolescent is likely to find it increasingly difficult to become emotionally involved with others. Alternatively, the adolescent may act out on the stage of the real world, the conflicts and anxiety that have been experienced. It is not unusual for adolescents who experience parental loss to become aggressive and disturbed at school. Because the causes of this disturbance may not be understood, the adolescent is not helped with the feelings of responsibility, guilt, and anger that lie behind his antisocial behavior. Misunderstood by his school, the adolescent's disturbance spreads into the community. This is a common cause of delinquency in adolescents.

Assisting a Child To Mourn

The adolescent who experiences the death of a parent can only mourn if helped by his environment. To assist this process is crucial for mental health. Sometimes no specific effort need be made, sometimes children seem able to use their environment unconsciously in a helpful way. Then trouble occurs only when their self-help is interrupted:

> Richard was eleven when his father died. The boy lived in a port; his father was a fisherman. Richard reacted to the death by going down to the docks every day after school and watching the ships go out. Because of the change in the family's finances, it was necessary for them to move to a town away from the sea. This, of course, interrupted the mourning ritual that Richard had established for himself. Inland he soon became delinquent.
>
> It is possible that as a newcomer to the district he found it easier to join boys, aggressive and disturbed themselves, who were all too willing to have a new recruit. But his delinquency was certainly associated with inability to deal with the feelings he found rising inside himself when his mourning was interrupted.
>
> The boy went through society's typical responses to delin-

quency—from juvenile court to probation officer. He landed at a
school for delinquent boys but ran away after quarrelling with
one of the staff. In another such institution he continued to behave
in an extremely disturbed and aggressive way. The principal asked
for a psychiatric opinion. During the interview when his father
was mentioned, Richard's eyes filled with tears. (This was some
three and a half years after the death of his father.) He was
thought to be suffering from an unresolved mourning experience.
Those staff members in the school who spent time with Richard
and knew him were asked to give him every opportunity to talk
about his father, if he voluntarily brought the subject up. If he
did not do this, they could appropriately raise the subject themselves—asking him what his father was like and what he might
have done in a given set of circumstances. With the combination
of genuine interest and the opportunity to talk about his father
with people who obviously cared about him, Richard became
less disturbed and a productive member of the school. He left
the school after six months. Two years later he remained a settled
member of society.

Richard was helped a number of years after his father died,
but often adults have to aid a young person who is suffering from
an immediate loss. The common assumption that children or
adolescents should try to forget and live life as father or mother
would have wanted is wrong. If a child has mixed feelings of
responsibility and anger, the suggestion that he live as the parent
might have wanted is likely to arouse stubborn resistance. To
talk about the dead parent helps the adolescent face the fact of
the death and share the experience of grief. It is not enough for
a helping adult to expect the adolescent to volunteer statements
about the dead parent. "What was your father like?" "What
might he have done in this situation?" are appropriate questions
to be raised. The mention of the dead parent will be painful, but
it is by sharing pain that the adolescent can grow out of the
traumatic experience.

Mourning adolescents constantly appear to be seeking

adults who will replace the lost parent; although they may experience the caring adults as not offering enough, they often apparently wish to repeat the experience of loss in their day-to-day life (Freud, 1933, p. 81). When bereaved youngsters become emotionally involved with an adult they seem to provoke a situation where they might lose him or her, as if, in order to convince themselves that they have control over the situation of loss, they try to provoke a helping adult into rejecting them—producing a loss they themselves have made. This is an attempt to separate the sense of being helpless from the experience of being deserted. Adolescents feel it is better to feel responsible for what happens in their world. The adult who is trying to help an adolescent disturbed by parental loss should have no expectation of gratitude. The young person in mourning is angry; some of the anger must be directed toward an adult with whom the adolescent has become involved. If adolescents, immediately after the loss of a parent, are given the opportunity both to talk about and to some extent play out their sense of despair, much subsequent suffering can be avoided. The adult who wishes to help the bereaved adolescent should be aware of the sense of confusion aroused by the death as well as his or her own feelings about death or separation. It is easy to overidentify with bereaved adolescents and, in helping them through their difficulties, to expect too little of them. The adult must use his intuitive understanding of how much to expect, too little may be as useless as the "snap out of it" attitude that expects too much.

Some common societal responses to death are misleading oversimplifications. When boys respond to the death of their father with aggressive, outwardly directed behavior, the tendency, particularly by juvenile courts and social agencies, is to point to loss of parental control. Sometimes the significance of parental loss is ignored; the decision of the helping authority to attempt to reimpose controls then represents only a partial solution. Often such young people, after a series of delinquent acts where symptomatic behavior is not understood, are separated from their known environments. Their experience of loss is then repeated, and they are sent to institutions where they will be controlled until they grow out of their difficult period. This tends to produce isolated, withdrawn human beings. At best such adolescents may make a social adjustment that is primarily an adaptation to life; but if they are not also helped with their confused feelings, they do not really live. At worst they swell the ranks of the criminal population. (It is perhaps inevitable that society should overvalue the controlling function of parents because this is the one that seems most easy to replace.)

Finally, a delinquent act that is a symptom of bereavement may also be gratifying; then, this type of behavior is reinforced. Similarly, when marijuana is smoked to relieve psychic pain, it can still give a pleasurable high.

Some adolescents respond to loss by withdrawal into themselves. They tend to be in a much more serious plight than those who respond aggressively (Menninger, 1963, pp. 200–261). The withdrawn adolescent is often considered by adults to be taking the whole thing so well; there is no awareness of the dangers. Withdrawal as a symptom of disturbance, seems almost wholly unrecognized by the American educational system. In the two years between July 1969 and July 1971 the Adolescent Service of the University of Michigan Medical Center in Ann Arbor, did not have one case referred to it because adults became anxious about overcompliant behavior; in the Adolescent Unit of the Tavistock Clinic in London, England, withdrawal and excessive compliance were fairly frequent reasons for referral, at any rate from sensitive and perceptive teachers.

Withdrawal is more usual as an anxiety symptom in girls than boys. If it is unrecognized, girls may continue to withdraw from others and become unable to make relationships with feelings. Alternatively, girls frantically needing emotional contacts may react by hoping for consolation in physical contact. Promiscuous behavior is an attempt on their part to contact another human being, to establish their own sense of femininity, and to resolve their feelings of hostility to men. Often intercourse is the price paid to be cuddled; sometimes, however, a purely physical relationship implies contempt for the total personality. It is an attack on both the girl's femininity and by identification that of her mother (Blos, 1962, p. 235). This is another way in which anger over loss may show itself, by an inner refusal to be really involved with another person. This reaction can also occur if young people perceive the adults in their world as distant and uncaring or if they feel at odds with their own age group. Acute emotional withdrawal then becomes chronic uninvolvement with people and things. This is not rare with those adolescents who are, in any case, unsure of the affection of those around them.

Adolescents and children should not be allowed to attack society or themselves as part of their grief. They need to have destructive behavior controlled, but they also need the chance to understand and work out in a positive way their sense of loss. This may be partly done by helping them to put their feelings into words to a helpful, interested adult. They also need the opportunity to use their environment to assist the mourning experience. When girls lose their mothers, they can, to an extent, work out their mourning experiences by occupying a helpful mothering role in the family both to other children and their father, as if to identify with their dead parent. When a girl takes over such mothering tasks, she is doing something that everyone will perceive as valuable. The risk is that she may be used by her family and unable to develop as a person in her own right.

Boys may attempt to take over the role of a dead father, but there are fewer socially acceptable ways in which this is possible for them. The schoolboy in Western society cannot easily earn wages to keep a family; younger children will resent attempts he may make to control them. Closeness to his mother is less tolerable for a boy than is the equivalent situation for a girl. When the mother of an adolescent boy dies, it is psychologically and socially inappropriate for him to take over housekeeping roles in the family.

Death of Friends

The death of friends of their own age is particularly anxiety provoking to adolescents. The mixed feelings aroused by parental loss can perhaps be more easily understood than the extreme distress that can be brought about by a friend's death:

> John was sixteen and was brought before the courts for indecent exposure; he was seen masturbating in a copse in a local park. He had no previous history of disturbed sexual behavior. Two days before the episode he had arranged to meet a friend after work and, to make this possible, had lent his friend his motor scooter. He waited in vain for his pal, who was killed on the way to meet him.
>
> It is not hard to see that John's masturbating might be understood as reassurance to himself that he was still alive. Although he had no conscious thought of exposing himself, the relatively public nature of his act might well have stood for his unconscious wish to be punished for his own part in his friend's death. The interpretation was made to John during the course of an initial interview, that it looked as though he had jerked off to prove to himself that he was still alive. John wept profusely, talked of how he was responsible for his friend's death, and said he deserved to be punished.

Typically, when two young people are together and one is killed, the survivor is guilty as well as grieved. It is common for one to feel that if they had acted differently the death might not have happened or that the better person did not survive.

Death poses another problem for adolescents: It reminds them of their own fragile destructibility. The necessity to deny this is the reason why some adolescents seem relatively untouched by the death of very close friends. This denial is often more apparent than real:

> Sally, a girl of thirteen, had a friend who died suddenly in the night after what appeared to be a trivial headache the day

before. This happened at the beginning of the Christmas holidays, and Sally appeared to be relatively untouched. Her parents noted later that she complained she was not sleeping well; on a couple of occasions she had reported nightmares and one night had been sleepwalking. On the first day of school, in class with her favorite teacher, Sally complained of a splitting headache, and she had to be taken home. It then emerged that she had been afraid to sleep during the holidays because she was afraid she would die; she waited until she was with an adult who mattered to her to develop the headache that finally led to the emotional first aid she needed.

Death of Siblings

The death of a brother or sister is a particular problem for an adolescent. Children feel intense rivalry as well as affection toward each other. The death of a sibling can cause intense internal and intrafamilial conflicts. Apart from the ambivalent feelings of the survivors, it is not uncommon for them to become the repository of two sets of parental feelings. On the one hand, the parents may split their own ambivalent feelings about their dead child; he is loved, and all the hatred over the loss is put onto a surviving child. This is, of course, unconscious, but the surviving adolescent experiences his parents as being both unreasonably angry and at the same time overcontrolling. It is a terrible experience for a son to be told by an angry, bereaved mother that "the best of you all was taken."

Effects of Chronic Parental Illness

Chronic illness in their parents, their immediate families or in boys or girls of their own age can also be very painful for adolescents. Illness arouses in the young a fearful feeling about the vulnerability of their own bodies. The pain, bewilderment, and anger that adolescents feel when a parent suffers from a chronic illness make it hard for them to be as considerate as involved adults would wish. Adolescents often need to withdraw from such a situation, and they may be overwhelmed with guilt because they feel they should be doing much better. The more painful and intractable the illness is, the more likely it is that the adolescent will be disturbed at school, showing poor work, constant troublemaking, or ready anger. The adolescent seems to need to demonstrate his own pain and deny the parent's agony, to ensure that he will be punished for his badness in not being loving to the ill parent. When a long illness ends in death, the adolescent is likely to be even more disturbed:

> Tom's mother was dying of cancer. She had been intermittently ill since he was nine, but as her illness reached its terminal stage and hope was abandoned he began to behave in an increasingly antisocial way in school. Tom was perpetually in trouble with the staff, and, presumably because the cause was not understood, he was suspended. At this point his mother died. The loss of his mother and the rejection and lack of understanding he felt at school drove him to larceny and assault and, after the usual interval of probation, placement, and various types of highly intermittent therapy, he was committed to a school for delinquent boys. The youth was overwhelmed; he was angry, sad, and riddled with guilt, feeling strongly that his mother's death was all his own fault because of his bad behavior. In his new school, he accidentally damaged a newly built wall that fell over on him and nearly killed him. Only after this probably unconscious suicide attempt was he given the opportunity of facing with an interested adult, whom he felt cared for him, his pain and anxiety over his mother's illness and death.

The disturbed behavior of guilt-ridden adolescents may occur because they unconsciously try to get their environment to punish them. They often seem to succeed all too well in this. The first response of society to the antisocial behavior of grief-stricken adolescents is usually sympathetic. When the behavior continues the response often becomes punitive.

Despite the almost inevitable response of adolescents to the loss of loved ones, adults who feel intimately involved in the care of the young may not be aware that a parental death or separation has occurred:

> In one school a fifteen-year-old boy began to steal repeatedly. This school had no tradition of communicating with the parents, and the first his mother knew about the problem was when she received a letter with the boy, who had been sent home. At no time during the discussions that had gone on between him and the staff over the thefts had the boy told them that his father had died during the previous holidays.

Extraordinary though this may seem, it is typical of adolescent behavior. During such a crisis the young take an attitude toward interested adults like that of the two-year-old to parents: One is supposed to know that the tragedy has occurred without being told about it in words.

Apart from the general disturbances of society, many specific environmental shifts can cause adolescent maladjustment, which is itself part of the attempt of the individual to deal with stress. The quality of the response may vary according to the genetic and environmental endowment of any given adolescent. Nevertheless, typical stresses do cause typical responses. Death and separation are some of the most painful experiences that happen to the young, fortunately, to relatively few of them. Those young people who are not helped over such crises are highly likely to become emotional cripples.

Caring adults available to young people need to be able to be sensitive to the underlying conflicts of their lives; to work with them in an emotional atmosphere that respects individual integrity, and to try appropriately to meet their needs. Adolescents may suffer today, but they can become part of the mature adult population of tomorrow if efforts are made to assist them through these acute conflict situations they cannot handle alone.

If these conditions exist, many can resiliently cope with severe stress. On the other hand, when an adolescent exposed to trauma is isolated from caring adults who can intuitively offer them help and emotional support, the best that can be hoped for is adequate, formally organized, psychological intervention. A failure to obtain this may produce a crippled, damaged, and damaging personality—both are too expensive for most societies.

References

Blos, P. (1962), *On Adolescence*. Glencoe, Ill.: Free Press.

Bonnard, A. (1962), Truancy and pilfering associated with bereavement. In *Adolescents, Psychoanalytic Approach to Problems and Therapy*, ed. S. Lorand and H. I. Schneer, 152–180. New York: Paul Hoeber.

Deutsch, H. (1944), *The Psychology of Women*. New York: Grune & Stratton.

Draper, E. P. (1965), *Psychiatry and Pastoral Care*. Philadelphia: Fortress Press.

Freud, S. (1933), Anxiety and instinctual life. In *New Introductory Lectures on Psychoanalysis, Standard Edition*, 22: 81–112. London: Hogarth Press.

Greenacre, P. (1952), *Trauma, Growth and Personality*. New York: Norton.

Jersild, A. T. (1963), *The Psychology of Adolescence*. New York: Macmillan.

Menninger, K. A. (1963), *The Vital Balance*. New York: Viking.

Miller, D. (1965), *Growth to Freedom, The Psycho-Social Treatment of Delinquent Youth*. Bloomington: Indiana University Press.

Robertson, J., and Bowlby, J. (1952), Responses of young children to separation from their mothers. *Courr. Cent. Int. Enf.*, 2: 131–142.

17

The Treatment of Adolescent Sexual Disturbances

Social Norms and Sexual Behavior

Nowhere is the interplay between environmental, intra-familial, and personal factors more evident than in the field of sexual behavior. Sexual attitudes, feelings, and activities shift with cultural and religious expectations, and conscious family effort may alter attitudes towards sexuality within a generation. A description of women's feelings about menstruation written in the 1940's in which concepts of dirt and shame are stressed, is now anachronistic (Deutsch, 1944, pp. 152 ff). Homosexuality is coming out of the closet, and a more liberal concept of sexuality that was previously present in history is returning. With sexuality, as other types of behavior, it is apparent that the definition of what is normal depends on criteria of social acceptability. The ancient Greeks saw homosexuality as normal; the Indians accepted every form of sexual activity, as is evident from their temple sculptures. A change in what society considers sexually acceptable and desirable relieves anxiety in some; with others, this may reinforce sexual anxiety, as guilt is less easily hidden by social constraints. Most young people are aware of the implicit and explicit sexual attitudes expressed in films, on the stage, and in contemporary books. Many have therefore come to expect a whole range of exciting sexual gymnastics from each other without any real awareness that some of these should imply great respect and love of one human being to another. Adolescents often believe that a girl's orgasm is inevitable, if only a boy is sufficiently skillful. They are not aware that sometimes this will occur only if a girl really feels in love and at one with her boyfriend. If some adolescent girls do not enjoy sex sufficiently, they may begin to feel that there is something radically wrong with them. Some become self-conscious, and then their chances of having a successful orgasm decrease. Others demand an orgasm as a right and bitterly criticize their boyfriends' failure to give them one. Because some boys feel that they are failures if their girlfriends do not respond with what they consider to be sufficient sexual excitement, security is not enhanced in either party. Nevertheless, an advantage of a decline in sexual prurience is that adolescents with sexual difficulties may now more easily seek help.

The increase in frankness in writing about various forms of preintercourse sexuality has begun to lead to a change in adolescents' awareness of what might be expected either of themselves or their partners. Many more boys than in the past are offended if a girl is not willing to kiss or suck their penis; others still feel this is a disgusting perversion (Messanger, 1971, p. 15). The frank discussion of fellatio and cunnilingus that has appeared in novels in recent years means that adolescents now talk of this much more freely.

It is abusive for one boy to call another a "cocksucker," but from the evidence of clinical practice boys who are anxious about being homosexual today talk about a wish for this type of sexual activity more frequently and more easily than they could in the past. Fellatio, which has always been accepted in some cultures (Altschuler, 1971, p. 55) is now written about as a common event and is shown by implication in films. Often little indicates that an intimate emotional relationship might be involved. Like cunnilingus, fellatio is frequently talked about, particularly by uppersocioeconomic adolescents, as if it were not more significant than any other type of petting (Gebhard, 1971, p. 209). A profoundly significant human activity with complex psychological significance may be treated as mild sexual frolic. Because in fellatio, a boy puts himself symbolically in the position of a feeding mother, he needs to feel great security about his own sense of masculinity. The boy who is fellated passively puts himself in a position of implicit trust in his sexual partner, a girl who takes a boy's penis into her mouth is conveying her immense love for her partner's sexual organ, which will give her ultimately such great satisfaction. The boy who tongues a girl's clitoris and vaginal opening similarly should convey great love.

Conscious parental attitudes toward sexuality have changed. The last generation of parents deliberately, the present generation more automatically, are less anxious about infantile sexuality. Clinically, masturbatory guilt associated with fantasy (Harley, 1961, p. 61) is still common, but conscious anxiety about the masturbatory act, except in certain small towns and rural areas, has almost disappeared in a decade. Working-class youth still describe the activity as infantile, and young adults who continue the practice may feel that they should have grown out of it (Woods and Natterson, 1967).

Sexuality and Autonomy

Many parents can now comfortably accept that healthy adolescents do not discuss the details of either sexual activity or sexual difficulties with them. Sexual intimacy is kept secret from parents, because this is a way in which adolescents develop autonomy and assert their separate identity. The privacy of sex helps prove to adolescents that they are no longer dependent children. Girls do not discuss what they feel might be orgasmic insufficiency with their mothers; boys do not discuss with fathers whether or not a particular sexual wish or activity might be perverse or whether they are sufficiently potent. This can cause particular problems in psychiatric adolescent outpatient clinics. It is increasingly common for boys of sixteen or seventeen to seek help for impotence in such settings. They come on their own and do not usually tell their parents that they are doing this. When these sexual problems do not respond to brief intervention and require a great deal of therapy, however, it may be illegal for the boy to continue to come without the knowledge of his parents. Therapy usually has to be paid for. In any case, if a clinic sees an adolescent over a prolonged time period without parents' knowledge, staff are agreeing by their actions that the parents are bad and persecutory; acting out with patients against parents vitiates against successful therapy. A good therapist will help an adolescent understand the need to tell parents that he has sought psychiatric help but still will guarantee confidentiality as to what he has been told. Parents then demand from either the therapist or a social worker the reason for their child's appearance at a clinic. The request made to a social worker may cause interdisciplinary problems, particularly with those who have worked with the families of smaller children; they find it hard to accept that the problem they have to discuss is that their children cannot be frank with the parents.

Parental responsibility for adolescent sexual feelings and attitudes depends on the implicit and explicit communications made during childhood and adolescence. Often, parental anxiety about their own role is deflected onto sexual issues, for example, what adolescents should see and read.

Pornography

Pornography is a current preoccupation for some. Exposure to knowledge about sexual techniques from books, films, and plays may modify behavior, just as exposure of small children to violence on television may affect their attitudes (Lefkowitz, et al., 1972, p. 153), but a healthy adolescent who is consolidating his identity in midadolescence does not change his fundamental attitudes on the basis of what is seen and read. An individual's capacity to be considerate and loving with others develops through childhood and is finally confirmed at adolescence. If young people have such a capacity, a film or book, however perversely it mixes sexual and aggressive stimulation, does not modify this. Early adolescents, who have less judgment, and emotionally disturbed older youth, who are less certain in their capacities to be loving, can be influenced by portrayals of sadistic aggressive sexuality, just as they can be influenced in their behavior by such individuals and the reporting of real events. Disturbed adolescents, whose capacities to be sexual and aggressive have become inextricably mixed, can take what is read in a book or particularly seen in a film as permission to behave in a disturbed and aberrant way, but the book or the film does not cause the confusion (Miller, 1969). The problem is that censorship, which is designed to forbid, also implies permission. If a film is given a certificate that says it may not be shown to adolescents under eigthteen, those over that age may assume what is shown is approved by the authority figures of society. This is a potent permission for the psychologically disturbed, although they may have acted out their fantasies anyway at some other time.

Adolescents who have been brought up in families with mutual love will not be changed by the entertainment industry. Secure people are not significantly influenced by what they may see on the stage or the screen or what they might read in books. All they gain is information. The less secure youngster, brought up in a less loving family with less mutual respect, is in greater difficulty. The increased sexual intimacy that can now be seen on the screen and on the stage may reinforce a preexisting lack of respect for the individual integrity of people. Very little may be wrong with two people engaging in intercourse on the screen as part of an act of love; however, the actors involved, even though they may portray it as an act of love, devalue this human activity by exhibiting themselves as part of an entertainment.

Society must decide how much freedom healthier sections

of the population will give up to protect those who are younger, weaker, or more disturbed; this problem exists in the arts, in the portrayal of eroticism and with drugs (if marijuana and other substances, for example, are made freely available to the young under the guise they are really only for their elders).

Effect of Early Seduction and Assault

Painful experiences inflicted on the adolescent may cause the appearance of disturbance in what appeared to be an otherwise healthy personality developing in a normal way. The most obvious difficulties are those associated with death and separation from a parent but other painful experiences can occur during this age period. A boy seduced by an adult homosexual or a girl sexually assaulted, even if they are unconsciously provoking, may have further maturation disturbed (Lorand, 1961, pp. 256–258). Boys may find it very difficult to trust adult males or may become homosexual by constantly provoking a situation in which they are likely to be seduced. Alternatively, they themselves may become the seducers of smaller boys, as if to put themselves in the shoes of the adult who seduced them. Both these responses are attempts to come to terms with the painful event. Girls who are sexually overstimulated are highly likely to behave in a promiscuous way but with little or no capacity to bring loving feeling together with the act of sex. On the other hand, they may withdraw from all contacts with men and repress all sexual feeling, often seemingly unaware of the emptiness of their lives.

Young people who are sexually attacked have often unconsciously provoked or consented to the incident. Most children are well taught that it is unwise to get into a car with strangers. Their forgetting this at the crucial moment, may indicate an unsatisfactory attempt to resolve unconscious conflicts, produced by disturbed nurturing experiences in their families as they grew up:

Mary was an only child. Her father who ignored her when he was alive, died when she was eleven. When Mary was fifteen, she was walking home from a movie and had a choice of going down a main street or taking a back road. Though it was no quicker than the main street, she chose the dimly lit road. A car with three boys in it stopped and offered her a ride home. She accepted and was later found bedraggled and frightened on a piece of wasteland some five miles away, having been sexually assaulted.

It is easy to abuse Mary for being a seductive child, but she had no conscious awareness when she got into the car that she was putting herself at risk. The episode was just as painful for Mary as it would have been if she had been a completely innocent victim.

Any help for an adolescent in sexual difficulty requires the helping adult, apart from assessing the etiology of the problem, to judge the normative behavior for the group from which the adolescent comes. Even typical behavior may represent an attempt by an adolescent to resolve either an internal or external conflict or a developmental difficulty. Outside help may be needed for either of these. Postpubertal completed heterosexual behavior may be quite normative in some parts of society, but vulnerable adolescents may still use it to help resolve their internal conflicts. Lonely adolescents may have sex to buy friendships, not as an act of love or even as part of human experimentation. An understanding of sexual behavior and its difficulties requires an understanding of the amount of sexual freedom adolescents can allow themselves. This varies between nations; within any given society in ethnic groups, religious sects, social classes; and from one part of a country to another.

Religious Ideology and Sexual Anxiety

Extremely orthodox Jews are not allowed any sexual contacts, not even kissing, until they marry; masturbation is forbidden. These were perhaps tolerable restrictions when adolescents married at puberty; in present-day society they present young people with intense conflicts about their own behavior.

> Karl, age sixteen, was sent to see a psychiatrist by his anxious parents because, before he obtained his driving license, he constantly took his father's car on long rides through the town. He was picked up twice for speeding, and the referral was precipitated because he crashed the car in a one-car accident. Since the father was a local family practitioner, the police took no formal proceedings, providing referral to a psychiatrist was made.
>
> The boy was a handsome sixteen-year-old, obviously mature physically, who showed no evidence that he needed to inhibit his sexuality. Nevertheless, being the son of highly orthodox Jewish parents he did not date, masturbate (he said), or allow himself any physical contact with girls. If he had attended an orthodox Jewish school peer-group social support might have made life possible for him. However, such a school was not available, and he went to the local high school. Because he was in grade eleven many boys were assessing their masculinity by trying to successfully have intercourse with a girl. Karl believed in the tenets of his religion but was aware of diffuse rage directed against his father. This he felt to be intolerable. He knew that driving his father's car made him less tense, particularly when he drove at high speeds.

The boy did not stay in psychiatric treatment. The anxiety about possible confrontations between his profound sexual wishes and his religious and intrafamilial morality was much too intense.

Some Christian churches cause similar problems to adolescents in present society: primitive Methodists, some Baptists, the Pentecostal Church, and others forbid any demonstration of tenderness and sexual affection outside of marriage. Puritanical Roman Catholicism continues to look upon masturbation as a mortal sin.

An apparent agrophobia in one sixteen-year-old boy was related to anxiety over masturbation. He thought that were he accidentally killed in the street before going to confession after masturbating, he would die not in a state of grace. The threat of purgatory had to be relieved before he was able to develop any sense of sexual freedom.

Social Class and Sexuality

Many blue-collar (Schofield, 1965) and black working-class adolescents are less inhibited sexually in some ways than the black or white middle class. Just as working-class boys and girls can allow themselves to be more impulsively aggressive physically than the middle classes and find verbal interchange tedious, the same applies to heterosexual behavior. Upper-upper-class groups of adolescents in both the United States and Europe are usually able to gratify themselves heterosexually with apparent ease, but in clinical practice little depth characterizes these relationships, which are often highly self-referent and unloving.

Sexual experimentation is natural among primitive societies (Mead, 1939), many of which institutionalize a period of relative license for their young. The puritan tradition among middle-class adolescents has inhibited this, but only some working-class groups have experienced this degree of control. In others, boys and girls from the the end of the pubertal stage of adolescence, usually fourteen or fifteen, are likely to be rather freely experimental with each other. Relatively early sexual intercourse particularly in poverty-stricken cultures is common and is considered, unlike the attitude of a typical, more affluent adolescent, experimental behavior that is not associated with a love relationship, as is often the case with marriage (Giver, 1955). Middle-class adolescents tend to expect a wider variation of sexual techniques even in their first heterosexual experiences.

A seventeen-year-old boy sought psychiatric help at the instigation of his parents because he had made a series of long-distance telephone calls with a false credit number. The calls had been made to impress his girl friend who was away on vacation.

The couple had begun to have intercourse some weeks earlier and in the first experience for both they had used "oral intercourse" (his phrase) prior to the actual sex act.

Clinically, this is fairly commonly reported among the middle-class group; it would be considered perverse by many working-class adolescents (Gebhard, 1971), perhaps because of its association with, what is for them an intolerable experience of passivity.

It was relatively safe for middle-class adolescents to take part in sexual intercourse at fifteen or sixteen. Boys believed that if a virgin was seduced, she would probably then become either promiscuous or pregnant. A double standard existed: If a girl had intercourse she would become unacceptable as a marriage partner to a male who might himself be sexually experienced. These attitudes are still fairly prevalent and often represent a projection of a personal conflict about sex.

Tom, a nineteen-year-old student, sought help for academic underachievement and depression. These complaints were only a ticket of admission for his real complaint: girls looked upon men's sexual wishes as disgusting and obscene; they put up with sex only in marriage. He knew this was untrue but nevertheless felt it to be accurate. These feelings were a direct projection of his parents' attitudes and the social norms, somewhat distorted, of the community in which he had been raised.

Middle-class white mothers still feel more prepared than those in other social and ethnic groups to order about their sons. They are readier to warn their daughters that if they engage in premarital sex, they will become less marriageable: Boys are not interested in damaged goods. General hostility is often expressed toward male sexuality; boys are thought to force their attention on girls, not caring whether or not the girl wants sexual intimacy.

On the whole, lower-socioeconomic-group fathers appear to

become closer emotionally to their sons than their middle-class contemporaries. The working-class boy is often in closer physical intimacy with his father than his middle-class peer. Often, male activities take place without women present. The unconscious homosexual wishes of the working-class boy are then perhaps, both more intense and more forbidden. Early heterosexuality is more necessary.

As a result, therefore, while working-class boys can seriously envisage having sexual intercourse at about fifteen years of age (probably most do not), middle-class youth, at the most, can consider a heavy petting session—wherein a girl might allow a boy to do everything short of penetrating her vagina—at a year or two older. Through adolescence, the typical working-class sexual attitude is that boys will seek intercourse if they can; they will be mostly experimental, and the girl will not be particularly valued. The stereotyped middle-class attitude is that virginity must be respected in all cases. Girls are sexually stimulated to the point of intercourse and do not experience complete sexual fulfillment; boys come to accept a basic frustration in their relationship with girls. These are probably still the most usual situations among young people.

Contraception and Adolescent Sexuality

A fear of pregnancy is still a potent bar to sexual intercourse among some adolescents, despite the birth control pill. Although it is common for midadolescent boys to buy contraceptive condoms, in the hope that the opportunity for intercourse will occur, most feel these to be unaesthetic, and many are aware of their statistical inadequacy. Most adolescent boys are convinced of their potent fertility; they fantasize that one sexual encounter will almost certainly produce pregnancy. They therefore carry male contraceptives more to impress their masculinity on friends than to use them. Less mature middle-class adolescents, and more usually working-class adolescents, are prepared to allow themselves to have intercourse, if they possibly can, irrespective of possible pregnancy. The legal age of consent does not appear to be greatly significant to many adolescents. Many who have intercourse are not particularly interested in whether or not they get a girl pregnant and make no effort to use contraceptives. The wish to "ride bareback," the British slang phrase to describe condomless intercourse, is very common among impulse-ridden youth. Most adolescent boys equate fertility and potency, and only a sophisticated and highly mature attitude looks upon the former as not too significant for male security. However, a significant number of adult males still have this internal equation, and it appears that this is a cause of some of the psychological complications of vasectomy. For many men as in adolescent boys, the ability to be fertile is essential to a masculine self-concept. Many boys will insist that intercourse feels better if their partner does not use the pill. What they really mean is that they experience it as more satisfactory because no one controls their fertility without their permission.

The cultural equivalent of this psychological state can be found in India. There the male Khama (spirit) gains immortality through the birth of sons. Contraception will not be practiced by poor Indian males, nor will they allow their wives to use it, until they have sufficient sons to ensure that at least one survives (Elliott, 1970). The implication for contraceptive problems in a poverty-stricken country, where death from malnutrition and its side effects are common, is obvious.

Problems of Male Potency

Impotence, absolute (Ferenczi, 1950, p. 29) or relative, is a common complaint of late-adolescent middle-class boys. Although most boys are aware that they may fail to penetrate a girl successfully the first time they have intercourse, this occurrence may cause great anxiety. If they are fortunate and have a male friend with whom they can discuss the failure, or if the girl is understanding, all may then go smoothly. Effectively, they seek consensual validation from another male about the transiency of the experience. Many boys need sex so that a girl will discount their internal image of a devaluing female, which they may have acquired in their nuclear family. The dominance of the American mother and the fragmentation of American society, both of which make it extremely difficult for the young male to develop a firm sense of himself, probably account for the prevalence of sexual anxieties. Even though black ghetto society is matriarchal, and clinically it appears that overt homosexual behavior is more tolerable to adolescent black males than it is to white; adolescent blacks seem less aware of sexual insecurity in late adolescence. This may be because black mothers do not appear to devalue masculine sexuality as often as their white sisters.

> A nineteen-year-old black youth was seen by a psychiatrist because of academic underachievement. He was totally dominated by his professional father. Of his mother he said, "When I go home for a vacation, mother is concerned that my brothers and I have time to go out with girls. She worries if we don't seem to be having a good time when we go out with them at night."

Black girl students, however, are often more puritanical about sex than their white sisters. The instillation of guilt about sexuality and a devaluation of masculine roles is a long-time quality of some white middle-class mothers.

The impotent adolescent may appear for help after several unsuccessful attempts at intercourse with the usual story that he can maintain an erection until he is about to penetrate the girl's vagina; at that point he loses his erection. This type of impotence, on the assumption that the boy can successfully maintain an erection and ejaculate when he masturbates himself, is often responsive to brief therapy.

In theory there are two possible psychological reasons for impotence just before vaginal penetration: the adolescent may be fearful of women and anxious that they will engulf him: alternately, he may be so unconsciously angry with women that at the moment of intercourse he refuses to gratify his partner. If a therapist interprets a boy's anxiety he implies, "I know you are an anxious fearful person who is not able to be much of a man." This invites dependent incompetence on the part of the client and years of therapy. If, on the other hand, an interpretation is made about the aggressive teasing implicit in such impotence, the boy is being implicitly told that he is a powerful male, desirable to women, who uses his sexuality potently, if with mutual lack of satisfaction. This may produce rapid resolution of the symptom. Two cases, one from Britain and the other from the United States, demonstrate the value of interpretations about hostility rather than anxiety:

> Peter was an eighteen-year-old student at one of the colleges of Cambridge University. His father had been in the Foreign Office and was now an industrial tycoon; his mother was a brilliant and witty raconteuse. Peter had been brought up surrounded at home by the world of arts and music, and his mother's wit was often used to quell both her husband and her sons. Peter attended a famous British school and at the age of sixteen met a beautiful girl of the same age with whom he attempted an affair. He took her to bed, and at the point of penetration he lost his erection. He reassured himself, by talking to his best friend, that this was reasonably common and thought little more about it.
>
> A brilliant scholar, Peter went to college at seventeen and within a few months tried to have an affair with a fellow student; the same pattern of impotence persisted. Becoming increasingly anxious, Peter failed his exams in the first term of his second year, and his academic tutor referred him for psychological help because of his apparent tension and anxiety.
>
> A quiet-spoken, charming, handsome youth, Peter told his story in his first psychiatric interview. The psychiatrist, having heard of the controlling mother and the exact nature of the

impotence, said "I think you must be one of the biggest shits I have met in a long time." The boy went white with rage, which did not abate when the therapist told him that he was "a reverse prick tease." This idea, however, obviously intrigued Peter, who agreed to return in three days.

He came back and with delight said that he had successful intercourse many times. During the first occasion he had thought to himself "I'll show that bastard." Feeling much better about himself, Peter decided he would come back only if he got into academic or sexual difficulties. The psychiatrist next heard of Peter three years later, when he was invited to the boy's wedding.

The technique had been deliberate. The use of vulgarities as interpretations were designed to present Peter inferentially with the picture of aggressive masculinity that he had to deny in himself. The interpretation about aggression made his masculinity potent. His thought about the therapist was in a sense, homosexual; nevertheless, the relief of his symptoms led to his ability to be himself both vocationally and sexually in the future.

In another situation a patient was to be interviewed in a one-way vision room before a medical school junior class who were being taught interviewing techniques. The patient had come in to the psychiatric outpatient clinic's walk-in service that morning. He was a nineteen-year-old student from the southern United States.

Jim was a pleasant, soft-spoken man with a pronounced southern accent. He complained of a completely unsatisfactory sexual life. From the age of fifteen to eighteen he had thought of himself as a homosexual. He said that he would masturbate or "blow" the other man, usually a pick up. However, he never got an erection himself, as soon as the homosexual behavior started, although he would get hard walking to an assignation and before the sex play began. He had met a girl in his freshman year, was in love with her, he felt, and wanted to marry her. However, whenever he tried to make love to her he always lost his erection when his

penis touched her vaginal orifice. He had tried alcohol and marijuana to see if this made him feel better and more successful,
but neither had worked. The psychiatrist said, "You don't give
anybody anything, do you? You tease both men and women and
pretend that you are going to give something of yourself but you
don't." The patient became defensive and anxious and said that
he never saw himself as a hurtful individual. Arrangements were
made for him to return the following week.

The discussion with the students was lively. They felt that
the psychiatrist had been overaggressive and did not really understand the point of the comment. The patient, rather than waiting
the week, returned to see the psychiatrist four days later. He
said, "I came to thank you. I am going to get married." He then
said that he had gone to bed with his girlfriend that night after
the interview. He had attempted intercourse and it failed. He
then, with great sadness, told his girlfriend that he did not want
to tease her, that he really wanted to make love to her. She burst
into tears and told him that she had thought there was something
wrong with her; they then proceeded to make love successfully.
They had done this several times since. The psychiatrist said that
he thought the patient was perhaps treating him psychologically
as he treated his male lovers sexually; he showed his potentiality
but refused to follow through. The patient was delighted with this
interpretation. He said he thought it was true, but he proposed to
use his energies to be a good husband and get through school. He
indicated he would let the psychiatrist know how things went.
One year later, he reported good grades, no more homosexual
conduct or interest, and a happy relationship with his wife.

Two short-term cases do not make a series, but it appears
in both patients that the therapist had both interpreted the crippling conflict and reinforced a sense of socially acceptable masculine aggression and sexuality. Neither boy had been so anxious
about his relationships with girls that he had been unable to make
some physical and emotional contact with them. Such an approach would not have been successful with boys who kept at a
distance from girls because they were afraid of their own

murderous hostility or because they feared being totally swamped by a devouring female, although both these fears may be in the genesis of some types of impotence.

Orgasmic Insufficiency

Both male impotence and failure to achieve orgasm in girls imply an unconscious devaluation of members of the opposite sex. Orgasmic insufficiency in girls, however, is harder to treat than impotence in boys. Boys get no erotic satisfaction from impotence, girls get closeness and warmth when they are unable to achieve orgasm. Orgasmic insufficiency successfully devalues both male and female sexuality. Girls who experience this may play out their hostility both to their own role as women and to the male and his penis with success—even though the victory is pyrrhic. One reason for the relative failure of the treatment of orgasmic insufficiency is that unmarried adolescent girls do not feel safe in their relationships with boys, even if they seek treatment. It is hard for a girl to be totally giving to a man when she has conflicts about this—when she is unsure of the permanence of the relationship.

Societies that believe that the roles of men and women in families should be the same, that take away from men an authoritative family status and give this to women, are likely to produce large numbers of sexually anxious boys who either are, or fear being, impotent. They may also produce angry women, unable to establish lasting heterosexual relationships. The momism initially described by Philip Wylie and then again by Philip Roth in *Portnoy's Complaint* causes problems to boys in reaching a comfortable sexuality. Similarly, if there is no obvious mutual love between parents, girls find it difficult to accept sexuality with all its sensitive emotional depths. As women, when they cannot achieve orgasm in a full, caring relationship, the devaluation of masculinity and femininity affects their husbands and children. Both partners may collude in an unsatisfactory marital relationship, and this reinforces the likelihood of emotional difficulties being perpetuated through the generations.

Etiology of Sexual Inadequacy

The still common sexual insecurity of both boys and girls seems to exist in relationship to fairly specific causes particularly of upbringing. Parental attitudes toward the sexuality of children are still often confused. If a little boy touches his penis, appropriate horror might still be expressed. The attitude that sex is dirty and disgusting is still too common, and many women still put up with sex with their husbands to appease and satisfy them (Rainwater, 1960). Early heterosexuality is pushed by the "halo" effect of the discussions about it in the various media. Adolescents are led to expect unique experiences without the necessity for a long-term, loving relationship. Many boys will not get too close to women, because they fear either their own loss of control or the over-control of their girlfriends.

Homosexual Anxiety and Its Treatment

Therapy for homosexual conflicts depends on the motivation of the patient for its success. If an individual wishes to retain his homosexual orientation, psychotherapy may be helpful with a variety of his conflicts, particularly those related to shame and guilt. Homosexuals who wish to become heterosexual are not usually helped by less than a complete psychoanalysis: behavior modification plays into the passivity of many homosexuals and may produce a pseudoheterosexual adjustment. If a man is incapable of feeling love and affection for a woman, he may behave heterosexually, but the sex act is not loving.

Many boys who seek help for homosexual anxieties are often afraid to become intimate with anyone. The typical paradigm of the overcontrolling mother and the distant father (Coons, 1971, p. 261), is more likely to produce this syndrome with essentially masturbatory relationships either homoerotic or heterosexual, than homosexual involvement with an emotionally meaningful relationship.

> Seventeen-year-old John sought treatment because he thought he was a homosexual. He was very attracted to boys of his own age who were handsome and muscular, as he was himself. He had an overcontrolling mother who allowed him no privacy; he was a very good son out of fear of her rages and hysteria. He hardly ever saw his father who was a busy attorney who played tennis each weekend. During the course of his therapy he described one of his three homosexual experiences as follows:
> "You would think that to come over another being is one of the most intimate things you can do. When this happened I just got up and left, I wanted nothing to do with him. It was not that I felt disgusted, I just felt nothing; I turned off."

Homosexual activity is markedly related to societal pressures, intrafamilial conflicts, and the level of personal maturity of the individual. Although the gay liberation movement has made the public discussion of homosexuality possible without criticism, anxiety about homosexuality is common to boys and their parents. Lesbian behavior is more tolerable still to Western society, and, as a result, parental and individual anxiety about lesbian activity among adolescent girls is less usual than concern about homosexuality in boys. Many more boys are seen in clinical practice with homosexual concerns than girls, although both are often actively colluded in by parents. The mothers of homosexual boys may actively provoke their son's homosexual relationships:

> Paul was hospitalized because of drug dependence. He was

fifteen, and he had become very dependent on marijuana in association with an active homosexual relationship with a man of twenty-three. Paul's physician thought that communication with his homosexual partner was disturbing to him. The mother smuggled letters from the lover to her son in her own letters.

Lesbian activity probably implies a greater degree of personal disturbance than does homosexuality in boys; it is also probably less common. This is because adolescent girls are less easily sexually stimulated than boys, often markedly fearful of bodily contact with other girls, and less needful of the physical release of sexual tension until they have actually been involved in meaningful sexual intercourse (Brunswick, 1968). A boy who obtains sexual satisfaction with another boy, is using his sexual organs to obtain gratification in a way that may be masturbatory and thus close to a natural developmental act. The nature of the homosexual act among adolescent boys signifies whether this is associated with a transient stage toward heterosexuality or whether the boy is becoming fixated at a homosexual stage of development. The culture and the environment in which the boy lives is relevant in assessing the significance of behavior. In adolescence, mutual masturbation does not necessarily indicate a fixation at an emotionally immature position: it is commonly associated with a general sense of loneliness and insecurity, sexual curiosity, intense sexual frustration, and social acceptability within a group. Fellatio among boys is more likely to indicate psychological immaturity in Britain, where it is a less generally acceptable form of normative sexual activity than in the United States. Sodomy almost always implies psychological disturbance either of a permanent or transient nature.

Etiology of Homosexual Activity

Homosexual activity may be primarily a function of situational pressures. It is common in single-sex, isolated, male boarding schools, in youth prisons, and in underprivileged urban areas. The type of activity engaged in may be a function of specific pressures: gang rape may produce sodomy; fellatio may be the price a boy pays for protection by a bigger boy in a youth prison. Lesbian activity is common in girls' juvenile institutions, the absence of any males in the environment gives particular status to the butch girl and is highly pathological.

Some homosexual activity is most clearly related to family pressures. The stereotyped situation involves a devaluing mother and a passive father who is nevertheless subtly seductive to his son. This can produce a homosexual orientation, and a family row in such a constellation can be the precipitant of such activity. Homosexual seduction is common; there is sufficient conflict about the activity that the sharing of guilt by proselytizing is fairly usual.

A twenty-eight-year-old camp counselor who was an overt homosexual did his best to persuade a seventeen-year-old boy with obvious homosexual conflicts to be his lover. He told the boy that treatment attempts were stupid, that he should accept his role. What pleasanter place to be broken into the activity than in the summer in the woods? The boy refused and told his therapist, "I don't want to be as pathetic as he is at twenty-eight, having to use all that effort to try to get me into the sack with him."

A mature adult male should not need to feel repulsion or disgust at homosexual behavior, although it may not represent his object choice. Thus, a heterosexual male who hates homosexuals is as conflict-ridden as the homosexual male who hates women. Despite the current argument over homosexuality as behavior of an immature male in Western society, boys who come from families in which there is mutual security between parents, in which a husband's role is valued by his wife, and a boy's masculinity is valued by his mother are not likely to become active adult homosexuals, even if they engage in transient homosexual activity as boys. An exclusive homosexual orientation in the male occurs when boys have been brought up in families in which there is sexual conflict between the parents and male sexuality is not respected. Lesbianism may be found in those girls who have been devalued by their fathers; just as exclusively homosexual boys implicitly are hostile to women and girls, so such lesbians devalue men.

Most homosexuals appear unable to create permanent love relationships with men. It has been argued that this is a result of the stress they experience from society. This pressure does exist, but many homosexuals are so intensely involved with themselves and their own needs that they are unable to be loving. It is decidedly easier for two homosexuals to perceive each other as narcissistic extensions of themselves than to be mutually giving. Sometimes homosexual partnerships, as those that are heterosexual, may last because the individuals meet each other's immature needs. A boy who is convinced of his own frailty may feel he receives the strength of his male partner when he incorporates the other man's penis into his body, either by fellatio or sodomy. Equally when he conquers his partner his own masculine potency may be reinforced.

Sexual Attitudes

Sexual inhibition is often related to parental attitudes about the sexual play of children, which is, of course, common. Children may closely examine each other's genitals, lie on top of each other, bang each other's bodies together, and generally act out fantasies of intercourse. Alternatively, they replay a sexual act they might have seen or heard their parents perform. If sex play is freely allowed in childhood, and the child's parents do not sexually love each other, sexuality in adolescence tends to remain experimental. Although it may be freely engaged in, it may never become loving.

There are two stereotypes of loveless sexual behavior: one more typical of groups that allow themselves impulse gratification; the other more controlled, characteristic of middle-class groups. Intercourse at the end of adolescence in the former retains an aggressive play quality, some do not feel it matters very much whether or not their partner enjoys the act and often talk of sex as being overrated. In this case sexual activity does more to release a physical need than to provide erotic and loving satisfaction. A boy in such a situation feels that the girl is lucky to have his penis inside her; the girl accepts this attitude. In both men and women, masturbatory sex play is seen as indicative of satisfactory masculinity and femininity. If maturation past this point does not occur, a loveless sexual attitude is found in married couples. Men may feel that they must have sex with their wives because it is expected of them, but actually they prefer to masturbate themselves. Women may feel that men have their sexual and other rights to which subservience is necessary. A woman in such settings may not like the sexuality of men and may not see them as loving, but her husband's and her son's sexual wishes are acknowledged without overt complaint. In such families activities in the house that are obviously feminine —making beds, washing dishes, cleaning—are never given to boys. This stereotype is probably still normative among a considerable sector of the population who remain relatively untouched by changing women's roles. Loving relationships are mostly fantasied; sexuality is seen as the outlet for men's erotic needs rather than as a mutually loving interaction.

A boy of eighteen, a trainee in electronics engineering, was in psychotherapy for a functional gastrointestinal disorder. He was discussing his weekend and talked of having sex with his fiancée. His therapist wondered if his girl had enjoyed the experience. The patient looked astounded and said that it never occurred to him that it mattered. "I fucked her; she should have been pleased to have that happen."

Among the middle classes, the normative attitude to sexual
activity has always been somewhat constricted. The close super-
vision of children, which is usual in more tightly structured
smaller families makes it more difficult for boys and girls to
take part in natural sex play. In adolescence a delay in anything other than autoerotic sexual activity is still commonly
associated with an expectation of academic achievement even
in socially mobile groups (Kinsey, *et al.,* 1968). This is not
surprising, for academic education demands more control of
impulsive behavior than vocational studies and a greater capacity to tolerate frustration. In academic tracks the opportunities
for sexual involvement of one child with another are considerably
reduced, if only because of demands of homework. Until high
schools began to go on half-day schedules because of financial
stringency, the opportunity for free unsupervised interactions
between children was rare; during the school day it is still at an
absolute minimum. This repression leads to a situation in which
adolescents go home having treated the school like a factory or
they sometimes behave in an overaggressive way to each other
until grade eleven or twelve. Middle-class families tend to be
smaller relative to the amount of available space than those of the
working class; physical intimacy between the family members is
less intense, and impulse expression less allowable than with other
social groups. When middle-class families are angry with each
other, they tend to shout or be tight-lipped; members of other
social groups tend to hit out. All antisocial behavior has roots
in both social and personal pathology. Incestuous behavior,
when it occurs in middle-class families, is associated with greater
personal pathology than is the case with the impoverished, when
the social pathology is greater.

Jennifer was eighteen and seen in a university student health
service after a schizophrenic episode that had occurred shortly
after she entered as a freshman. She had a history of regular
intercourse with her father since she was twelve. Her brother

was seen at the adolescent service of a nearby city because of academic underachievement and being too quiet for the comfort of his teachers. His father had been practicing fellatio on him since he was nine. When the father was interviewed by a social worker, he explained that he felt it his duty to show his son what a vagina was like, "He needs not to be hurt on its teeth." The situation was complicated by the fact that the whole family needed the father's salary as an engineer to survive economically.

Complications of Sexual Freedom

The double standard of sexuality has disappeared among many adolescents, if not among their parents. Most boys do not now feel that girls who have had intercourse with someone else are unacceptable; girls who have had pre-marital sex do not feel that they are loose women.

The attitude that sexuality should be enjoyed is now widespread and no longer considered by young people unacceptable outside marriage. There is, however, a tendency to oversell sexual intimacy; boys and girls come to believe that intercourse should automatically, without equivalent emotional intimacy, be a unique experience. It is not unusual for a boy to feel that he is in some way deficient if his partner does not automatically have an orgasm. Mutuality of love is not considered as essential as expert sexual gymnastics for fully satisfying and gratifying physical intimacy.

Kenneth's father called up a psychiatrist and said that his eighteen-year-old son was in urgent need of help. Kenneth was a well-built, lithe young man who suffered from an acute anxiety state. This was partly related to a recent operation for a benign tumor that for a while had convinced him that he was going to die. It was also related to his feeling of total sexual inadequacy. Kenneth had done a great deal of psychological reading and said, "My mother is a castrating bitch. My father does not care about

me, all he does is make money." The source of the boy's anxiety
preceded his operation. He said, "I have always felt shy with
girls but last spring Judy got me to go to bed with her. She didn't
have an orgasm so I felt absolutely useless. Whatever I did, she
did not enjoy it enough. I am a failure, I have a girl now who
wants me to sleep with her, but I won't because I know I won't
do it properly. I am impotent, I think."

Although some adults now realize that their adolescents are
likely to have premarital sexual intercourse, there is still intensely
mixed feeling about this. Attitudes vary from one part of a country to another and among different ethnic, social, and religious
groups. In clinical practice, it is now more usual for adolescents
of about sixteen from all social groups in both the United States
and Britain to report having had intercourse once or twice. Academically involved youth will report intercourse much more frequently than they would have ten or fifteen years ago. It is by no
means certain that all tell the truth, although this is more likely
in an interview with a doctor or social worker than in answering
an anonymous questionnaire. Adolescents fill up forms on the
basis of what is expected of them; therefore, despite figures produced in the United States and Britain, there is no way of knowing
how common premarital intercourse among adolescents actually
is. The idea that premarital intercourse is acceptable offers both
support and stress to the individual. All adolescents tend to believe that sexual intercourse among their age group is usual; apart
from those with obvious conflicts, many young people who do
not engage in premarital sex may feel that they lack a satisfactory
identity. The idea that everyone has intercourse has led to change
in the quality of human relationships between girls and boys.
Boys feel justified in pressing their sexual demands. Girls begin
to feel that if they do not have intercourse they are missing out on
an important human experience, an attitude that is reinforced
because many of their girlfriends claim to have had sex. Some
girls now demand that boys have intercourse with them.

The shift to extramarital intercourse, as a satisfactory social norm, has a varying effect on the emotional health of the population in general. Although it will probably lead to happier sexuality in marriage, difficulties can be caused for those who engage in such an activity. Ignoring anatomy, neurophysiology, and endocrinology it has been argued that the differences in the psychology of men and women are due to social conditioning; nevertheless, their emotional needs are not the same. Men can, perhaps, act promiscuously without impairing their capacity to be tender and loving (though this is debatable), but women do not adapt easily to a sexually promiscuous life. Promiscuity is no more normative now, at any rate from clinical evidence, than it was in the past, but prolonged and transient mating now seem common. In those tender, loving, sexual relationships girls are generally more dependent than boys, they are more future-oriented, they have a greater need to build nests, and feel that if their boyfriend really loved them, he would want this. Boys are much more creatures of the present; they do not want to rear children until they are aware of their own mortality. This recognition, perhaps, led to pressure from women for premarital celibacy as a socially acceptable norm. This provided a safeguard against illegitimate pregnancy and also protected girls from feeling failures as women because they were rejected by a less psychologically mature male. Love relationships in which there is full sexual activity with no intention of marriage are likely to cause problems, particularly for girls. One essentially feminine contribution to a meaningful relationship between a boy and girl, one of the factors that makes the bond secure, is that the girl feels a desire for permanency. Then she feels that along with love, is a wish to have children. This aspect of feminine psychology is not felt by the young male; who, if he considers the long-term future of his present emotional commitment, is likely to fear the responsibility.

The irresponsibility of late adolescents was noted by Shakespeare. In the *Winter's Tale* he wrote, "I would there were no age between sixteen and twenty-three. There is nothing but getting wenches with child." The Elizabethan situation still exists. The expression of a girl's normal feminine needs for permanency, when they are expressed as a wish, are often felt by a boy to be unreasonably demanding. When a late adolescent girl, feeling the flowering of love, allows herself to be and say what she feels, she is likely to be rejected by her boyfriend; the young male does not yet feel ready for long-term, caring responsibilities. An unplanned pregnancy is thus likely to break up a long-term, apparently satisfactory, sexual relationship. The boy irrationally feels that a girl has trapped him; the girl feels abandoned and let down by the boy's cold response to her news.

Sexual Promiscuity

Most young people do not respond to the removal of psychological barriers to sexuality by promiscuously moving from bed to bed. This common fantasy of adults produces anxiety based, perhaps, on how they would have behaved as adolescents, if only they had been less constricted sexually.

Promiscuity—relatively indiscriminate, loveless sexual intercourse—is a symptom of the more disturbed immature adolescent. Nevertheless, there is some implicit group and societal pressure to behave promiscuously. Not rarely a sexually curious girl will be seduced at a party, because enough of either alcohol or marijuana is taken to lessen internal controls. The pressure of group sexuality is evident at necking or petting parties. The presence of adults at early and middle-stage adolescent parties is a sensible constraint. Young middle-stage adolescents unsure of their own identity and with poor impulse control are particularly vulnerable to this type of pressure. The absence of adults at parties is often taken as permission by the young people to behave impulsively. Too much freedom given to adolescents before they are mature enough to make appropriate judgments becomes license; adults are felt not to care. Young people who feel rejected by parents, who feel isolated, lonely, or empty, are likely to plunge into premature loveless sexual relationships. Partly they are seeking love, often regressively infantile, from someone. Sometimes this activity represents hostility to members of the opposite sex; girls may seek cuddling from boys and the price they are prepared to pay is intercourse. Boys also seek to be cuddled, but since masturbatory activity is acceptable to the male his act of intercourse may be performed more willingly. It is not rare, however, for a boy to have intercourse because it is expected of him, and, some boys play out their hostility to girls by using their penis as a weapon.

> She groaned and writhed as I made love to her as if I was hurting her. She made me so mad I thought, "Fuck you!" and so I did it as hard and as long as I could. I didn't care whether she enjoyed it or not.

Some girls collect penises and neither know nor care about either their own feelings or the feelings of the boys involved. Promiscuous sex is a way of devaluing the individual's sexuality and that of the sexual partner; it also punishes the internal image of parents and effectively punishes parents in reality. Conscience is appeased by a feeling that one is unloved anyway.

Promiscuous adolescent girls are not usually treatable by formal outpatient psychotherapy. So much hostility and regressive satisfaction is contained in their sexual behavior that no therapist or therapy can titrate the level of frustration and contain promiscuous acting out. This behavior often gives unconscious vicarious gratification to mothers of promiscuous girls who are conflict-ridden about their own sexuality; this is particularly likely with sterile mothers of adopted daughters who replay the conflict about their own sterility and adopting a child by reliving the whole episode through the promiscuous behavior of their children.

The sexuality of adolescents cannot be controlled by adults, and many parents find this an almost intolerable burden. When their adolescent has a lover, parents face the fact that they may have lost a dependent child, as well as wonder whether the young couple can accept long-term responsibility for one another. If this is unlikely, parents will find themselves having to help heal their children's psychological wounds. Parents of late adolescents are similar in some ways to parents of small children who must allow their children a degree of physical risk if they are to grow up as physically secure people. The former may have to watch their children take equivalent psychological chances in human relationships. In order to grow adolescents have to match their judgment against the reality in which they live. A society that closes off other outlets to confirm identity, freeing itself of an obsessive overpreoccupation with the idea that extramarital sex is dirty—an attitude that leaked over into the marital state—will have adolescents who test out their own personality strength by behaving in sexual ways.

Illegitimate Pregnancy as a Symptom of Emotional Disturbance

The greater availability of contraceptive techniques and advice means that girls become pregnant, usually as a result either of their unconscious or conscious wish. Alternately, pregnancy may result from religious belief, intellectual inadequacy, or a willingness to go along with a boyfriend's need to prove his potency. It may sometimes be an attempt to force the hand of reluctant parents to allow marriage or it may represent a wish to obtain a fantasy stability from home making. Some girls have magical beliefs about not becoming pregnant or they accept the statement of the boyfriend that he will ensure she does not become pregnant. The techniques at the boy's disposal, however, are not particularly safe: He may use a condom, he may practice *coitus interruptus,* or he may quite cynically satisfy himself at the expense of the girl's peace of mind. The use of the contraceptive pill makes it easier for a girl to have intercourse promiscuously, but easy contraception poses problems both for adolescents and their parents. Parents may be tempted to encourage their daughters to use the pill or to be fitted with a diaphram. Similarly, doctors may make the same recommendation to their adolescent patients. This represents adult approval of, and collusion in, extramarital sex. Adolescents may not want this adult invasion of their privacy and may feel it as devaluing. On the other hand, adult failure in this respect may lead to illegitimate pregnancy with all its complications.

Easy contraception also brings to the fore a typical adolescent conflict between the wish to experiment with sex and to discover a physical self and the human need for the physical expression of tender loving feelings. This conflict is not inevitable, a first sexual affair may be, but often is not a love affair.

The illegitimacy rate among adolescents continues to be high, and the relative ease of abortion now provides problems of its own. Pregnancy for adolescent girls represents an attempt to feel whole and valuable as women though this is less true for mature women (David, 1972). When a pregnant girl goes to an obstetrician she may be asking this man, whom society values, if he thinks she is worthwhile as a person and a woman. This question may be couched as a request for an abortion, but granting the request may imply a devaluation of the girl's role as woman; this must be understood. There are no psychiatric indications for an abortion; there are only social pressures. A useful question to ask a girl requesting an abortion is whether she would want it if there were no such pressures upon her.

Many girls who become pregnant do not really want to have babies. They are thinking of playing house, with no idea of the demanding greed of an infant and often they are quite unable to cope with this. Physicians tend to be too willing to accept the content of a girl's statement at face value; an illegitimately pregnant girl may arouse the rescue fantasies of doctors who come to accept a girl's statement that she has bad parents. But a pregnant girl may project her own angry feelings about her state onto her parents and insist they will be punitive when this is not so.

> A sixteen-year-old high school girl went to a free clinic to ask their help in obtaining an abortion. She said her parents must not be told and a physician wrote a referral letter to a clinic in New York saying the girl was eighteen and requesting an abortion. The girl had to raise $250 and she borrowed the money from all her friends. She got the sum, but her older sister found out what was happening and sought help from the school social worker. This woman persuaded the girl to tell her parents who were kind, supportive, empathic, and helpful.

The physician broke the cardinal rule of good adolescent psychiatry to be on a child's side but not against the parents. Moreover, he did not recognize the area in which she really wanted help. Adolescents may not mean what they say.

Sexual Exhibitionism

Some degree of sexual exhibitionism has always been typical of adolescent boys and girls. Its social acceptability has varied from time to time. For a while women had to hide the fact that they had legs and ankles; men that they had a penis.

In the Middle Ages affluent males wore an elaborate codpiece that covered and called attention to their genitals. Clothes were colorful until the nineteenth century, and bawdy sexuality was constantly seen in the theater. After a period of approximately 120 years, men in the last two decades have once again been "allowed" to be more exhibitionistic. Many adolescent boys shrink their jeans skin-tight, thus outlining their genitals. Stylish adolescent boys' slacks now have buttons, which are no longer hidden, to replace a zip fly. The unacceptable can become erotically stimulating, and rapid changes in fashion can cause anxiety to some. Girls who do not wear a bra may stimulate pubertal boys and be felt by them as teasing. Sometimes young women social workers or physicians wear revealing clothes that may disturb immature adolescents with whom they have contact. Similarly, a young male doctor who wears "with it" clothing may be felt by his young patients to indicate something about his sexual and drug-related attitudes.

In general, among young people, prurience is slowly being removed from nudity, but exhibitionism as a symptom of sexual immaturity is still fairly common and is a measure of personal immaturity of the adolescent (Kaiser, 1961). It is natural for a little boy to show people that he has a penis and that he is proud of it. An adolescent who exhibits his penis to girls or women and who masturbates in front of them demonstrates an infantile level of sexuality. Such boys and adult men are afraid of women and at the same time contemptuous (Christoffel, 1956). Although women become extremely anxious about such behavior, it is not dangerous. Exhibitionists are not able to form close relationships with girls; neither do they attack girls. Some very disturbed aggressive boys will strip off their clothing, however, as though to attempt rape; hence, the common feeling that an exhibitionist is dangerous.

Women too may be provocatively exhibitionistic. The girl who undresses in front of an open window in an apartment block needs to be safely aggressive to males. It is an intriguing double standard that a naked girl who behaves this way is not liable to legal penalties, while a boy who strikes a naked pose in front of a window where he might be observed commits an offense. Both suffer from similar levels of psychological maladjustment. There are, however, exaggerations of normative behavior. The boy who wears skin-tight jeans is exhibitionistically trying to encourage the voyeurism of girls, although an even more unconscious homosexual provocation may also be present (Fraiberg, 1961, pp. 84–85). The display of a well-muscled body has the same intent. Girls who dress to encourage the sexual interests of males also encourage their voyeurism.

Voyeurism

Just as exhibitionism is an exaggeration of a natural human tendency, so is voyeurism, the act of looking at someone else's genitals to obtain a feeling of sexual gratification. It is common and usual for small boys and girls to be interested in each other's genitals. Initially, voyeurism is part of a normal developmental stage of human sexual development. Postpubertal boys, particularly in a gang, may be involved in episodes in which a girl's pants are taken down; alternately a girl may exhibit herself to gratify a group of boys. The boys may also demonstrate their erect penis to each other. In deprived communities sexual exhibitionism and voyeurism coexist when a group of boys all have intercourse with a more or less willing girl in a "gang bang," as the boys stay to watch others perform the sexual act. Such a situation is also homosexual because the boys become sexually stimulated from watching the sexual excitement of their peers. It is also quite common for male spectators of pornographic films to become sexually excited by watching and identifying with the man on the screen.

In Western culture many men gain gratification from being able to see a girl's genitals or her pants, and this can be part of natural sexuality. This titillation of men's sexual appetites was routine in the can-can. All these types of voyeurism can be present in boys, but true voyeurs are always severely disturbed. Men and boys who engage regularly in Peeping-Tom activities, lurking around houses to try to see women and girls undressed are as disturbed as the girls and women who haunt parks and lovers' lanes to see if couples have intercourse. Many adolescents who accidentally see others having intercourse will be sexually gratified from the experience and will often stay to watch, but this stimulation of voyeurism is not the same as a substitute for natural sexual relationships.

Transvestism

Unrelated to environmental pressures but associated with intrafamilial conflict is transvestism. A boy who wears women's clothes, whether or not he masturbates while doing so, is convincing himself that he needs no one. When the clothes are those of his mother, the apparent masturbatory activity is highly pregenital, the boy is doing the equivalent of sucking his thumb while being held in his mother's arms. Such a boy in fantasy is being both a man and a woman at the same time; he is, at the same time, seeking to return to an omnipotent oneness with his mother. Those who steal the clothes of strange women are actually not as regressed, but no transvestite ever grows out of this conflict situation and reaches adult sexuality without treatment. Transvestites are commonly found out because they are caught stealing women's clothing. The type of theft demonstrates their general emotional immaturity; they do not basically *feel* that such thefts are wrong, even though they may know that they are. They are aware of the penalties society will extract but always feel they will not be caught.

Some transvestite boys wish they were girls. They enviously feel that girls have every advantage in life because they do not have a penis. A small percentage of transvestites become murderous during sexual intercourse. In the act of sex, it is brought home to them that women have a vagina and they do not. Their envious rage of women then overwhelms them, and the men who mutilate women's sexual organs are these men. The diagnostic issue in transvestism is to establish whether or not the individual is murderous. In a skilled interview, murderous transvestites will become lost in their erotic and aggressive fantasies and talk freely of their murderous intentions (Miller and Looney, 1973).

Transsexuality

There are some who are brought up as infants in such a way that they really feel themselves to be members of the opposite sex. It may well be that because of circulatory hormonal stimulation prenatally a girl is born with a boy's body or vice versa (Yalom, *et al.*, 1973). Distorted upbringing around the issue of sexuality may then be a result of the child's response to the parents, not parental psychopathology in itself. True transsexual boys are very rare, and there is no known psychological treatment for them; they are transvestites because they do not see themselves as men at all. They continue to demand mutilating operations often until they find a surgeon prepared to do these. Transsexual girls cannot obtain an artificial penis that will become erect and often they appear indistinguishable from lesbians. A typical lesbian despises men and does not wish to have a penis; a transsexual girl uses lesbian behavior to fantasy herself in a male role with a penis.

Most psychological upset is not hereditary. The foundation stones of personality development are laid in childhood, but adolescence is a second chance for mature development. In the psychological and social turmoil of puberty and adolescence the plasticity of the human personality makes new perceptions of the world possible. The incorporation of these into the personality helps modify conflict, and the increasing freedom from childish emotional ties makes the adolescent less vulnerable. Society is less preoccupied with the sexual difficulties of adolescents but all too often conflicts about sexual identity and either an incapacity to be a loving person or a doubt that one can ever be an object of affection from others lie behind the drug problem and delinquent activity.

Sexual maladjustment is usually a symptom of fairly severe personality disturbance. Some symptoms respond to brief conflict-focused psychotherapy; others are immensely difficult to treat because sexual behavior, even though aberrant, is a source of such instinctual gratification that its abandonment becomes difficult if not impossible.

References

Altschuler, M. (1971), Cayapa personality and sexual motivation. In *Human Sexual Behavior,* ed. D. S. Marshall and R. C. Suggs, 38–50. New York: Basic Books.

Brunswick, R. (1968), The pre-oedipal phase of libido development. In *Psychoanalytic Reader,* ed. R. Fliess. New York: International Universities Press.

Christoffel, H. (1956), Male genital exhibitionism. In *Perversions, Psychodynamics and Therapy,* ed. S. Lorand and M. Boliut. New York: Random House.

Coons, F. W. (1971), The development task of the college student. *Adolescent Psychiatry,* 1: 261, New York: Basic Books.

David, H. P. (1972), Abortion in psychological perspective. *Am. J. Orthopsychiatr.,* 42: 61–68.

Deutsch, H. (1944), *The Psychology of Women.* New York: Grune & Stratton.

Elliott, D. (ed.) 1970, *The Family and Its Future.* London: J. and A. Churchill.

Ferenczi, S. (1950), *Sex in Psychoanalysis.* New York: Basic Books.

Fraiberg, S. H. (1961), Homosexual conflicts. In *Adolescents, Psychoanalytic Approach to Problems and Therapy,* ed. S. Lorand and H. I. Schneer, 84–85. New York: Paul Hoeber.

Gebhard, P. H. (1971), Human sexual behavior: A summary statement. In *Human Sexual Behavior,* ed. D. S. Marshall and R .C. Suggs, 209. New York: Basic Books.

Giver, G. (1955), *Exploring the English Character.* New York: Parthenon.

Harley, M. (1961), Masturbation conflicts. In *Adolescents, Psychoanalytic Approach to Problems and Therapy,* ed. S. Lorand and H. I. Schneer. New York: Paul Hoeber.

Kaiser, S. (1961), The adolescent exhibitionist. In *Adolescents, Psychoanalytic Approach to Problems and Therapy,* ed. S. Lorand and H. I. Schneer, 113–132, New York: Paul Hoeber.

Kinsey, A. C., et al. (1948), *Sexual Behavior in the Human Male.* Philadelphia: W. B. Saunders.

Lefkowitz, M., et al. (1971), Television violence and child aggres-

sion: A follow-up study. In *Television and Social Behavior*. Vol.
3, ed. G. Comstock and E. A. Rubinstein. Washington, D.C.:
Government Printing Office.

Lorand, R. L. (1961), Therapy of learning problems. In *Adolescents,
Psychoanalytic Approach to Problems and Therapy*, ed. S.
Lorand and H. I. Schneer, 256–258. New York: Paul Hoeber.

Mead, M. (1939), *From the South Seas: Studies of Adolescence
and Sex in Primitive Societies*. New York: William Morris.

Messanger, J. C. (1971), Sex and repression in an Irish folk community. In *Human Sexual Behavior*, ed. D. S. Marshall and R. C.
Suggs, 15. New York: Basic Books.

Miller, D. (1969), *The Age Between*. London: Hutchinson.

————, and Looney, J. (1973), The prediction of murder by adolescents. Paper presented at American Psychiatric Association
Meeting, 1973.

Rainwater, L. (1960), *And the Poor Get Children*. Chicago: Quad-
rangle.

Schofield, M. (1965), *The Sexual Behavior of Young People*. London: Longmans Green.

Woods, S. M., and Natterson, J. (1967), Sexual attitudes of medical
students. *Am. J. Psychiatr.*, 124: 323.

Yalom, I. D., Green, R., and Fisk, N. (1973), Prenatal exposure to
female hormones, effect on psychosexual development in boys.
Arch. Gen. Psychiatr., 28: 554–561.

18

Drug Abuse in Adolescence

Incidence of Drug Abuse

It is extremely difficult to assess the extent of the problem of either drug use or abuse in adolescence particularly because young people themselves are not reliable witnesses. In school pupils may exaggerate the incidence of drug taking, and those who take drugs believe they must stick together and not tell tales. Studies of incidence are, however, possible with reliable cross checking as to validity (Robins and Murphy, 1967), and the conviction figures for drug offenses and clinical evidence still suggest that drug taking among adolescents of all ages is still high, even if the number of drug-toxic adolescents seen by doctors and others is apparently decreasing.

The frequency of drug taking in adolescence varies from experimentation to regular and progressive drug abuse that becomes dependence and, in some cases, physical addiction. Figure 1 illustrates drug-taking behavior and its variations (J. E. Villareal, personal communication).

Drug experimentation need not be considered evidence of psychopathology. It can be defined as the self-administration of a drug (which may be taken to the point of intoxication) to discover its psychological, physical, and social effects. Even though the experience may be perceived as gratifying, intoxica-

439

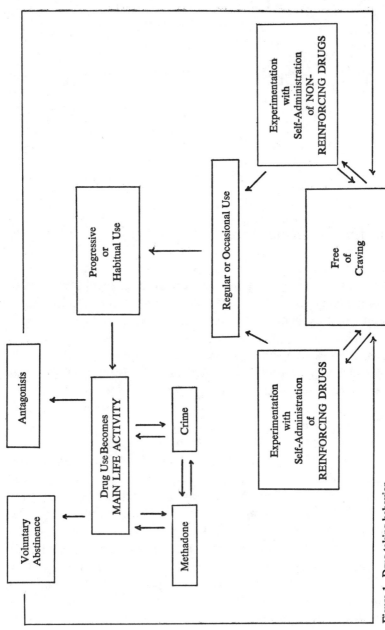

Figure 1. Drug-taking behavior.

tion, with its consequent ego regression and conscious awareness of lack of control, is felt by many adolescents as psychologically threatening. In order to restore a feeling of self-mastery and a sense of control of ego functions, drug experimentation is likely to be repeated four or five times after an actual intoxication experience.

Although drug experimentation in itself may not be pathological, drug responses are likely to be unpredictable and idiosyncratic. In general, experimentation with reinforcing drugs, which are addictive in that they specifically influence hypothalamic centers, are indicative of greater personal or social pathology affecting the individual. In addition, intoxicant effects related to the use of hallucinogens may be felt as intensely psychologically threatening and ego disintegrating.

Both early and midadolescent drug experimentation are vulnerable to a halo effect; the more drugs are talked and taught about, the more likely adolescents are to use, if not abuse, them. Identification with a valued non-drug-using adult is more likely to lead to abstinence than the content of antidrug propaganda or classroom teaching about the subject.

Regular drug usage is the occasional more or less regular use of drugs because of their sedative and/or intoxicant effect. This category includes the regular use of tobacco, alcohol, barbiturates, marijuana, any hallucinogenic or mood-changing drug, whatever its frequency. The regular user may be psychologically dependent on a drug or may intermittently crave its use to relieve tension. The fact that an individual may be able to withdraw from a drug with no apparent ill effect does not mean that its use is other than pathological.

Progressive drug usage with its equivalent—the habitual use of one drug—implies a variation of drug use from "softer" to "harder" drugs: for example, cigarettes to alcohol and marijuana, or in some social groups to glue sniffing. A variety of synthetic or natural hallucinogens, stimulants, and sedatives, and ultimately heroin, other opium derivatives, or cocaine may be taken. Adolescents who take cocktail mixtures of drugs in an effort to avoid the toxic effects or addictive qualities of any one of them are progressive drug users. Commonly, but not necessarily, such individuals ultimately change from taking drugs by mouth or sniffing them, to their injection, either intravenously or subcutaneously. Any chronic drug abuse, either regular or progressive, that may lead to drug dependence can best be understood as an unconsciously sought ego regression.

The terminology of drug abuse is confused. The term "addiction" has been defined as a "chronic intoxication produced by the repeated consumption of a drug." Its characteristics are said to include a compulsion to continue taking a drug, a tendency to increase the dose, and psychological and sometimes physical dependency on its effects. "Habituation" is said to differ from addiction in that it creates a desire, but not a compulsion, to continue taking a drug because of the increased sense of well-being it may produce.

This sense of well-being although often diffusely mixed, can be broken down into three divisions, some of which are more obvious in any one individual than others. Dependence may be on the high of drugs. This is particularly obvious with marijuana and, in early adolescents, with their greed for new experiences and urgent wish to escape in a pleasurable masturbatory way from the frustrations of the age period, it may occur very rapidly:

John was the tall fourteen-year-old son of divorced parents. He had been an early developer and had both sexual experiences, having had intercourse four times, and had also used grass since the age of twelve. After he was caught stealing to get money to buy more, his father and stepmother moved to the country, and he was kept under more control than he had been when he lived with his mother. He said, "As soon as I can get back to marijuana I will. I like its effect and would use it daily. It's not dangerous, so why not? It's better than sex since you don't have to hassle with someone else to get it. Besides sex is not as good as everyone said it would be, grass is better."

The dependence may also be on the regressive experience (Weider and Kaplan, 1969). One girl talked of how "warm and cosy" downers made her feel. Alternately, the implicit permission of some drugs for impulsive loss of control may be sought. This loss of control may be psychological, as with such hallucinogens as LSD and is particularly appealing in a society that alienates emotional from other experiences. It may also be an outlet for physical aggression, not uncommon in highly controlled individuals who intermittently abuse alcohol.

Obviously, there is no clear distinction between the meaning of habituation and addiction, and in 1965 the World Health Organization recommended the term "drug dependence" be substituted for both. Nevertheless, in 1966 the United Nations Commission on Narcotic Drugs decided to keep the old definitions.

The liability of drugs to generate compulsive self-administrative behavior obviously varies. Precise information is lacking, although age seems significant: Adolescents for example, probably are less likely to be involved in this way with opiates and more likely with cannabis than adults. The commonly available reinforcing drugs that specifically influence the hypothalamus for adults rank in the following order (after J. E. Villarreal):

1. *Cocaine*
2. *Parenteral heroin, dilaudid, morphine, methadone— "snorting" the above*
3. *Intravenous amphetamines*
4. *Intravenous barbiturates*
5. *Oral narcotics*
6. *Oral barbiturate-like sedatives with quick onset of action, Nicotine (inhalation)*
7. *Oral alcohol*
8. *Oral amphetamines, Solvent sniffing in some adolescent social groups*
9. *Cannabis (high doses) (?)*
10. *Oral barbiturate-like sedatives with slow onset of action*

Nonreinforcing drugs are not necessarily less dangerous. Hallucinogens such as LSD do not affect the hypothalamus; nevertheless, any motivation not to use them is dissolved after a variable intake in different adolescents.

Psychological Effects of Different Drugs

Unsuccessful attempts have been made to equate various types of pharmacological effects of drugs with different levels of ego regression, for example, the results of taking opium (Mahler, 1968) with the psychological state in the characteristic behavior pattern of the second half of the first year of life. It is probably impossible to draw hard and fast lines as to what the psychic effect of any one drug might be, particularly as their psychologi- and toxicological effects often seem idiosyncratic.

Adolescents are particularly likely to become dependent on the psychological effect of drugs, and this dependence may occur with or without physical reinforcement and hence addiction. Those who are dependent on the drug experience show a significant degree of total personality involvement with drugs and the people who use them. They may crave either the relief of psychic tension that the drug gives them or they may seek a specific psychological sensation. (Chein *et al.*, 1964). When they take drugs, adolescents seem to be seeking satiation and contentment in the same way a baby demands its bottle. The concept of the drug-dependent adolescent who is intolerant of frustration and is unable to make affectionate and meaningful object relationships would appear to be valid (Hartman, 1969).

Etiology of Drug Use

Drug use can be understood, as can all other adolescent behavior, by looking at the interplay of personal, social, and intrafamilial factors. Like sexuality, drug use tends in the early part of adolescence to be hidden from parents and society generally; by the middle stage of adolescence use is more overt and possibly defiant of society's norms.

Early adolescents in Western culture first experimented with mood-changing drugs. It is ironic that as an attempted step to adult behavior early adolescents identify with the infantile and sometimes dangerous habits of their parents. They use, in particular those drugs about which the adult world has mixed feelings, drugs adults use to induce some degree of infantile regression; typically these are alcohol and tobacco, although now marijuana and sometimes sedatives or stimulants may be added to this dyad. Any drug about which adults have mixed feelings, that induces the infantile experiences associated with ego regression, and that is widely and easily available is likely to be tried by early adolescents.

Smoking and drinking are both related to peer-group expectations as well as adult behavior, but alcohol, other than wine, is usually rejected because the early adolescent does not like the taste of beer or spirits. Wines, particularly those with a sweet, fruity flavor, are often enjoyed but are rarely abused by adolescents for many reasons: Wine drinking is surrounded by many cultural controls, especially because it may be taken as part of a family, religious, or mealtime ritual. Although its use is increasingly common in midadolescence, wine is rarely used by early adolescents as part of a rebellious acting out of angry feelings directed at parents. Furthermore, the unpleasant hangover associated with excessive wine drinking spoils it as a way to reaching a state of psychic infantile bliss.

Although its taste may not be initially enjoyed, tobacco may be abused more or less regularly from early adolescence onward. Like drug taking, cigarette smoking is related to parental behavior (Emery *et al.*, 1967). Parental attitudes about cigarette use are similar to those toward sexuality; it is said to be acceptable only as adult behavior. Furthermore, its equation with danger in the future allows adolescents to reinforce their own sense of immortality with what has come to be felt as death-defying behavior. Because to smoke is to seek after an infantile experience both early adolescent boys and girls, with mothers who smoke, are more likely to become dependent on cigarettes than those who have nonsmoking parents. Because it also represents a step to adult status, early adolescents with older brothers or sisters who smoke are more likely to use cigarettes than those with nonsmoking relatives. Adults who smoke cigarettes during the childhood of their children up until the time when they are ten or eleven are likely to discover that the chances of dependence during adolescence are considerably increased. Because of pressure from children, parents may stop smoking when their children reach puberty. It is not unusual for twelve- and thirteen-year-olds, who read newspapers and watch television, to feel that their parents are being suicidal when they smoke. One boy wrote over all his parents' cigarette packets "nicotine kills." The paradox of the situation is that the very children who in early adolescence were pressuring their parents not to smoke, may themselves smoke heavily as adolescents.

Early-adolescent drug experimentation is associated with early adolescent experimentation with sexuality. Just as the pubertal child deals with the reawakening of sexual impulses by reexperimentation with the masturbatory activity of infancy and childhood (Miller, 1969), so drug taking is associated with the revival of the omnipotent dependent wishes of infants.

Psychological Significance of Infantile Behavior

Early adolescents who do not experiment with smoking, drinking, or other drugs do not necessarily have particularly strong personality controls. On the contrary, failure to experiment with any drugs may be understood, particularly in boys, in the same way as the failure to masturbate.

Before significance is ascribed to the fact that an adolescent cannot allow any self-experimentation that induces an infantile psychological state, environmental and intrafamilial attitudes must be taken into account. A powerful parent who does not use drugs and thus gives children a consistent message may make early adolescent drug experimentation impossible. Others may not experiment with drugs because they are very dependent on a peer-group that itself forbids the use of drugs. Some delinquent groups refuse to allow any drug taking and this habit is, of course, forbidden in older adolescents by such groups as The Children of God and The Process.

The personality style of adolescents may forbid experimentation with intoxicants. Some individuals do not try drugs because of religious convictions, either their own, those of parents, or those of other important adults with whom they have meaningful emotional contacts. Those religious groups that cannot allow infantile experiences—autoerotic sex or drugs—may substitute for these with intense religious experiences. Alternately, they may force individuals within their sect to attempt to resolve conflicts with various types of reaction formation, often including excessive puritanism.

Some cultural and religious groups cannot allow regressive sexual activity. When adolescents are forbidden to experiment with infantile types of sexuality such as masturbation, many solutions are sought. The interdiction may be ignored; repression may be intense with consequent affective isolation: In some the need is met by early intercourse. Masturbation is then replaced by an apparent heterosexuality, which is, in reality, masturbatory in nature. A girl may become the vehicle for a boy's demonstrating to himself his capacity to control his own ego regression and also his feelings of sexual excitement. In other adolescents a failure to masturbate may be associated with late development into puberty.

Drug Experimentation in Midadolescence

After the flurry of experimentation early in the pubertal period, there is a new episode of drug reexperimentation toward

the end of the first year of midadolescence (Miller, 1969). Environmental pressures play a significant role in this. Early adolescent drug experimentation that uses "parental" drugs can
be an initiation rite to the adolescent group; the midadolescent
who becomes a regular user of intoxicants, often those of which
parents disapprove, may do this to reinforce a tenuous sense of
personal identity by continuing intense peer-group involvement.

> Douglas was a fifteen-year-old boy who was seen by a psychiatrist
> because of intense overdependence on marijuana. He smoked four
> or five joints daily, used the drug while in school, and began to
> make D's and E's, having been an A student. Diagnostically, he
> was suffering from a failure to develop a firm sense of identity,
> and he went, therefore, to a small boarding school with close
> relationships between staff and students. Of this setting he said,
> "The staff actually cares about you. It matters to them who and
> what you are and what you do. In high school there were a few
> good teachers who might have cared but they had no time."
>   Douglas desperately wanted to belong to a new peer group.
> He said, "They put me in a room with a boy who got high on shit
> all the time. I did not want to smoke, but some of the kids used
> alcohol so I started that. I get stoned on wine about twice a week.
> I get sick, but I need to belong."

This middle-stage adolescent felt impelled, largely because
of social pressure, to seek out what was to him a new drug. The
type, as always, depended on a current peer-group fashionable
norm. Douglas' parents did not drink and, as is usual with drug
use at his age, the drug chosen was less significantly related to
parental behavior and attitudes than might have been the case
in puberty. It was, however, significantly related to the behavior
of older adolescents in the group, another typical aspect of drug
use at this age. Adolescents are vulnerable to what the peer
group–at–large perceives as fashionable: There is a feeling today
that trying drugs is the thing to do. In cultures where alcohol is
the drug of choice, for example in part of Scandinavia, many

middle-stage adolescent boys feel that they ought to get drunk. Those British working-class groups who take stimulant pills feel that they should get "blocked"; those middle-class groups who use marijuana feel that they must get turned on or smashed. In the United States legislation allowing eighteen-year-olds to purchase alcohol will produce an increased incidence of alcoholism in fifteen- to sixteen-year olds.

At one time a middle-class youth tried drugs and sex about two years later than his working-class counterpart, but this now appears to be changing. From clinical evidence the end of the pubertal stage of development, about fifteen in boys, is becoming the peak age in all social classes for starting to experiment with drugs other than tobacco.

Early adolescent drug taking tends to imitate adult norms; midadolescents who abuse drugs act in defiance of them. Socioculturally, drugs may be used as part of a phony war against adults; adolescents who group together to use drugs often appear to believe that they are a group of nonconformists fighting a corrupt and conformist adult society that wishes to attack them. It is, however, ironic that the adolescent who is least sure of his capacity to be independent is most likely to take drugs and become dependent upon them.

The difference between the use of alcohol and marijuana appears to be that adolescents often take alcohol not to get drunk but to participate in what they see to be an acceptable adult ritual. They may also like the taste. Marijuana is rarely used in low dosage when its intoxicant effect is mild, unless joints are handed around at pop concerts and the like. It is mostly used in greater dosage although some adolescents attempt to titrate the degree of intoxication they may experience (Hollister, 1968). Those adolescents who try alcohol and cigarettes at the beginning of puberty and then stop may become regular users of either or both at midadolescence. Those young people who are regular users of cigarettes in early adolescence may become intensely dependent on them as midadolescents.

Drugs Used by Adolescents

The type of drugs used by adolescents depends on their personal history of drug taking. Early adolescents who become regular users of marijuana seem more likely in midadolescence, or sooner, to try other hallucinogens. For example, midadolescents who use LSD all seem to have a history of more than a previous experimental use of marijuana. The drug used also varies from one year to the next, from country to country, within institutions in any given society, and between different social groups. Drug abuse appears to vary with fashion; amphetamine derivatives may be preferred at one time and in one culture; sometime else hallucinogens appear to be the drugs of choice. Lower socioeconomic-group black and white early adolescents may use glue and paint thinners for their intoxicant effect in parts of the United States and continental Europe. In Britain their use is rare, except in penal institutions. Marijuana was used in Sweden for many years before it was used in neighboring Finland. From clinical observation its use is common among middle-class students in Britain and in the United States. Deprived and black adolescents in the ghettos of American cities, and the British working class, have been likely to abuse amphetamines for years. Only more recently have these groups begun to use hashish, and LSD usage is rare compared to its middle-class incidence.

STIMULANTS

Stimulant pills used by British working-class youth have special names, such as "black bombers" (durophet) and "purple hearts" (dexamyl). In the United States stimulant pills are "bennies," "dex," "crystals," "dominoes," "minstrels," "purple hearts"; dexamil pills are known as "Christmas Trees." In the United States all stimulants carry the generic name of "speed." In Britain this name is reserved for methedrine. In the United

States those young people who inject methedrine are usually known as "speed freaks." In Britain speed is always injected. When methedrine ampoules were taken out of the pharmacopoeia in Britain, those individuals who used it injected the powdered tablets.

When the use of mood-changing and mind-bending drugs spread out of the black ghetto and the world of jazz music in the United States to the white population, the first drugs to be widley abused were the stimulants; in particular, amphetamine derivatives. Prior to 1955 these drugs had something of a vogue among students who used them to cope, they felt, more adequately with examinations, a habit that still continues. In America stimulants began to be pervasively used among middle-class white adolescents at about that time. About three years later they began to be the drug of choice among working-class British youth. By 1960 the use of amphetamine–barbiturate mixtures was common in large cities and in new towns that had not been designed to meet emotional needs. Since the use of amphetamines was more culturally aberrant by the middle class than by the working class, the few academic middle-class young people who used them were more likely to be severely psychologically disturbed.

Initially, the amphetamine derivatives were prescribed by physicians mostly for middle-aged women as antidepressants and appetite supressors. The women passed them on to their children; family practitioners did not apparently recognize that particularly in lower socioeconomic groups a good drug given to mothers is implicitly prescribed for the whole family. Adolescents who felt unsure of themselves and complained of boredom, emptiness, and depression have often been given their mother's pills. The underworld rapidly discovered that adolescents could take stimulants in excessive dosage and that there were enormous profits to be made. Those people who steal pills and methedrine, which sold to adolescents for a profit of up to 3000 percent, either from factories or distribution points, get considerably less than the usual retail price for them. Methedrine for injection (twenty-milligram ampoules) was legally used to facilitate psychiatric abreactions and in the treatment of the coma caused by alcoholism; the tablet (five milligrams) was also given as an appetite suppressor. Methedrine is abused specifically for its side effects, which include restlessness, euphoria, and extreme talkativeness. Up to eight injections a day are taken by addicts who go on jags lasting up to six days. Individual doses may be very large, and while on the jag the subject does not eat or sleep. Each injection sends an intense pleasurable orgasmic flush throughout the whole body, and the user becomes fascinated with his own thoughts and feelings.

In the aggressive and sexual activity of disturbed adolescents, there is often a relationship between the implicit and explicit messages parents give their children and the latters' explicit behavior. The same is true for drug abuse. Parents say that they do not wish their children to take drugs but act as if they do.

> Larry, a fifteen-year-old schoolboy, was hospitalized because of his aggressive antisocial behavior; he began to abuse amphetamines at age thirteen. He was first given them by his doctor father because he slept excessively when having to work for an examination. The boy felt that his father was "always giving me pills," and he used this behavior to justify his own drug abuse. The father was told about this by the psychiatric social worker and asked not to give the boy drugs. During a visit the boy complained to his father of headaches. The latter immediately gave him some aspirin. The same day the boy absconded from the hospital and was picked up by the police one week later in a commune of boys, all of whom were drug toxic.

The typical symptons of amphetamine use in large doses are tachycardia and peripheral vasoconstriction with dryness of the mouth. Along with a transient euphoria, sleeplessness is quite common. If amphetamines are taken over several days, their psychic effect seems to be similar to that experienced when any individual stays awake past the usual barrier of fatigue. Preludin (phenmetrazine) and the amphetamines both can cause psychosis. Cases of individuals who became psychotic after a single dose, as well as after several, of amphetamines have been reported (Connell, 1958). The capacity of an adolescent to tolerate the physical abuse of large toxic quantities of stimulants is remarkable. Some individuals die from methedrine overdosage, but most adolescents appear not to suffer permanent damage to their circulatory system. Nevertheless, abnormal electrocardiographs have been reported in adolescents on such stimulants, and endarteritis has recently been reported in those adolescents who abuse amphetamines. After overdosage stimulant users may be restless, overexcited, and difficult to control some twenty-four hours after the last dose has been taken.

In a toxic psychosis due to an overdose of amphetamines the individual is typically paranoid:

A fifteen-year-old ran away from a school for delinquent boys and was later picked up by the police blocked on speed. The police called the principal of the school, who collected the boy in his car. As he was driving back, the boy suddenly tried to wrench the steering wheel from his hands, screaming, "We must get out. We are being attacked by a gang of murderers who are firing machine guns at us from the sidewalk."

One effect of drug use, insofar as there is a need to obtain a network of human relationships, is demonstrated by adolescents who become involved in pushing drugs. In order to obtain money drug users often develop a special relationship with an adult pusher and get security from this grown-up or older adolescent.

Rob, a seventeen-year-old boy, suddenly got the feeling that he must have some amphetamine pills. Having no money, he went to a local cafe, notorious for its drug scene, where he knew he would find the man who could find him a supply. He found the adult pusher who offered him a drink, gave him a sandwich, and then went off to make a telephone call. He then drove Rob across town to a club, again gave him food and drink, and shortly appeared with the pills. Rob was told how much he should ask for the pills and how much he was to give the pusher.

Most adolescents who regularly use drugs discover that it is easy to find an escape from anxiety and frustration in this way. They develop the notion that under no circumstances should they suffer psychological pain. The intermittent urge to use drugs as a medication to relieve psychic pain, a method similar to that implicit in the prescriptions of many family practitioners, can become total dependence:

> Sixteen-year-old Michael was referred to a psychiatric clinic because he was dependent on marijuana. Two years earlier, when he was leaving school with his best friend, the latter dashed across the road ahead of him and was killed by a passing car. Michael was upset and unable to talk to anybody about the death. Two or three days later he wandered to a section of town where drugs were readily available. In a coffee bar he was offered marijuana, which he smoked. This relieved his tension. He began to take the drug on weekends, then even more frequently. His school work steadily deteriorated and by the time he was seen by a psychiatrist, he was constantly toxic and high.

If Michael had not discovered that marijuana relieved his tension, life and the passage of time might have helped to solve his problem. Instead, he began to use the drug as self-medication.

The relationship between drugs and sexual anxieties is fairly clear. Shakespeare wrote in Macbeth:

> What three things does drink especially provoke? Marry sir, nose painting, sleep and urine. Lechery, sir, it provokes and

unprovokes—it provokes the desire but it takes away the performance.

The amphetamine–barbiturate pills taken in high dosage lead almost universally to a situation in which boys become impotent and cannot get an erection. For the boy who is unsure of his own potency anyway or who has problems of control, the ability to make oneself impotent and then potent is obviously important. One boy said, "I don't care about the chicks at all when I am blocked on Saturday, but it's wonderful to fuck on Monday." Another talked of how exciting it was to find that he could again get an erection. Some boys justify their inability to get a girl by quoting the fact that on pills intercourse is impossible.

The use of stimulants is as particular to the age range of adolescents as is juvenile delinquency. Statistically (Gibbens, 1968), it has been shown that those adolescents who engage in delinquent acts for the first time at the end of puberty are likely to be conforming to the accepted social norms of society by the time they are twenty-one. Delinquent acts are typically associated with the struggle for a secure masculine identity in a socioeconomically underprivileged boy. On this basis, an experiment in model building showed that a penal setting in a social system designed to enhance a boy's feelings of masculine identity produced less recidivism after discharge than the usual more punitive setting (Miller, 1965).

Providing they are able to make meaningful emotional relationships with others, most disturbed adolescents with identity problems tend to consolidate some more or less secure feelings of self by young adulthood. There is apparently a built-in recovery process to antisocial behavior, although as adults ex-delinquents may replay conflicts with their children. Like delinquent activity, drug abuse, particularly of stimulants, appears to be related to a search for a secure identity.

Many adolescents who abuse amphetamines in their adolescent years may give them up in association with some type of adult adjustment and more secure identity at the age of nineteen to twenty-one. Thus, just as many adolescents grow out of criminal activity, many appear to spontaneously recover from drug abuse.

SEDATIVES AND ALCOHOL

Sedatives and alcohol are both used by adolescents mostly after the middle stage of the age period. Tolerance to both these drugs develops apparently as rapidly with adolescents as adults, at any rate from clinical evidence. This differs from the hard drugs, in which, it appears harder for adolescents to develop a tolerance, and it seems to take higher doses to become addicted. Short acting barbiturates are typically used as downers along with hypnotics such as methaqualone (Quaaludes). Librium (chlordiazepoxide hydrochloride) is also used in this way. Adolescents, in taking sedatives, hypnotics, and alcohol seek not sedation but a high; most are not aware at all of the dangers of either barbiturates or methaqualone. The young alcoholic behaves like his adult peer; he denies his dependence and is reluctant to seek help.

HALLUCINOGENS—MARIJUANA

Marijuana, whose active principal is tetrahydrocannabinol (THC), is derived from the hemp plant *Cannabis sativa* and has been the subject of controversy since ancient times. It remained in the United States pharmacopoeia until 1937 and was used for a variety of psychosomatic complaints, in particular, asthma, dysmenorrhea, and migraine.

Drugs prepared from hemp vary in potency depending on the climate, the soil, the type of cultivation, and the method of preparation. The drug is obtained almost exclusively from the female plant. In Britain, where most marijuana comes from the Middle East and is of fairly similar potency, the terms "grass" and "hashish" were used fairly interchangeably for some time. In the United States, where much of the drug is obtained from the leaves of the uncultivated plants, marijuana tends to be called grass. The extract of the plant resin, hash, is usually more potent than grass; the best hashish is thought to come from Mexico.

Marijuana is historically a drug of protest. Its abuse to dependence is currently associated with a peaceful dropping out from an overcentralized society, but among young people marijuana has long been associated with a withdrawal from the established norms of society. In the Middle East in the eleventh century the protest was violent. Hasan Sabah formed a secret society of Mohammedan Ismaelites to spread a new doctrine through an authoritarian, yet loosely integrated, environment. A compact force that could strike suddenly at the authority of the state would lead to its disintegration, and the new doctrine would take over. This group, with its grand master, terrorized Persia and Egypt for centuries by its sudden and effective assassinations; it became a state within a state. Hasan motivated the young members of the group by feeding them hashish after their murderous attacks. The intention was to give them a glimpse of the sensual joys that awaited them in heaven; ultimately they obeyed him with robot like obedience.

The Crusaders came into contact with this group in the twelfth century and learned to know them as assassins (hashishim) from the part that hashish played in the life of the young novice. The analogy with the present century is more than apparent. Marijuana is the drug of the rebellious young in all Western societies in which it is used; in itself, it is not normally associated with violence, but it was commonly used after the violent outbursts of the late sixties by those involved in this type of radical protest.

When marijuana is eaten, its effects seem to last about twice as long as when it is smoked—five to twelve hours. The cigarette or joint usually gives an effect lasting about two to four hours. The amount smoked affects the degree of intoxication, but, unlike wine, it is rarely used only for its taste, which is thought by some to be quite revolting. One boy said, "Now I know why it is called shit." The price of marijuana varies depending on the available supply. It is very often given by adolescents to each other rather than sold, and it is usually smoked in groups. It is not unusual for young adults to give marijuana cigarettes to younger adolescents.

The flushed face of the stoned early adolescent is easier to notice than with older individuals. There is a distinctly sweet smell to the drug that can be noticed on the breath and clothing of smokers, sometimes for a day after it has been smoked. If the drug is used by adolescents inside school or in their parents' automobile it is reasonable to assume that they have an unconscious wish to be caught.

Marijuana intoxication typically is initiated by an anxious period that lasts for about ten to thirty minutes. Because of this, many individuals who suffer from nonspecific anxiety attacks use marijuana as a way of giving themselves a reality reason for their anxiety. One boy experienced intense anxiety just before going to bed at night; he therefore began to smoke marijuana nightly: "It makes me even more anxious, and I get very paranoid and think the police are after me. But I know what it's about and strangely I feel better." After initial anxiety the individual may become calm and euphoric; the body may feel light, and visual and auditory perception is sometimes enhanced. Just as with alcohol, the individual may feel that his conversation is particularly brilliant. This is a type of chattering, and the individual who is high on marijuana is often not making a meaningful emotional communication with others. Time sense is distorted, and depersonalization and splitting are common. Paranoid ideas are not unusual, yet the individual may appear quite bland about them. Under the influence of marijuana, adolescents often appear dreamy and uncaring, although they can also feel impotent. Marijuana leads to a psychological withdrawal from involvement in the world outside the self, a withdrawal associated with a preoccupation with a fantasy world of daydreams.

The psychological effect of marijuana depends on whether or not it is taken as part of a group experience and on the mood of the user. When adolescents feel depressed or anxious before taking the drug, marijuana is often said to make this worse. Occasionally, adolescents report vivid, aggressive fantasies while under the influence of marijuana. One boy insisted that he had stabbed another to death, another that he had drowned a girl in the local river. In neither case was there any evidence that this had happened.

The effects of marijuana are highly variable and the results of studies of its effects contradictory (Grunspoon, 1969). The drug has less effect on driving skills than does alcohol; but clinical studies do not take note of a volitional disinclination to pay attention, an aspect of driving that is reported by many patients. The drug has not been studied on people who have used it in large quantities over a long period of time, and the amount of active principal in any joint is, of course, variable. Intellectual functioning and motivation to study, when marijuana is taken repeatedly, seems to be impaired as measured by academic progress. Some students, however, appear to do better in their school work when they are chronically intoxicated; these are often very disturbed young people who use the drug as a tranquilizer.

Adolescents who become dependent on marijuana may spend most of their days in a state of intoxication, and they can make no satisfactory relationships with anyone. This total drug dependence is associated with an inability to cope with the complexities of life. It has been said that marijuana is less habit forming than tobacco, but the clinical evidence suggests that this is not true for adolescents.

Eighteen-year-old Robert smoked six joints daily, ate inadequately, and dropped out of school. He was hospitalized because of his inability to care for himself for a period of three weeks. He was not able to smoke marijuana and his intense passive–dependent needs were automatically met by being in the hospital. Diagnostically he was thought to be a borderline psychotic and his EEG showed abnormalities typical of marijuana overdosage with rapid beta waves. He had no obvious heterosexual wishes but experienced an intermittent craving to "get blasted on hash." Three weeks after discharge from the hospital, while in twice weekly psychotherapy, Robert began to smoke grass again. Within two more weeks he was back on large doses of hashish and he sought rehospitalization because he felt he could not stop taking marijuana without such support.

There is no evidence of physical dependence on marijuana, but emotional dependence on the high can be intense. Marijuana use may be symptomatic, as with alcohol, when emotionally vulnerable human beings use it as an escape from conflict. Alternatively, it may be essential when it fulfills a personality need. In many ways its use is then psychologically very similar to that of a perversion.

It would appear from clinical evidence that once marijuana is regularly smoked, dependence on it becomes more likely. It was used, for example, by a moderately depressed boy of eighteen for thirty-six hours each weekend because "I find the strain of life intolerable." Its use as a transitional object (Winnicott, 1953) to meet profound emotional needs is demonstrated by a fifteen-year-old boy who smoked grass once following an acute traumatic episode and then began to smoke five joints of hashish daily. He was noticed because of a sudden decline in his school work.

The belief that marijuana is not addictive may mean that adults do not take adolescent requests for help, implicit when they get themselves caught with drugs, sufficiently seriously. The following example illustrates this as well as the tendency for girls who use promiscuous sex to try to solve their emotional difficulties to use marijuana also.

Anne began to smoke marijuana when she was eleven; at that time a friend of hers was killed in a road accident, her parents had separated and her mother was ill in the hospital. Anne liked the effect of the drug, and by the time she was twelve she was promiscuous and smoking three times weekly. She was either given joints by older boys or bought the drug fr m pushers. At thirteen she tried some pills that she thought were heroin but gave these up, and at fourteen she tried LSD once. Anne was frightened by the effect of this, although she was tripping with many other youngsters, and so she continued only on marijuana. She also borrowed sleeping pills that had been prescribed for her mother.

Anne asked for help in the following way: She was caught smoking cigarettes in the school toilet and as a punishment was told to write an essay on the evils of tobacco. She wrote one full of incomprehensible jargon, and when seen by her teacher she described her marijuana smoking. The teacher warned her of its harmful effects but, apparently, thinking the drug was not very dangerous because it was nonaddictive, did nothing. Three weeks later, in a state of severe confusion Anne was seen by a psychiatrist. She revealed a whole network of fourteen- and fifteen-year-olds in a similar state to herself, and she was hospitalized. Diagnostically Anne had never really reached the psychological state associated with adolescence for she was suffering from a severe hysterical personality disorder.

HALLUCINOGENS—LYSERGIC ACID DIETHYL-AMIDE, PHENCYCLIDINE (THC), PSILOCYBIN AND MESCALINE

The most commonly used synthetic hallucinogen carrying the generic name acid has been LSD 25. It was synthesized in 1938, and discovered to be hallucinogenic in 1943; it is one of the most potent mind-affecting substances known. One hundred to two hundred fifty micrograms given by mouth causes symptoms in thirty to forty-five minutes; if it is given intramuscularly symptoms appear in fifteen to twenty minutes. In small doses, LSD seems to act as a psychic stimulant; in larger doses it ultimately becomes a depressant. The experience associated with taking LSD, whether as a clear liquid, a tablet, or as an intravenous injection, lasts from one to six hours. Psychotic episodes lasting three to four months and then apparently totally remitting have been seen. Repeating the dose of LSD 25 while still on a trip does not enhance the hallucinating experience, although it may increase the duration of its effect. After a "trip" a mild fatigue is common (Hoffer and Osmond, 1967). Specifically, the effects of LSD 25 have been divided into six stages, but these grossly overlap. In general, the experience varies from a flight of ideas, with tension, irritability, and perceptual changes, to a state of preoccupation with somatic discomfort. This is often followed by confusion, perceptual distortion, and paranoia, all of which may elide into a stage of dual reality, in which the patient feels as if his inner world is being explored. The effects of LSD can be summarized by saying that the drug basically impairs the ego functions, followed by a burst through of primary-process thinking.

There is an apparent connection between the hallucinatory state induced by LSD and schizophrenia, and it was for this reason that it was used experimentally for a period of time on volunteer subjects to try to induce schizophrenia chemically. LSD had a vogue during the early 1960s in a type of abreactive therapy, but the results did not justify the initial enthusiasm. It now appears to be the treatment of choice in few, if any, psychiatric illnesses, and the drug is banned from legal production in both the United States and Britain. LSD was first used illicitly in the United States, followed by Britain and Europe. Sometimes a mixture of LSD and strychnine is taken; supposedly this gives especially vivid hallucinatory effects. Other hallucinogens reported in common use are psilocybin and mescaline. It is probable that street drugs sold as these contain neither. None have been found in Maryland, for example, for two years. Psilocybin, used originally by the Aztecs, is very similar to LSD and is the active psychotomimetic of a Mexican mushroom. It is likely to produce a chronic toxic psychosis, and the visions it generates are rich in color patterns. Psilocybin is, however, notable in that there are never reports of erotic experiences. Its usual dose is 10 milligrams for 135 pounds of body weight. A cross tolerance to psilocybin and LSD may develop. Mescaline was isolated in 1896 from mescal buttons, which are used in South and Central America, and is also used as part of Indian religious rituals in the form of peyote, of which it is the active principal. Its typically toxic effect is that it allows the individual to feel removed from earthly cares. The hallucinations are concerned with perceptual changes, particularly in the areas of hearing, smell, and taste; quite often these are pleasant. The usual dose of mescaline is from 400 to 750 milligrams and very prolonged reactions are common. A relatively recent drug which seems to be replacing LSD is phencyclidine. Wrongly called THC, used as an animal tranquilizer, it gives a peculiar warm, cozy physical effect, "like being cuddled." Steadily increasing doses are often taken.

RESPONSE TO HALLUCINOGENS

The hallucinogenic drugs are dangerous and their effects idiosyncratic and unpredictable, apart from the fact that drugs purchased on the street are often mixes of strange chemical combinations.

The use of hallucinogenic drugs is most common among late adolescents, often university students and drop-outs, but it is not rare among thirteen- or fourteen-year-olds, and regular users aged nine have been seen. Often philosophical constructs are given to hallucinogenic usage: Many adolescents who take LSD and other drugs begin to be intensely preoccupied with a type of pseudoexistentialist philosophy. Hallucinogens are particularly associated with a conscious desire on the part of adolescents to opt out of society because of its corruption. Often these adolescents appear to suffer from somewhat passive-

aggressive personality styles, but it is difficult to know whether
a chronic user of hallucinogens could have dealt with the complexities of societies in any case. Many hallucinogenic fantasies
are highly unpleasant; pleasant fantasies, erotic and otherwise,
are relatively rare depending on the drug used. The latter may
last for only a short period of time in any hallucinogenic experience, which in itself may last for hours or even longer.

> On his seventh LSD trip sixteen-year-old Kenneth was grossly
> psychotic for three days showing every evidence of an acute
> toxic psychosis. He showed a classical schizophrenic picture. He
> heard the voices of angels and the devil, believed everyone was
> about to kill him, and became dangerously aggressive. On the
> fourth day he had occasional nightmares.
>   Psychological tests one week later showed no evidence of a
> borderline state; presumably Kenneth had experienced a toxic
> psychosis.

Some adolescents, perhaps as an idiosyncratic response, perhaps
because they were previously suffering from a borderline psychosis, appear to suffer from a prolonged psychological disorder
after taking hallucinogens. One symptom noticed in adolescents
who have taken many trips (some patients claim to have had up
to 300) is a quite affectless appearance. This can be seen when
they are talking, even though they have not taken the drug
recently. It becomes extremely difficult for these adolescents to
make meaningful emotional contacts with others. One described
this as an experience of feeling "like a tape recorder." Often
they suffer from a subtle confusional state, which the interviewer
recognizes because the patient's thoughts do not hang together.
Of all the drugs on which intense psychological dependence is
possible, the hallucinogens appear to be the most dangerous for
two reasons: First, the users of hallucinogens, particularly LSD
takers, are one of the few groups of young people who have no
wish to stop when they do become drug dependent and are
aware of it; secondly, a marked aftereffect that may last for

years, a flashback, is quite common. One doctor, for example, reported getting a flashback effect for a year on hearing the same piece of music that had been playing on the one occasion when the drug was taken.

Clinical evidence of organic brain damage after many trips may be seen. One youth reported that he could no longer multiply six times six but had to add the sixes together. Highly concrete thinking becomes common, and the capacity to make abstractions appears to be impaired. On the other hand, adolescents who were dependent on LSD, may appear to be making satisfactory life adjustments with no treatment some two to three years after they have stopped taking the drug. Suicide on LSD trips is not rare, and bursts of wild maniacal excitement have been observed:

> A seventeen-year-old boy was having intercourse with his girlfriend while under the influence of LSD. He suddenly became extremely violent and attacked her and then completely destroyed the furniture in the apartment (his father's) in which he was staying. The girl locked herself in the bathroom for several hours, and the boy was in a catatoniclike stupor for two to three hours after having ingested the drug. The apartment had to be broken into in order to help him and his girl.

As might be expected, the chemical effect of the drug brings preexisting pathology to the surface of consciousness. Diagnostically the above patient was suffering from acute identity confusion. The destruction of the family furniture is a well-known phenomenon in this state.

OPIUM DERIVATIVES

An unknown number of adolescents involved in progressive drug usage move from marijuana or stimulant pills to methedrine injections and opium derivatives. There is no evidence that marijuana causes heroin addiction, although almost all heroin addicts have previously been regular, as distinct from experimental, users of marijuana. Since almost all adolescents experiment with cigarettes and alcohol, a previous experimental use of marijuana would not in itself be significant. Emotional dependence on marijuana may follow addiction to heroin after its withdrawal; many heroin users withdrawn with methadone substitute marijuana for heroin.

Heroin addiction may lead to physical deterioration and ultimately to the death of the addict, although the rate of physical deterioration is idiosyncratic to the individual. It also appears to depend on the technique by which heroin is used; its degree of purity, and the use of clean or dirty syringes.

> A twenty-year-old youth was offered and took heroin while under the influence of marijuana. He liked the effect and began to think he could safely use heroin. He was brought by a friend to a house full of people who were on the drug. He called a psychiatrist who had seen him previously and said, "I must have help. I cannot become like them."

It is not possible to predict the dosage of heroin that will lead to physical dependence on drugs such as heroin and other opium derivatives. Some adolescents claim to have injected two or three grains of heroin daily for a period of weeks, either under their skin (popping) or into their veins (mainlining), without being dependent on the drug. On the other hand, addiction with one sixth of a grain daily has been observed. In Britain, where the heroin is pure, some disturbed adolescents will know of one person who has taken himself off the drug with no apparent ill-effects. They may then reject the risk of heroin addiction as a reason for avoiding the drug. In the United States, where the heroin is cut to a varying degree, when an adolescent comes off a dose of eight to ten caps a day (a cap equals one dollar's worth of the drug) with no withdrawal symptons, it may well be the dosage of heroin was small. Addicts usually can tell the strength of their cap from the type of high that they obtain when they inject the drug. It is usual, for example, for the popularity of any one dealer to decrease if the heroin cut becomes weaker.

Britain has a particular problem with hard drugs because it is possible to become a registered addict. Since there is no way of telling the exact amount that any one addict may need, and since addicts are very often unable to mobilize themselves to earn a living, such addicts tend to live by selling the spare drugs they obtain by claiming a dose greater than their need. Sometimes adolescents in Britain are introduced to drug taking by registered addict friends who give them heroin.

> A fourteen-year-old boy who had taken heroin only once insisted that he managed to get himself registered as an addict. He said that he was given two grains of heroin and four ampoules of methedrine daily by a drug clinic.

Heroin addiction in Britain is not associated with widespread and pervasive crime to sustain the habit as is the case in America.

In the United States adolescents commonly graduate to heroin from methedrine because speed is known to be so dangerous. As younger adolscents become involved in regular and then progressive drug use, the spread of addiction to early adolescents becomes inevitable, although the preferred drug may turn out to be alcohol rather than heroin.

The Family, Social Networks, and the Profit Motive

The etiology of drug abuse can be understood if intrafamilial, social, and individual factors are considered. Only when these are taken into account can treatment plans be adequately formulated for the chronic drug dependent adolescent. Apart from the etiology of disturbed character formation, which finds its roots in the emotional deprivation of infancy (particularly multiple handling, parental inconsistency, physical and emotional abuse), families can convey to their children either an attitude

that all pain must be magically relieved or that some frustration
can appropriately be borne. The drug scene, other than in
severely deprived groups, was created in the relationship between family practitioners, their adult patients, and their children.

The profit motive is, not surprisingly, at its maximum on
the drug scene. The underworld has rapidly discovered both that
adolescents could take drugs in high dosage and that there are
enormous profits to be made.

Many admired figures of the youth world boast of their
drug taking, particularly marijuana, and thus offer adolescents
a model. Young teachers may make no bones of this type of
drug use. Besides the drugs given by older adolescents to each
other adolescents who deal in drugs to support their own habit,
have usually little hesitation in selling to a younger age group.
In universities it is not unusual for some staff to offer drugs to
students as they might alcohol. One psychology professor regularly invites students to his house to smoke hash with him.

Many adults are quite unaware that obvious drug intoxication in younger adolescents is a request for help with more
than intoxication. The obvious fact that adolescents are high
is ignored by others because they are unsure what to do. Some
parents choose not to see the toxicity of their children; one boy
regularly would talk to his mother when he was tripping on
LSD; she never noticed. Many drug-help organizations unconsciously collude with drug abuse; they look after adolescents
while they are drug toxic but make no effort to assist with the
problems that led to the abuse. As the young helpers in these
organizations usually do not deny their own drug use, and the
organizations are adult supported, the message to adolescents
who use the service is generally clear. Some parents may be
anxiously obsessed with the fear that their children of sixteen or
seventeen will use drugs such as marijuana, LSD, cocaine, or
heroin. They may seek constant reassurance from the adolescent
boy or girl that they will not smoke. Yet such parents may be
aware of neightborhood houses in which marijuana is smoked,

or where acid is pushed; they may know the local source of a drug but do nothing. If parents do behave in this way, their children then get the message in action: drug usage is accept- able. The same attitude is reinforced if parents are themselves chronic drug users. These parents who rush to the aspirin bottle at the slightest tinge of a tension headache, or who take pep pills to control their appetite, should not be surprised if their children medicate themseleves as well.

Drug-Maintenance Clinics and Adolescent Drug Dependence

Western society has not made up its mind how to handle the problem of drug dependence among the young. The usual response is to be puntive or to concentrate on individual treat- ment, but the social implications of the latter course are not always seriously considered. If, as in Britain, the giving of addic- tive drugs can be legal when an addict is registered, a clinic set up to treat such adolescents becomes highly inconsistent. On the one hand, the explicit message to the youngster is that drug tak- ing is bad; on the other, society is saying in effect: "If you register yourself as an addict, we will give you drugs." Such contradictions make more disturbed behavior almost inevitable. Some drug addiction centers, moreover, appear prepared to register young addicts without telling their parents. This confi- dentiality encourages disturbance: the doctors are agreeing by their actions with the adolescent's idea that parents will not help. For early and midadolescents this is poor treatment. It is never of use to young adolescents to agree, implicitly or expli- citly, in action or words, that their parents are bad. In the United States the same process goes on in methadone centers. In one state in 1971 the National Institute of Health authorized a physician who works alone to give methadone, he then addicted adolescents to this drug. At least one methadone treatment

center offers methadone maintenance to adolescents between
sixteen and eighteen.

Problems of Identity and Drug Abuse

Drug use may be an attempt to facilitate maturation and
to free the self from infantile dependence on parents or parent
figures. Some adolescents, without drugs, may experience feelings
of loss of individual autonomy in relationship to authority figures.
Such young people also tend, when off drugs, to complain of
feelings of depression, anxiety, or emptiness. Before the present
pandemic of drug abuse, those adolescents who suffered from
identity diffusion (Erikson, 1968) behaved symptomatically in
different ways: They were often delinquent, sexually promiscuous, or academic failures due to underachievement.

The most usual cause of a failure of psychological maturation in adolescent is isolation from extraparental adults. The
most common reason for adolescent inability to make significant
relationships outside the immediate family is not just the personal
psychopathology of the individual. Social instability due to the
vertical and horizontal mobility of society contributes to the
increasing difficulty of obtaining stable extra-parental adult relationships. When important human relationships are made by
early adolescents especially with a teacher, school counselor, or
social worker, the structural organization of the school system
makes it highly likely that this adult will be lost. The pupil may,
like a two-year-old who experiences parental separation
(Bowlby, 1971), then forego his attempt to make an attachment.

Individual psychopathology can, of course, be significant
in a failure to make extraparental adult and peer-group relationships. Those children whose early attachments within the family
were impaired are, as adolescents, likely to find it hard to establish a trusting relationship with anyone. A stable network of
extraparental relationships may protect adolescents from a dis-

turbed parental relationship, but it is less likely to protect them from the effects of severely early deprivaion.

Those adolescents who do not make significant emotional relationships with extraparental adults whom they and society value, find it difficult to develop a sense of personal autonomy. Without attachments to such grown-ups, adolescents may remain overdependent on parents. More usually such young people continue to be overdependent on peer relationships through the whole of adolescence in a manner that is more usual in early adolescents.

A typical group process of early adolescence is to seek awareness of commonly held feelings with peers. It is not unusual in some cultures for groups of early adolescent males to masturbate together; they thus become aware that others can obtain the same feeling of sexual excitement as they themselves. This awareness may also be acquired through the intensive intimacy of early adolescent friendships. In midadolescence, if psychological development is proceeding satisfactorily, a group of young people may use alcohol not to get intoxicated but to facilitate interpersonal relaionships. Depending on its strength and the amount used, marijuana, which is often used with the same intent, may instead produce an essentially masturbatory type of relationship. The adolescent toxic on marijuana with his peer group is more preoccupied with his own internal imagery and the feeling that others have a similar experience than he is with an emotionally meaningful interpersonal relationship. This behavior parallels the passivity of television watching, and midadolescents who do not develop a satisfactory sense of self continue by the use of such drugs the early adolescent type of interpersonal group relationships. It is also reasonable to hypothesize that the regular use of marijuana by early adolescent groups may reinforce masturbatory types of relationships and so inhibit the development of more mature types of interpersonal communication.

Within groups some individuals who may have difficulty

establishing relationships and establishing a sense of their own
identity may not become drug-involved, even if drugs are available. People whose psychological orientation is more passive are
likely to graduate to drugs alone; some, on the other hand, may
become "radicalized." Still other high school pupils seek an
identity by becoming greasers (or in Britain skinheads), who
may anathematize drug taking. Adolescents without adult relationships are extremely vulnerable to group contagion; a changing fashion of drug usage is likely to be as rapidly transmitted as
is a variation in language, dress, or delinquent activity.

Adolescents in an acute identity crisis who are introduced
to drugs may deteriorate because of the drug, rather than
because of their fundamental emotional instability.

Sexual Conflict and Drug Abuse

Drugs may be used in an attempt to resolve conflicts about
sexuality: They may be used to substitute for sexual intercourse,
to allay anxiety about possible impotence, to potentiate masturbatory activity, or to resolve conflicts about heterosexuality.

Dan, age seventeen, was referred to a psychiatrist because he had
run away from home three times. He described his parents as
compulsively straight; they did not smoke or drink and rarely
went out. The boy was academically motivated, denied any personal problems, and saw the difficulty only in that he had overrigid parents who made him terribly angry. He said that he got
"stoned on grass" every Friday and Saturday night with his
buddies, and he saw no problem in this. He had no interest in
girls but was aware of feeling horny from time to time. The
comment was made that surely Friday and Saturday were the
nights when boys his age sought dates. He said, "Do you suppose
I use drugs to avoid girls?"

Marijuana appears to reduce the push toward resolving

conflicts about sexual activity. Marijuana does not generally seem to affect sexual excitement, although boys say that girls who are turned on are less sexually inhibited. Some boys will talk of how pleasant it is to be satisfied with just necking with a girl and not to need to be more sexually aggressive: "Both of us are satisfied." On the other hand, some boys with homosexual conflicts report having been seduced by other males while they were turned on:

> Tom came to see a psychiatrist on his own because he was worried in case he was queer. He had been away camping with a friend of his who was two years older than he. They had both smoked marijuana, and after going to bed he had let the other boy sodomize him. "The terrible thing was that I think I enjoyed it, although I am not sure."

Some boys with sexual conflicts typically take large doses of amphetamines on the weekend. In American and European culture this is the typical time for dating, so boys with sexual anxieties can use the chemical impotence of amphetamines both to save face with their peers and to avoid the anxiety they might experience because of sexual incompetence or disinterest. Some adolescents who are consciously aware of sexual anxieties, which the processes of psychological maturation might have resolved, without drugs, may deliberately use amphetamines and methedrine to inhibit potency. It therefore becomes possible for these young people to say that they use drugs and therefore do not need sex. In small doses amphetamines are said to enhance a boy's capacity to maintain a penile erection; in large doses no erection is possible. The association between the use of stimulants and sexual anxieties in girls is also evident.

> Jane was a seventeen-year-old suffering from an infantile personality disorder with many hysterical features. Initially, she took many drugs and was also sexually promiscuous. When she caught syphilis, she took seriously the injunction that she should

not have intercourse. Then she began to inject drugs, saying that the feeling she obtained from the injection was like the feeling of having intercourse. Jane was hospitalized for a short time and then absconded. She went to live with a boy who, when she angered him, would punish her by refusing to have intercourse. Whenever he did this, she would go and buy some speed and take it by mouth.

The price paid by the individual is almost certain inhibition of psychological maturation but not necessarily permanent impairment. Without other treatment than intermittent supportive psychotherapy, Jane had given up drugs by the age of nineteen, finished her high school education, and established a semipermanent relationship with a stable young man of twenty five.

Heroin and cocaine are often associated with homosexual fantasies in both sexes. Heroin may produce prolonged erection during intercourse for the male, with an inability to ejaculate. Women may behave with less inhibition when "done up" with heroin. Although there is an apparent relationship between mainlining and sexual activity, to a girl with a hysterical or infantile personality the phallic injection has the same meaning as the use of a penis; what is really being sought is the omnipotent oneness that is obtained with infantile sucking.

Among the hallucinogens, LSD is sometimes described as giving special erotic parameters to sexual intercourse; more often it appears to be associated with masturbatory activity. Psilocybin and phencyclidine obliterate erotic experiences and so psychologically have a similar effect to the chemical blocking of large doses of amphetamines.

Relief of Intrapsychic Pain With Drugs

Drugs are commonly used by adolescents as a defensive medication to avoid the experience of anxiety. With this type of behavior young people are very directly imitating the behavior of the adult population. Drug taking in adolescence may often occur following the traumatic loss of a love object: parents by death or divorce, loved adults, or peer-group members. Since the awareness of death is a threat to an adolescent's necessary feeling of immortality, the toxic effect of a drug defends against this by allowing a return to omipotent infantile feelings. Since excessive drug usage is dangerous to life, adolescents may also use drugs self-destructively, playing a game of Russian roulette with their bodily and psychic health. The injection of morphine derivatives was used in this way by one seventeen-year-old patient, both of whose parents died when he was ten. He said, "When I shoot up, I feel at first as if I am going to die. Then I feel sleepy and warm and comfortable." Thus drug taking can be an attempt to work through a mourning process.

Those adolescents who suffer from severe chronic ego disintegration or who diagnostically suffer from a variety of borderline states may use drugs as tranquilizers. If they use hallucinogens, such as mescaline and LSD, or stimulants, their overt clinical condition worsens, although they are apparently less aware of psychic tension. Those adolescents who take large doses of marijuana, for example, three or four pipes of hashish daily, and who continue to function with a high degree of competence in academic or other work, clinically often appear to be suffering from either schizophrenia or borderline psychotic states. Although it is said to produce psychosis, the toxic effect of marijuana may also provide a defense against ego disintegration.

Drugs can also be used as a defense against severe chronic feelings of deprivation. In adolescents suffering from an anaclitic type of depression, in which they cannot make object relationships because of early traumata, drug toxicity may become a substitute for a loving mother or act as a transitional object. A patient's description of his LSD trip clearly symbolized his omnipotent wish to be mothered.

I feel as if I am in a room manufactured by the government given to all its citizens which will take care of all my survival functions: eating, air, living. It will prevent me from hurting myself, and it can even hold my hand. In the room I have nothing to worry about, everything is done for me. I have no fear of bodily harm; it is a great place to trip.

A seventeen-year-old boy who came into treatment because of heroin addiction was dried out from the drug by the use of methadone. He then became highly dependent on hashish, which he smoked each evening. The following interchange occured in his therapy, as he described having taken heroin:

He said, "I feel when I take smack as though I am hugging a teddy bear." While making this statement, he was playing with his mouth and the therapist said, "I guess you really want to feel loved." The reply was, "I cannot bear to be pushed around." The therapist said, "No, I did not mean that, I meant loved as your mother might love you as a small child." The boy answered that he wanted nothing better than to be able to curl up into a small ball and be looked after.

Complication of Drug-Abuse Treatment

Treatment for drug abuse is complicated because adolescents find it so difficult to give up the easy solution to a feeling of frustration. The social and educational organizations to which young people belong can be very helpful. Youth centers that have managed to produce a setting in which there is no drug taking provide a haven for the adolescent. This environment can be maintained if such organizations refuse to admit regular drug users or pushers. Schools can create the same environment by sending away those young people whom they know take drugs. With schools, however, the situation is more complex.

If schools expel adolescents who use drugs, their further education is destroyed. The logic of the individual school's position is clear: If they do nothing when they discover adolescents are taking drugs, they will be seen by other boys and girls as colluding in such actions. It would probably be better to see that young people got adequate treatment, if this were available. The realistic thing would be to create a social environment in schools that enhanced, rather than impeded, environmental growth.

If adolescents trust adults with whom they have a relationship, it is worthwhile to try to show the unreality of generational conflict. Young people might then see that their use of drugs may make them victims of adult greed; they can also be helped to understand the addictive needs of mankind in general. When a man cannot tolerate pain and frustration, he is likely to become addicted. The first addiction, which all humanity experiences, is for the magical relief from pain that a loving mother gives an infant. Those people who retain an infantile need for relief may become addicted to food, drugs, or sex; these can all be used in an unthinking impulsive way. The people who are vulnerable may be of any age.

In an editorial, the *British Medical Journal* (1967, p. 692) wrote to "a large extent the solution to drug abuse lies in the hands of local health authorities and hospials, general practitioners and voluntary bodies: Imagination, energy and good organization are needed in the many local communities where drug addiction is established or beginning to be seen." The clinical evidence is that the drug-taking problem among the young will not be solved while their other difficulties remain. It cannot be dealt with simply by the provision of treatment services. The answer must lie in more effective organization of society so that the needs of the young are met.

References

Bowlby, J. (1969), *Attachment*, Vol. 1 of *Attachment and Loss*. London: Hogarth Press.

British Medical Journal (1967), Editorial. 3: 692.

Chein, I., *et al.* (1964), *Narcotics, Delinquency and Social Policy*. London: Tavistock.

Connell, P. H. (1958), *Amphetamine Psychosis*. London: Chapman and Hall.

Emery, F. E., *et al.* (1967), *Affect Control and the Use of Drugs*. London: Tavistock Institute of Human Relations.

Erikson, E. H. (1968), *Identity, Youth and Crisis*. New York: Norton.

Gibbens, T. (1968), *The Psychiatric Offender*. London: Routledge, Kegan and Paul.

Grunspoon, A. (1969), Marijuana. *Sci. Am.*, 221: 17–25.

Hartmann, D. (1969), A study of drug taking adolescents. In *Psychoanalytic Study of the Child*, 26: 348–399. New York: International Universities Press.

Hoffer, A., and Osmond, H. (1967), *The Hallucinogens*. New York: Academic Press.

Hollister, L. E. (1968), *Chemical Psychosis—LSD and Related Drugs*. Springfield, Ill.: Charles C Thomas.

Mahler, M. S. (1968), On human symbiosis and the vicissitudes of individuation. In *Infantile Psychosis*. New York: International Universities Press.

Miller, D. (1965), *Growth to Freedom, the Psycho-Social Treatment of Delinquent Youth*. Bloomington: Indiana University Press.

———— (1969), *The Age Between*. London: Hutchinson.

Robins, L. N., and Murphy, E. G. (1967), Drug use in a normal population in Negro men. *Am. J. Public Health*, 57: 9.

Weider, H., and Kaplan, E. H. (1969), Drug use in adolescents. In *Psychoanalytic Study of the Child*, 26: 399–432. New York: International Universities Press.

Winnicott, D. W. (1953), Transitional objects and transitional phenomena. *Int. J. Psycho-Anal.*, 31: 89–97.

19

The Treatment of Drug Abuse

Adolescents need to assert themselves, to form judgments, to prove bodily competence, and to prove adulthood. The adolescent must also find a place for himself or herself in relationship to the opposite sex and to society-at-large (Zachary, 1945). Drug abuse has added a complex parameter to adolescent therapy; it has made some, but not the majority of adolescents apparently unreachable. Because of its danger to young people, society naturally seeks the simplest, least expensive, and most magical solutions to the problem. Drug education is the politician's dream of omnipotence: it allows people to think that something useful is being done, although there is no evidence that it is of value. Education about cigarette smoking has been pervasive since the 1950s, yet at the present time, cigarette usage among adolescents is at a peak.

Prevention of Drug Abuse

The appropriate way to prevent drug abuse is to build social networks for adolescents, providing them with anchor points

for development. This, however, implies making difficult social
changes in schools and other organizations that are of service to
youth. Adolescents should only be educated about drugs by
adults whom they value, for there is always the chance that they
will model themselves on the speaker. In talking to groups of
adolescents about drugs, however, the speaker's respect for their
capacity to make decisions should be conveyed. Ultimately, adolescents must decide for themselves on the basis of the knowledge
they are given. Although marijuana is illegal, it is hardly more
difficult to obtain than if its use were not condemned. In large
cities' and small towns even a moderately determined youngster
can obtain it. The negativism of adolescence has led some to believe that if the sale of marijuana was legalized abuse would decrease. It is true that attempt at control, particularly if it is inadequate, is a costly error. It makes adolescents feel that they
are being treated like babies. The youth may then try to prove
that they are grown up by defiance and rebellion, becoming vulnerable to the very thing from which the adult is trying to protect
them. Legalization poses this problem: Inadequate controls perhaps provoke some to smoke marijuana; the absence of any controls may provoke a pandemic among early adolescents.

Legalization of Marijuana

Some people maintain that they should be permitted to do
what they wish to their own state of consciousness and that all
drugs should be legally available. Many more, including certain
prominent figures, assert that marijuana should be legalized since
it is safe and not addictive.

Adolescents assume that society accepts their use of a drug
that is legally available to adults. The laws restricting the use of
tobacco to adults do not impress adolescents and there is widespread use by early adolescents. If marijuana were legally available to adults, it would certainly be smoked even more often by

twelve-year-old children, particularly since it lacks the built-in control of creating unpleasant aftereffects, as does alcohol.

Adults who smoke marijuana—or tobacco—but tell young people not to do so seem inconsistent; children and adolescents identify with what is done rather than what is said.

If drug education is to be attempted it will do least harm if information is factual about the drugs, in particular about their here-and-now effects. Overstressing danger may provide denial. It also appears useful to tell adolescents how they are being used by certain segments of society when they take drugs. But there is no point in pretending that the argument against drugs is stronger than it it. Much of the evidence about various drugs comes from clinical reports, and although a drug-dependent youth may appear superficially very sick, it is often difficult to know whether a disturbed adolescent who uses a drug would have been less disturbed without it, although his accessibility to therapy is certainly lessened. Moreover, only those who are disturbed are likely to be seen by a psychiatrist; we know much less about those drug takers who are not disturbed enough to be seen by a clinician. We do not know enough about the effects of many drugs, including marijuana. This, however, does not justify using the young people of today as guinea pigs for the malaise of society. With drugs, as with many other corruptions of society, youth is the victim.

Paramedical Treatment

Acute drug toxicity has always been a problem in emergency medicine. The advent of the drug scene of the last two decades has lowered the age of drug-toxic individuals who require urgent treatment, necessitating a change in medical care delivery and leading to the widespread use of paramedical treatment settings—drop-in centers, drug help services, storefronts, free clinics, and the like. These have been created for a service area in which orthodox social medicine fails to deliver. Their very presence offers disturbed adolescents a refuge, although the quality of care is often not the best, and sometimes they may be a provocation to behave in a self-destructive way. These centers are often based on the fantasy that adolescents mean what they say; for example, wishes to be separate from adults are believed. Alienation from adults is partly a result of the latter's refusal to listen. A seventeen-year-old who denies a wish to communicate across the generations is much like the adolescent who, in the middle of a family fight, rushes to his room and slams the door.

If ancillary treatment centers are to be used, such services need to be upgraded to provide first-rate care. Paramedical solutions are often looked upon by society as the magical answer to the problem of drug abuse, but so far adequate follow-up from these centers rarely exists. This problem is true for all social–psychiatric endeavors. Compliance in the establishment of a relatively low level of care is nevertheless unjustified, for this merely perpetuates rejection of adolescents. The centers sometimes make it possible for runaway adolescents to get back in touch with their families. Adolescents who are being exploited sexually or otherwise by their more aggressive peers may find a haven. They are a signpost to more orthodox treatment clinics, and they often provide food, shelter, and immediate care for drug toxic youth. The centers may also provide the only nontoxic human contact that can demonstrate caring for nonmotivated drug-abusing youth.

Society is now preoccupied with the issue of heroin abuse. In its acute stage such drug abuse is less common in adolescents than acute toxicity due to sedatives such as barbiturates, other hypnotics and alcohol, hallucinogens, and stimulants.

Medical Management of Heroin Overdosage

The management of acute heroin overdose requires recognition of the syndrome. The patient may be in severe shock, and death may occur due to respiratory failure. Typically, a continuation of needle track marks, coma, pinpoint pupils, and respiration depressed to two to four breaths a minute with consequent cyanosis make the diagnosis. Treatment apart from measures to support circulation and respiration, consists of three to five milligrams of nalorphine intravenously. This may have to be repeated in twenty to thirty minutes. As a side effect of the use of nalorphine, the patient may recover from the acute respiratory and circulatory distress and develop the acute withdrawal symptoms of abdominal pain, lachrymation, yawning, and painful muscle spasms. Furthermore, if the heroin is impure and contains sedatives respiratory failure as a possible side effect may have to be coped with. Physicians should be particularly prepared to deal with this. Naloxone, which has no effect as a respiratory depressant if a mixed drug toxicity is suspected, is the drug of choice. One hundred milligrams blocks twenty milligrams of heroin for up to ten hours. Since both these morphine antagonists are short-acting, the patient must be observed in case coma returns.

The acute phase is ended with the withdrawal of the adolescent from heroin by methadone substitution. An initial dose of fifteen to twenty milligrams of methadone is given orally; ideally, one milligram of methadone is then substituted for two of heroin. Since the exact dose of the latter is rarely known, the initial dose of methadone probably is slightly larger than really necessary. It should, however, be withdrawn at a 20% dose reduction daily. Nothing indicates that adolescents should be on a maintenance dose of methadone—it is the underlying pathology that requires treatment. Similarly, there is no evidence that group homes for drug-dependent adolescents or programs such as Synanon, Lexington, and Daytop Village help this age group once these centers have been left. The treatment of the young heroin addict is the treatment of their basic character problems and the social pathology that helped create this. Realistically, society has neither the resources or the will to undertake such a task. Testing the urine of young soldiers is not the equivalent of undertaking the complete treatment techniques that would be needed (Aichorn, 1969).

Therapy for the Addicted Personality

Heroin addiction poses a psychotherapeutic problem apart from the issue of drug withdrawal. If the adolescent is genuinely addicted and highly motivated, both relatively unusual in this age period, outpatient withdrawal is possible. If, as is usual, motivation is in some doubt, a socially acceptable regressive experience meets many adolescents' needs, or there is a question about genuine addiction, hospitalization is necessary. Preliminary observation, without physicians or nurses, suggesting drug withdrawal symptoms, may indicate that little need be done medically. Sometimes librium (chlordiazepoxidehydrochloride), in doses of twenty-five to fifty milligram tablets three to four times daily, effectively makes withdrawal a smooth process. Unless liver function tests can be given, it is probably unwise to give chlorpromazine to abate the possibility of cold turkey. Only if physical addiction is certain is methadone withdrawal justified.

Barbiturate Intoxication

Adolescents who become dependent on barbiturates need to be withdrawn in hospital at the rate of one-tenth of a gram daily. A number of young people die each year in status epilepticus from the result of the acute withdrawal of downers. Sometimes in injecting themselves or their friends with barbiturates, adolescents inadvertently pierce an artery and cause severe arteriospasm. This occurs relatively frequently because the high of downers is, of course, the exact equivalent of alcohol intoxication, when judgment is not likely to be at its best. Liver disease due to syringe hepatitis is a complication of barbiturate injection as with all other injectable substances.

Acute Alcoholism

Acute alcoholism is still unusual in adolescents; clinical evidence points to increasing abuse of alcohol among middle-stage youth. This is to be expected; adolescents are still conformist to the norms of society-at-large, and alcohol remains the drug choice of adult society. Furthermore, lowering the age of majority means that middle-stage adolescents feel that society is reinforcing this drug as desirable for their age group. The treatment of acute alcoholism in adolescence is the same as in adults and includes the replacement of vitamin deficiencies, attention to fluid balance, the giving of antibiotics and use of cross-dependent drugs such as pentobarbital (0.6–1.2 grams) daily, paraldehyde (60–80 cubic centimeters daily), or librium (300–500 milligrams daily). The latter is the drug of choice.

Acute Hallucinosis

The most common form of drug intoxication seen among adolescents is probably due to LSD. It is now generally agreed that tranquilizers should not be used for the acute hallucinosis of a bad trip, for these may hide the effects of other drugs such as strychnine, that are commonly mixed with street drugs. Similarly barbiturates, which are potentiated by the phenothiazines, may be mixed in with acid. The optimum treatment of acute hallucinosis is to talk down an adolescent. If this is to be done satisfactorily, it requires adequate handling of the patient in a safe, comfortable, nonthreatening environment. The more womblike the surroundings the better. The average emergency room, with its bustle, surgically oriented rooms full of instruments, and so on, is a frightening place for drug-toxic adolescents. Nevertheless, because of the toxicity of many street drugs, numbers of adolescents on bad trips end up in these areas as part of adequate overall treatment. The street scene has, therefore, implications for hospital design, particularly emergency and walk-in areas. Adolescents on a bad trip should preferably be under the care of physicians or paramedical personnel who can spot effects of drugs other than hallucinogens and who can monitor vital signs within the context of the acutely diagnosed intoxication.

Talking down is done by two primary techniques: accepting the attitudes, words, and feelings of the patient and moving to a generally supportive stance. It is helpful to make clear to the individual that he exists apart from the effect of the drug. A patient's attempt to hurt himself needs to be prevented by gentle, firm, physical control by other people, not by physical restraints. Often body-image boundaries become highly fluid and physical contact such as holding and stroking is needed. This may sexually threaten the patient and produce anxiety. Boys who are anxious about homosexuality may become frightened of either sexuality or aggression. One boy who became wildly anxious when his best friend tried to be physically reassuring said:

> I felt he was putting my arms and legs through a meat grinder. Then I thought he was going to do that to my cock and balls— it's funny I felt all that because he is my best friend.

The acute hallucinosis may be over in about six hours, but particularly after a bad trip episodes of acute flashbacks are common for weeks or months intermittently. It is not unusual for perceptual distortion, commonly a feeling that the world looks flat, to be present for some weeks thereafter. The anxiety produced by this may induce the individual to perpetuate the state of being strung out by taking small doses of hallucinogens. The adolescent's attempt to control the helplessness of a painful experience by deliberately reexperiencing it is obvious.

The duration of a trip varies, but when patients are high on a hallucinogen these are always finite states. Because of the time it takes to talk a patient down from a bad drug experience, some are tempted, once they are sure other drugs aside from LSD have not been taken to arrange for chemical intervention. An assurance of adequate liver function is needed, particularly if the patient has a history of heroin usage with the possibility that previous syringe hepatitis has caused liver damage. Valium (diazepam) in small doses of five milligrams by mouth relieves the tension associated with a trip but does not oversedate the patient. Many patients in a toxic confusional state may be hyperanxious, if not paranoid, about any pills that may be offered them. They may refuse this or any other medication by mouth. Furthermore, a physician has to decide the implicit message given to a patient when the individual who has set himself up to be helpful becomes the dispenser of downers.

Parents and Drug Abuse

Chronic drug abuse, regular or progressive, is a symptom, not a disease entity in itself. This is ignored by society in general and by many who wish to be helpful to youth. Underlying drug abuse is significant emotional disturbance in all adolescents who behave this way, although family and societal pathology may be highly significant. A particular problem is the collusion and unconscious provocation by parents and society in the drug abuse of adolescents, which is very like that found in sexual perversions and in symptomatic aggression. (Eissler, 1958).

Many parents do not understand that drug experimentation needs to be defiant and secretive. They destroy this adolescent attempt at autonomy with permissiveness, producing either a swing to increasing drug use or, if all attempts at externalization of aggression are blocked, some degree of ego disintegration:

Peter was the fourteen-year-old son of parents who highly valued understanding the norms of modern youth. When he experimented with marijuana at twelve, they gave him permission to do this providing he did not smoke excessively. Peter became a regular user being high two or three times weekly. He then externalized his aggression by seeing his role as making peace between black and white factions in his local high school. He began to feel less and less able to relax and became increasingly tense with a press of ideas and some hallucinations. He called his parents from a friend's home one night and said he was insane. They immediately called a drug-help organization thinking he was on a bad trip. He was acutely schizophrenic.

Meaning of Drug Abuse

Adolescence is an action-oriented age and significant communication is often nonverbal. Being caught smoking may be a request for control, help with emotional difficulties, or a test of whether the individual is cared for by the adult world. If neither help nor control is offered—and there is either no response other than words or a tariff reaction—an increase in symptomatic disturbance is likely. Adolescents need to feel adults care what they do; they may also need to produce in others the experience of helplessness that they themselves experience. The constant repetition of symptomatic behavior, when its causes are understood and an appropriate response given, means that drug abuse is covering very severe characterological difficulty.

Rarely do adolescents ask for help in words; this implies a loss of independence and is a threat to autonomy. Antisocial activity from academic underachievement, to theft, running away, promiscuous behavior, taking drugs, leaving joints of marijuana, pills or letters describing drugs or sex around for adults to see, and becoming intoxicated in front of authority adults are ways of asking for help. Similarly, smoking marijuana in school parking lots and returning to classes high is a desperate, if unconscious,

request for assistance. Many such adolescents are not helped because the meaning of this behavior is not recognized or ignored.
A drug-toxic adolescent may be taken home and nothing else may
be done. Alternatively, punitive control may be attempted. When
adolescents misbehave as part of an unconscious request for help,
the agency used often depends on both symptom chance and who
catches them. Disturbed adolescents may thus see a member
of a family service agency, a psychiatrist, or a juvenile court official. Pediatricians and family practitioners other than those who
become known for their interest in adolescents are usually involved by parents.

Some people misperceive adolescent drug abuse as symptomatic of the norms of a disturbed society and adopt the attitude
of many adolescents that it is normal or part of growing up.
Adolescents involved in drug experimentation or occasional or
even regular use as part of an identity crisis and an ensuing acute
conflict with parents may grow out of it. If they have never really
reached psychological adolescence and suffer from basic characterological defects, the situation is more serious. Parents, in particular, want to believe that their children are no different than
others or that episodes of drug use are at worst part of a transient adolescent crisis. A pertinent issue in middle and early
adolescence is whether the drug use is associated with the individual's being out of the parents' control. Young people may secretly misbehave but, when confronted with a parental demand
or request, adhere to it; failure to do so means that an adolescent
with few inner controls lacks the support of control from outside.
There is then an escalation of disturbance:

Patricia, age fifteen, defied her parents successfully on three separate occasions. She refused to stay home when told and ran away
from home. On the first occasion, she stayed at a friend's house;
on the second, she arrived at a local runaway center for youth
who played the game of being on her side against her parents.
After a third runaway, she was overheard talking to a friend on

the telephone; she indicated that she had intercourse several times, might be pregnant, and had snorted cocaine.

This indirect request for help gives some indication of what might be done. If the etiology of the disturbance is not associated with difficulty in making relationships with extraparental adults, outpatient therapy is possible. Some agencies can provide the adults to offer controls on the basis of a human contact. This will help contain self-destructive behavior; it is unlikely to resolve personality difficulties that have roots in childhood conflicts. If Patricia perceived the whole adult world as persecuting, evaluation of the difficulties in a setting that provided a controlling network of human relationships, often a hospital, would be necessary as she could not be contained in an outpatient evaluative situation. The success of these approaches depends on the quality of the services offered; poorly staffed adolescent units in inadequately equipped state hospitals may be as pathological as certain aspects of the penal system.

Methadone Maintenance

Some adolescents have so damaged a capacity to relate to other human beings that even with every conceivable effort, little apparently can be done using the usual psychiatric techniques. There is little point in keeping such young people in traditional psychiatric hospitals; often the only way to stop them from absconding is by chemical restraints. Methadone maintenance, with the justification that adequate psychiatric treatment is not available, or would be refused, is offered adolescents without real effort at serious rehabilitation having been made—the sequence of foster home, juvenile detention center, intermittent social work, and youth prison is not adequate trial of therapy. Very often, if such adolescents are treated in an environment with positive implicit mores and in which a network of human relationships is available, improvement does take place (Miller, 1966), although treatment may be stormy and many are damaged by drug use. Some boarding schools for maladjusted children in Britain both contain and help adolescents with severe personality damage (Shields, 1962).

Hospitalization

There is justification for hospitalizing adolescents who are severely drug dependent for a brief period of four to six weeks to see whether, when they are detoxified, they are able to make meaningful emotional relationships with others. Some may be found to be sufficiently intact as personalities so that they work at their difficulties either in groups or individual psychotherapeutic relationships. Others, without being able to use formal psychotherapy, may be able to utilize human contacts:

Cathy, age fourteen, was hospitalized in an adolescent unit because of severely disturbed promiscuous and drug-abusing behavior. Her parents rejected her and wanted her permanently institutionalized. After four months of intensive therapy with a psychiatric resident and a full milieu program including school in the hospital, she absconded and fled to Toronto. After six months she was picked up by the police there and returned to her home. The court social worker wanted to arrange for further hospitalization since she was intermittently delusional.

In Toronto she had lived in a commune in which she earned her keep by washing dishes and living with one of the male members in a pseudo-marital situation. Each morning she would go to one free clinic to rap with the staff, in the afternoon she would go to another. She was picked up by the police only because she asked her way and accidentally gave her correct name. When she returned she had gonorrhea, which was appropriately treated.

Instead of hospitalizing her she was allowed to live in a

group home and each day went to a day hospital where she attended school for two or three hours daily. Occasionally, she
would fail to turn up and then would go to the local free clinic to
talk to the staff. She reduced her drug taking and her promiscuity
and had a flirtatious relationship with a psychiatrist who saw
her for five to ten minutes daily.

With this type of regime other similar adolescents appear to be
able over the years to slowly mature and gradually decrease drug
intake.

As adolescents progress into maturity they may be able to
ask for help, depending on the way of life in their social environment, the availability of helping people, how they are perceived
by local youth and the quality of care available. If magical solutions are offered, adolescents are quick to perceive these as pre-
tentious and no better than the solutions they themselves try.
"All you want to do is get us strung out on your thing rather
than mine," said one angry late adolescent to a family practitioner
who offered him tranquilizers for his drug dependence. The ability
to ask for assistance in words also depends on an adolescent's perception of the value of helping adults as people. To assess this,
adolescent drug takers, like delinquents, attempt to corrupt helping adults. One technique is to manipulate them so that they appear to collude with drug-taking activities.

A juvenile court probation officer was approached by a drug-
taking, heroin-dealing boy of sixteen who requested admission
to the juvenile detention home. The boy was on probation for
being a previous runaway. He handed the worker four packets
of heroin worth about $200 in order to be admitted on the basis
of breach of probation. Apparently, he was seeking refuge from
the vengeance of some larger dealers whom he had crossed. The
court worker admitted him to the detention home. When the
boy told a sad story of deprivation to the juvenile court judge,
the latter was prepared to have him placed in a foster home,

providing he agreed to come in for a daily urine test for heroin. The boy was reported to have had a $75-a-day habit.

The boy succeeded in his manipulative efforts. Nothing was done about his illegal possession of heroin as the court worker "forgot" to turn it in to the police. The message to the youth, and his peers in the local drug scene, was that the juvenile court authorities did not take dealing in drugs very seriously.

Peer Counseling

The fashionable belief is that only people with similar problems can help each other. Thus, black people alone can assist black people; only youth can really understand youth. Adolescents therefore often use informal so-called peer-group networks for assistance. These rarely are able to offer highly technical help; they are supportive and useful for some, but the helping peer often acts out his own internal conflicts with his client. The desire to relate only to one's own age group is an aberration produced by social pathology, but it is easier and perhaps less expensive for adult authority figures to sponsor peer-group counseling than arrange for well-trained workers to be available. A particular belief is that individuals who have had a bad drug experience will really understand this and thus be able to be helpful to others. The problem is that such an individual may constantly relive his own anxieties through the pain of others and perhaps gain vicarious satisfaction. Furthermore, there is little evidence that an episode of acute toxic confusion necessarily leads to an attempt to stop drug use in those people who are regular or progressive drug users. Many of those who are involved in drug help organizations are still themselves users. By apparently assisting others some adolescents prove to themselves how invulnerable they are. Far from being a deterrent to further drug use, fear may actually precipitate it. Some adolescents may change the type of drug used; others do not even react this way. Particularly with LSD and the various animal tranquilizers that are passed as THC, chronic use may lead to such an impairment of judgment that even repeated flashbacks do not lead to a cessation of the habit.

Acting Out with Drugs

Drug toxicity is a problem for those already in individual or group psychotherapy. An adolescent may appear for a session intoxicated on one of a variety of drugs. The therapist then must decide whether specific medical intervention is necessary. The type of drug taken may not be known, either to the therapist or the adolescent. Young people may not know what drug they have taken because, just as many adolescents have an irrational distrust of adults, they may also have an equivalent irrational trust of their peers: Many seem as trusting toward the latter as infants with their mothers. Others have apparently such low self-esteem that they do not care what drug they buy; they tend to try anything they are offered. Drug dealers often lie about what they are selling.

The mix of social and personal pathology means that when a patient appears toxic for a psychotherapy session, a therapist must have doubts about the safety of the patient. For nonmedical therapists, particularly, the possible complications produced in a transference neurosis do not justify a failure to take an individual to the nearest hospital emergency room, if there is any doubt as to what might have been taken or its possible effects. For the patient who has taken a large number of downers, hospitalization is necessary because withdrawal in a nonmedical setting is dangerous.

Apart from complications associated with dangerous toxicity, since the "observing ego" and personal controls are interfered with by drugs, a therapist has to decide whether or not to continue a session from which the patient has partially removed himself. Although a patient may come to a psychotherapy session high in an attempt to relieve anxiety, appearing toxic also shows contempt for the therapy and the therapist: To continue the session may be to collude with an attack on a process designed to be helpful. This, in turn, may lead the patient to conclude that the therapist does not really value what he claims inferentially to be a worthwhile effort. Because an LSD trip requires someone to be with the patient and to be generally supportive until the episode is over, and since therapists are time-bound because of their commitment to other patients, the implications for manipulation of the therapist if patients have a bad trip in psychotherapy are obvious. If the therapist tries to talk the patient down himself there may be an active change of role, with all its implications. The need, in drug intoxication, to have one's body touched and stroked is equivalent to cuddling a frightened child; patients who regress in psychotherapy may act out their infantile wishes in the therapeutic situation. A psychotherapist may become involved in a counteraction that may turn out to be unhelpful. He may also seem to be playing favorites; time spent talking down an adolescent on a bad trip may force mass cancellation of other patients. On the other hand, the therapist's finding someone else to talk down may be felt as an intense rejection. In psychotherapy a patient who becomes high on acid is acting out a regressive fantasy in which the therapist is cast in a maternal role, that becomes either accepting or rejecting but is not interpretable at the time.

There are other specific complications of drug abuse that are particularly relevant in psychiatric treatment. All drugs produce transient or permanent chemical toxicity, and this may potentiate underlying psychological disturbance. Drug withdrawal is necessary before the underlying psychopathology can be treated; paradoxically, the causes of drug dependence often cannot be treated until drug withdrawal has occurred. The symptom must be contained before its underlying cause can be treated.

Motivation and Treatment

In all the emotional problems of adolescence that require treatment, the motivation of the adolescent and his family is always a crucial issue. Before the drug scene spread pervasively through society, the most difficult adolescent treatment problems were those connected with sexual perversions and promiscuous behavior. (These activities seemed to offer a magic solution to difficulties and, by infantile behavior, helped in the flight from the experience of psychological tension.) Now drugs provide a regressive solution to conflict, and motivation for therapy is adversely influenced. Furthermore, adolescents who were initially motivated to seek assistance and are in ongoing psychotherapy for another problem may discover drugs and become relatively inaccessible.

Hallucinogens, barbiturates, morphine derivatives, and other mood-changing drugs may be used by adolescents as a resistance in treatment as alcohol is used by adults. Providing there is no idiosyncratic response to the drugs, and the abuse can be controlled in psychotherapy, the situation needs to be dealt with by interpretation, like any other resistance. However, drug toxicity may be the storm center in which otherwise successful psychotherapy may flounder. Accurate and well-timed interpretations do not necessarily control acting-out behavior in adolescence, and drugs may destroy therapy that would otherwise have been successful.

Before the present pandemic of drug abuse, conscious motivation for therapy became more likely in midadolescence and was very likely by late midadolescence. As the complexity of society has increased, however, in particular, as social networks have deteriorated, individual adolescents have tended to isolate themselves more and more from adults. Without adult support, middle- and late-stage adolescents who are psychologically disturbed find it increasingly difficult to separate themselves from the regressive dependency needs of childhood. They are likely to see psychiatrists as the hostile representatives of an alienating world. These adolescents also tend to involve themselves in the drug culture and particularly if they are dependent on marijuana, or are regular users of LSD, often become consciously unmotivated for therapy even into young adulthood. Many parameters of therapy to involve such adolescents in a treatment situation may have to be used. The psychiatrist may have to be prepared to arrange for the protection of the young person with all the complications of taking over a magical, omnipotent role.

Psychotherapeutic Problems in Drug Abuse: Inpatient Care

Many drug-dependent adolescents are consciously satisfied with their ways of handling reality and making interpersonal relationships. Adolescents who have learned to medicate themselves with drugs thus appear to prefer ego regression to the frustration inherent in psychotherapy. An initial goal of therapy is to help them become consciously motivated to change. One aim of the opening stages of therapy is to show the patient, affectively as well as intellectually, that his style of personality functioning is not helpful to him. This requires of the patient a capacity to make a positive relationship with a therapist and a preparedness to suspend destructive acting out.

However, drugs of abuse change the adolescent's capacity for self-observation in a complex way. This varies with the extent of personality muturation and with the capacity to make a meaningful emotional relationship with others. A boy or girl who has made many LSD trips or is constantly strung out on any drug may be quite incapable of making such relationships for a long time, unless offered other emotional support, usually hospitalization. Those who have used LSD may take weeks or months to be really approachable.

These are adolescents who are only potentially able to make object relationships, and they are not consciously motivated to abandon drug dependence. They remain psychotherapeutically inaccessible unless authority figures other than the therapist, either parents or representatives of society-at-large, are primarily responsible for entry into treatment. The superegos of such drug-dependent adolescents tend to be harsh and weak. They are rarely powerful enough to control impulse discharge. Neither is the ego capable of handling regression without its functions being overwhelmed. If early in therapy the therapist becomes identified with this harsh, weak superego by being realistically responsible for the patient's entry into treatment, then the patient will attempt to escape from the therapist as he does from his own superego pressures. Therapy then becomes impossible.

When parents have made arrangements for the treatment of their adolescent child, with or without the support of legal processes, such a step threatens the intrafamilial libidinal equilibrium (Spiegal, 1951). After the immediate crisis is over it is often very difficult for a parent to support the continued hospitalization of a drug-dependent adolescent (Miller, 1958). The therapist needs to keep the responsibility with the parents and refuse to accept the role of forcing the adolescent to stay in the hospital. In any case, a hospital psychiatrist is likely to become a representative of the early omnipotent mother in the patient's mind and psychotherapeutic movement may not take place. Like the person who is drug toxic, the hospitalized adolescent may have no motivation to move from a state of idealized dependence. Probably successful psychotherapy in that situation is possible only with a therapist who first works interpretively with the patient in his life space and is prepared to intervene with a continuation of administrative therapy and psychotherapy. If the therapist also has been responsible for the hospitalization this work becomes impossible. The idea that the therapist is responsible for everything cannot be given up and the therapist cannot move from direct involvement with the patient's lifestyle. The transitional point, which has the same hazards as the abandonment of an idealized transference figure in outpatient therapy, when the patient must agree to exercise his own controls without the therapist acting as an external ego for him, will not take place. The patient may appear to become integrated in the hospital setting but this does not carry over into the world outside the hospital.

Because of the chemical and psychological insults to the personality involved in drug abuse, not all drug-toxic, drug-dependent adolescents are able to make affectionate and meaningful object ties (Rado, 1926) when drugs are removed and they dry out. The severity of the symptoms in drug dependence does not necessarily indicate the degree of underlying personality disturbance. In particular, adolescents may become heavily involved with drugs as part of a developmental crisis or painful experiences produced by reality. Those suffering from an acute identity crisis and ensuing identity diffusion may be significantly helped by once-weekly expressive–supportive, individual psychotherapy, which may last over a period of two or three years.

Outpatient Care

Many adolescents who appear drug dependent, even though they may suffer from severe personality disturbances, do still retain a capacity to make a meaningful emotional relationship with a therapist (Miller, 1968, pp. 625–628). Although outpatient pyschotherapy is particularly hard for those individuals who find it difficult to make object relationships in any case, significant drug abuse may be suspended because of the initial idealization of a therapist. To make ongoing therapy possible, however, the adolescent must begin to understand that his projection of an idealized mother onto the therapist is unreal; it represents the patient's wish to retain his own omnipotence. The frustration involved in this recognition is the point at which efforts at psychotherapy break down and destructive acting out of the wish for omnipotence restarts. On the one hand, the therapist must use the omni-potence given him by the patient as part of this idealization; on the other, he must carefully titrate the ending of this phase of treatment. Otherwise, the patient is exposed to an intolerable level of psychic frustration, as the therapist becomes the repre-sentative of a frustrating world that denies him satisfaction. The patient needs to be able to abandon the use of drugs because of his infantile, loving feelings for the therapist; he needs to feel self-love, not just self-preoccupation, which is no bar to self-destruction.

In the initial stages of individual therapy, drug-dependent adolescents may have to be seen daily if they are able to give up drug abuse. At the same time it is necessary to interpret both the patient's wish to have an omnipotent therapist and the patient's hostility to the therapist because he is not omnipotent. The goal is therapy valued at a more mature level, therapy that will be worth keeping and not lost in a fog of drug toxicity. The non-motivated delinquent adolescent with a character disorder, simi-larly has to abandon the gratification of his impulse-ridden be-havior to avoid the risk of a jail sentence and so preserve therapy. Once the problem of idealization has been worked through, the frequency of psychotherapy can be reduced to more manage-able proportions. Depending on the extent of the patient's char-acterological difficulties, this may vary from three times weekly intensive psychotherapy to psychoanalysis. The particular diffi-culty is interpreting the patient's feelings of rejection at the time he perceives a rejection. A therapist's vacation will almost cer-tainly be catastrophic in these patients, since they are likely to return to drug toxicity.

John came to see a psychiatrist at the age of seventeen at the instigation of his parents. He had a long history of LSD use and was a heavy smoker of marijuana. He was confused, circum-locutory, and relatively affectless. In the first three weeks of therapy, when he was seen four times weekly, his drug use effectively ceased. He became more coherent and emotionally more appropriate. He then insisted on going on a previously arranged visit with his girlfriend and during this reverted to his previous drug-taking habits. His opening words when he saw his psychiatrist after the return home were: "Why weren't you there when I needed you?"

Network Therapy

The adolescent character disorder, even if accessible to individual (or group) psychotherapy, needs many parameters to treatment. Young people should be spending a large part of their day in a social system that provides a network of potentially caring adults and a stable non-drug-taking peer group. For those who cannot use individual intense relationships because pre-existing personality damage is too great, a network of therapeutic relationships in a social system with a meaningful lifestyle is the treatment of choice. In modern society this is inordinately difficult to find. Some good small private boarding schools are able to do just this.

Brief Therapy with Drug-Dependent Youth

Adolescents who become drug dependent as a result of a psychic traumata late in childhood or early in adolescence may be significantly helped by brief focal intensive psychotherapy once they are withdrawn from drugs.

Sixteen-year-old John was referred for outpatient assistance from his local high school because of a fairly acute falloff in his grades. He was a tall, gangly youth whose clothing had the typical sweet smell of grass. He, at first, denied drug taking, and it was interpreted to him in the first session that maybe he wished it was that way but, by the smell on his clothing, he was indicating otherwise. He then said he smoked seven joints daily, seven days a week. "You must deal then," said the therapist. John then gave a two-year history of intense marijuana usage that followed a car crash in which his friend who was driving was killed. John had escaped with only minor injuries.

The therapist's ability to pick up the nonverbal communication of John's drug abuse and his "omnipotent" comment about drug dealing were both designed to have John perceive the therapist as a perceptive and valuable person. Arrangements were made to see John the next day only on the condition that he himself wished to come. John was apparently sufficiently intrigued to do this; he arrived stoned. The therapist interpreted this as contempt and refused to spend time with John, offering him the chance to return the next day sober. "But I don't expect you can make it. You are after all a pot head." This made John furious, and he came back at 9:00 p.m. the next day, saying he had no dope since 11:00 a.m. The actions of the therapist were designed to show John that:

1. Like dope, the therapist required some effort to be used.

2. The therapist was sufficiently sure of his value to behave towards the patient like Tiffany's: He had valuable things to offer, but the patient had to wish to buy.

3. The therapist was as capable of the same arrogant omnipotence as the patient himself.

In subsequent sessions, the therapist focused on the death of John's friend and, in particular, John's use of marijuana to avoid getting involved with people. John's affective isolation, loveless sexuality with other freaks at school, need to be criticized, and destruction of his own goals were all interpreted in relationship to John's guilt about the death. Fifteen sessions later John was only a rare dope smoker, had found himself a "straight" girlfriend, and the parting from the therapist was interpreted as yet another important separation.

John represents the group of drug-taking adolescents who are the most treatable. Their drug taking is a ticket of admission for help; their statement that they are "into dope" does not negate the fact that they are people. Initially, the therapist is used as a substitute for the drug. If there is an acute underlying conflict, the prognosis of such individuals is excellent. If the underlying pathology is a profound emotional deprivation, extra-hospital therapy is not possible, because the psychotherapeutic relationship in itself is insufficiently gratifying. The patient will then initially take flight into the regressive solution of the world of drugs.

References

Aichorn, A. Quoted by Eissler, R. S. (1955), Scapegoats of society. In *Searchlights in Delinquency,* ed. K. R. Eissler, 288–306. New York: International Univerities Press.

Eissler, K. R. (1958), Notes on the problems of techniques in the psychoanalytic treatment of adolescents, with some remarks on perversions. In *Psychoanalytic Study of the Child,* 13: 223–255. New York: International Universities Press.

Miller, D. (1958), Family interaction in the therapy of adolescent patients. *Psychiatry,* 31: 277–284.

———— (1966), A model of an institution for treating delinquent adolescent boys. In *Changing Concepts of Delinquency and Its Treatment,* ed. H. Klare, 97–117. Oxford: Pergamon.

———— (1968), Principles of psychotherapy in adolescence. *Wis. Leitschuft Univ. Rostock.*

Rado, S. (1926), The psychic effects of intoxicants. *Int. J. Psycho-Anal.,* 7: 396–413.

Shields, R. W. (1962), *A Cure of Delinquents.* London: Heinemann.

Spiegal, L. A. (1951), A review of contributions for a psychoanalytic theory of adolescence. In *Psychoanalytic Study of the Child,* 6: 375–395. New York: International Universities Press.

Zachary, C. B. (1945), A new tool in psychotherapy with adolescents. In *Modern Trends in Child Psychiatry,* ed. L. N. Pacella, 79–88. New York: International Universities Press.

20

Treatment of Delinquency

Meaning of Delinquency

Most adolescents have the urge from time to time to behave in an antisocial way that will get them into trouble if they are caught. Only when this happens is the label of delinquent behavior properly applied. Probably the most common form of antisocial activity in which adolescents engage nowadays is the illegal use of cigarettes, alcohol, and marijuana. These socially defined crimes are often followed by theft. Offer (1969, p. 67) reported that the middle-class teenagers he studied rated the control of antisocial tendencies as among the three most difficult problems faced by a teenager. During the psychosocial moratorium allowed by society (Erikson, 1959), the breaking of some rules is common, but theft, presented as an outburst of early adolescent gang activity, is not really accepted in that category. Nevertheless, it may not be taken too seriously. The fact that many stores put up notices indicating to adolescents that if they are caught stealing, the police will be called, indicates that there is an assumption that this will not happen. Thus delinquent behavior is socially defined, and what is classified as an offense in one culture may not be so in another. Even within social class and ethnic groups in one country, definitions of the word delinquent vary (Jersild, 1957, p. 311). Nevertheless, generally the individual delinquent can be understood as an individual who may obtain relief from tension, actual or potential, by attacking society. An attack on family standards, or the self, is not generally looked on as delinquent, and legally it is not so defined, although its etiology may be the same as behavior that carries this definition. The attack is designed to help avoid the tension produced by the stimulation of an internal conflict by external frustration. However, the individual, in addition, is gratified either by acquiring objects, or by the excitement of avoiding capture or directing aggression at others.

Delinquents may sometimes be able to be social because they like the adult who is trying to be helpful to them; sometimes, they abstain from antisocial behavior for fear of punishment, although this is rarer than is commonly supposed. It is a judicial fantasy that deterrence is a significant aspect of crime prevention. Most delinquents are convinced that they will not be caught, or they never consider the possibility. An adolescent who has been a highly successful thief, and who finds that crime does pay, is satisfied by delinquent behavior and can only give it up when appropriate control is available. The problem is quite different from that of an individual with basically similar emotional difficulties who has not discovered that antisocial behavior can be gratifying. The delinquent has discovered that relieving intrapsychic tension can be pleasurable, the nondelinquent's symptomatology may, in and of itself, be troubling. The delinquent then needs more environmental control than the nondelinquent. Alternately, special parameters are needed in any possible psychotherapy so that such a relationship will maintain intrapsychic equilibrium without the necessity for antisocial behavior.

The use of the judicial process both to assess whether or not a crime has been committed and to prevent cruel and unusual punishment under the guise of treatment is entirely justified. Furthermore, judicial process, when an adolescent is found guilty, is an important technique of indicating to adolescents, who have behaved in a way of which society disapproves, that what they did was not acceptable. Disapproval of an action does not necessarily mean being punitive or arbitrary, nor does it vitiate against empathy with the child's underlying difficulties. As with other symptom pictures, delinquents who are unsure of their identity may use a court appearance with its consequences as a label in an attempt to define a sense of self. The answer to "Who am I?" may be "I am delinquent." Delinquent behavior also has the same three main etiological roots that exist in homeostatic balance in any other given set of symptomatology. Whichever of these provides the principal source of stress playing on the individual provides a basis for a diagnostic classification of delinquency. This can make for more rational treatment approach in that the weight of efforts to be helpful can be appropriately placed (Miller, 1965).

Situational Delinquency

Situational delinquency has its major determining factors in the environment (Sutherland and Cressey, 1955). There are a number of these:

1. *In high delinquency subcultures in the larger cities, delinquent behavior conforms to the mores of the social system. This is not unlike the system that used to exist historically in certain tribes in India, the Dacoits for example, where antisocial behavior was accepted as a way of life. A state of cultural and social conflict, when old values are no longer wholly accepted and adolescents no longer get support from the implicit and explicit norms of society produces this type of subculture. Theft may become part of the way of life of a social system; it is not rare in the average high school, in university dormitories; it*

*is very common in army units with poor morale and in penal
settings.*

*2. The breakdown of the extended family and consequent
alienation from adults and authority figures.*

*3. Rapid social change, for example, in newly developing
countries, and the abandonment of emotional prejudices in older
societies. This may mean that one way of dealing with aggression, the projection of hostility onto an out-group is no longer
possible. The attack is then made on individuals who technically
belong to the same social group. Prejudicial behavior is in some
societies labeled delinquent.*

*4. The most common cause of adolescent crime in the cities
at the present time is probably drug dependence. A decade ago
it was not unusual for a psychiatrist to see an early adolescent
who was dependent on cigarette smoking steal in order to buy
an increasing quantity of tobacco. The frequency of theft in
association with the use of other drugs of abuse has considerably
increased. Clinical evidence indicates that there is a correlation
between drug dependence and the necessity to deal in drugs to
finance the habit. This is as common with marijuana as with
other drugs.*

Sometimes situational delinquency is related to society's
promising objects and gratification but failing to deliver; the
implication of television advertising that goods are easy to obtain is an example of this.

Not all individuals who are exposed to situational pressures become delinquents, so it is unusual for these to be the
sole cause of the behavior. The behavior of an individual adolescent is a function of a group process insofar as it affects the
individual personality. If the neighborhood adolescent code generally requires theft, it is not only the well adjusted who stay
home, the most severely disturbed may also fail to join in the
activity. Isolated, withdrawn adolescent boys may not take part
in gang thefts because they cannot make contact with their peers.

Group contagion (Redl, 1955, p. 315) when numbers of
adolescents, impelled by a common conflict and situational pres-

508   ADOLESCENCE

sures, act in an acute antisocial way, is another determinant of
situational delinquency. A riot arising during a political demonstration may involve otherwise law-abiding people who are
lured away by the situational pressure under which they find
themselves.

For most situational delinquents no special treatment is required, but individuals brought up in a delinquent subculture may
have a personality structure which the larger society finds intolerable. If this happens, society applies pressure on these people to
get them to accept the larger views, usually by being punitive.
Whether a subculture's way of life is labeled "delinquent" depends on the attitude of the larger group. Sometimes as a way
of dealing with this, people are incarcerated under the guise that
they are mentally ill. But even in family units of people whom
society at large would label "delinquent," some behavior is antisocial and perceived as psychologically disturbed.

> The nineteen-year-old daughter of a gangster was given a mink
> coat by her father for successfully lying to a congressional com-
> mittee about his whereabouts. He later referred her to a psy-
> chiatrist because she lied in an inveterate manner to him and
> her whole family. Although he controlled the local prostitutes,
> he could not tolerate his daughter's promiscuity.

Situational delinquency may occur in adolescents under stress.
Its unacceptability may lead the behavior to be labeled pejora-
tively as delinquent because the authorities in a social system
cannot accept their place in the etiology of the behavior: A
group of six patients on an adolescent psychiatric ward in a
general hospital were noted one evening to have wantonly destroyed large quantities of furniture. The etiology of the episode
was as follows:

> None of the physicians concerned with the group had interpreted
> to them their transference hostility. By discussing only their
> reality situation they had reinforced anger with environmental

staff. The furniture episode began because the staff stopped a sixteen-year-old boy from absconding from the ward to obtain some stashed marijuana. He stirred up a group with conflicts similar to his own, and one of the male staff became frightened and thus provocative. Another retreated to play checkers with some quiet patients. The boys began to throw books around, and the doctor on call came to the ward, stood, watched the episode, and said he didn't think it mattered, as no individual was being hurt.

With no external controls more and more furniture was destroyed until some new staff came on duty who stopped the episode with firm behavior. Some angry staff members tried to find a leader to scapegoat. The episode was however primarily a function of poor staff morale; the ward had been undergoing much social change. Thus, it was situational; although some of its etiology was related to the internal conflicts of individual members of the group. The episode would not have occurred in a more stable environment. Chronic theft, like chronic drug abuse and racial tension, can be a symptom of poor interpersonal relationships between adults and their young charges; it is then a type of situational delinquency. A side effect of conflict in the staff room may lead to institutional tension and then theft. In all these situations, staff prefer to look for scapegoats rather than at the tensions within the system or its organization as a cause of the malaise.

Intrafamilial Delinquency

Intrafamilial delinquency occurs when the significant determinant of an individual's antisocial behavior is conflict within the family. Its appearance depends on the balance between the psychosocial resilience of the individual and the emotional pressure that is experienced. The pressure may be applied in a variety of ways. An adolescent's antisocial behavior may be reinforced by his parents because it satisfies their unconscious needs (Szurek, 1942, p. 1).

> A boy was referred to a psychiatric hospital because he had destroyed a new housing development with a bulldozer. In discussing his son, the father got evident, if unconscious satisfaction out of the behavior. He then described how he, as a boy, used to enjoy putting sleepers across railway lines.

A more direct reinforcement of delinquent behavior occurs when adolescents steal clothes, stereo equipment, and other goods, and their parents fail to notice this new acquisition. A middle-stage adolescent boy may tell his parents that a collection of stolen goods have been acquired as the result of a successful gamble. Willingness to believe such a story is taken as permission to continue stealing. Parental collusion, particularly about clothing, is often reinforced by society; it is very rare for a juvenile court magistrate to order stolen clothes returned. Court social workers may be aware of expensive drug habits and never inquire seriously as to where the money was obtained.

Certain families are traditionally antisocial and have occupied this community role for generations.

> A fifteen-year-old boy was seen by a psychiatrist at a school for delinquent boys because the principal was concerned about the amount of illegality in which the boy had been involved prior to his admission. The boy was apparently well adjusted for his age and rather proudly indicated that he was doing what his father and brothers did. He gave a family history of antisocial behavior that went back for three generations.

Some families are so rigid that the structural organization of the family may be such that the individual is unable to play out the aggressive impulses that are aroused by family tensions. The children are forbidden to act out their conflicts when they are put under stress. These families that do not allow young people to show their anger and despair in the home fail to meet the developmental needs of their young. The constriction forces the spill out of aggressive impulses onto the larger community, if it is not internalized, producing a variety of individual stress responses. In situations like this, help for an antisocial early adolescent is unlikely to be successful unless the family conflict is resolved. In the middle and late stage of adolescence autonomy from the family is a reasonable goal, and once the adolescent has reached this maturational position, that the family is unlikely to change has to be accepted. The therapeutic issue for such young people is why they are so influenced by the behavior of their parents:

> A seventeen-year-old boy described how he had begun to break and enter houses when he was fourteen. He then stole electronic equipment from radio stores, became a dealer in drugs, and eventually developed a racket in which he persuaded his friends to steal Volkswagen cars that they then dismantled and sold. He was charming and a perpetual liar.
>
> He rationalized his behavior because he had to get away from his controlling and domineering mother who used tears as a weapon whenever he was untidy, late, verbally aggressive or did poorly at school. It never occurred to him that he could have defied her in many socially acceptable ways, nor was he aware that his contempt for all girls could relate to his maternal relationship.

This boy's passive aggression was further justified by him because he was angry with his powerful intellectual father.

Personality Delinquency

Personality delinquency should be diagnosed when an individual, by reason of his personality structure, attempts to relieve or abort the psychic tension, produced by conscious and unconscious conflicts, by acting out his anxiety and rage on society. Ego functions may be so weak that the pain of frustration and anxiety cannot be tolerated. Impulse release and gratification are then sought, irrespective of the pain inflicted on others. This can occur in people who suffer from mental deficiency, psychosis, character disorder, or neurotic illness; in all these syndromes the demands of reality produce greater tension than the personality can tolerate and it has to be relieved by antisocial behavior.

In another type of personality delinquency organic brain damage due to chemical toxicity or intercurrent physical illness is the cause; in another group growth problems may produce transient misbehavior. Typically in early adolescence the personality may not be sufficiently mature to deal with the psychological upsurge of aggressive and sexual impulses; in angry or inappropriately sexual ways these spill over into the community in an antisocial way (Winnicott, 1971, pp. 48–49).

Acute emotional trauma is a common cause of personality delinquency, typically, such a response may occur in a prepubertal child or early adolescent following parental death. If mourning is not possible, owing to either the age or the social position of a child, the anger at parental loss may appear in antisocial behavior, and the request for punishment implicit in this may be an attempt to expiate guilt.

Personality delinquency falls into three main psychological syndromes:

1. There may be a failure to develop an adequate conscience. The adolescent may feel entitled to steal and temporarily abstain normally only for fear of the consequences. Such an adolescent requires a prolonged and intensive period of help, which may have to be in some type of therapeutic setting.

2. There may be a transient psychological disturbance associated with an imbalance between the strength of the personality and the pressures put upon it by society or the conflicts of puberty. Auto theft is a typical example. Often boys who engage in this are unsure of their own masculinity and need to prove to others how powerful they are. If the lack of certainty is developmental, the chances of a boy becoming honest, whatever is done, clinically appear excellent.

3. Finally, personality delinquency may be due to feelings of profound deprivation of love and affection (Aichorn, 1935). *This type of delinquency appears common among girls and is often associated with sexual promiscuity. These are symptoms of a failure of personality development, and recovery is unlikely without highly competent assistance.*

Theft

In Western countries a common delinquent occurrence is theft. The preoccupation of society with property and the sense of the importance of material goods is great. In many countries the penalties for offenses against the person are often less than for those against property.

From an early age children are taught that only some objects belong to them. The boundaries of acceptability are, however, blurred. Many consciences, both for children and their parents, are elastic. "Finders keepers, losers weepers," chant children in some parts of England, and in society-at-large stealing by finding is common. Many people are surprised if lost valuables are returned, implicitly recognizing that honesty is rare. Children deny that they have stolen some object by insisting that the article was borrowed and would be returned. The concept of diluting the significance of theft begins in childhood to avoid parental punishment. In adolescence boys who steal scooters and automobiles to joy-ride, insist that their taking the vehicle was not really stealing, as they intended to return it.

A sixteen-year-old boy who had hitchhiked to a resort area with some friends realized that they were short of some camping equipment that could only be obtained from a town thirty miles away. He stole an automobile that had no plates from a used-car

ADOLESCENCE

lot, and he was picked up by the highway patrol. He knew he had every intention of returning the automobile and, although he understood that he had broken the law, did not really feel this to be the case.

Automobiles taken in this way are often returned to a place near their original location.

When a group, usually boys, steal small objects from a department store as part of a gang activity, it usually indicates an attempt to prove masculinity to one's peers. Dare-devil activity, especially that which is relatively safe, is difficult in cities and small towns, but it has in it an appropriate defiance of authority. Usually this type of theft will disappear with a response that clearly demonstrated disapproval but there are two exceptions to this assumption: if the individual within a group that steals in this way has previously stolen from a mother's purse, that type of theft usually represents anger at emotional deprivation. Early adolescent gang theft reinforces this solution to deprivation, so symptomatic treatment is usually of little help in itself. When a theft is highly successful and becomes one of a series, this convinces the youngster that crime does pay. In such situations, unconscious parental collusion or corruption by another adult is almost always found.

A boy or girl at the end of early adolescence may be found to be stealing. If a school, for example, reacts to the thief in its usual way and the stealing persists, disturbance is almost certainly indicated. This because adolescent stealing from other children in school, or from teachers, is typical evidence of difficulty in developing a sense of self. This is particularly likely when the adolescent is always caught. The theft appears to be an attempt to establish a relationship with a stable extraparental adult. These young people do very well, providing they are given the opportunity to have this without theft as an intermediary. Such a relationship must often last for up to three years. When it is with a psychotherapist, the latter will often comment that his role is only to be interested. If such a relationship is terminated too soon, the adolescent will almost certainly return to theft. These adolescents, when treated by court social workers, are then seen regularly during episodes of stealing; as soon as these stop, the frequency of contact is reduced. If thefts are an attempt to obtain an adult relationship, such behavior reinforces antisocial rather than social conduct.

The often inadequate approach on the part of society to the treatment of theft is possible, because most adolescents who engage in such activity spontaneously desist. Probably, of all caught delinquents acts, for every action taken by society, half the children will never reappear at any rate until the stage of institutionalization is reached. This applies to everything from warnings by policemen to probation with a court social worker. Good therapeutic settings for delinquent adolescents should have an 80 percent recovery rate; most have an 80 percent recidivist rate. This is more a measure of institutional inadequacy than of a psychological disturbance in most of the adolescents.

The Psychological Basis of Theft

Family attitudes have much to do with the development of a sense of possessions. However, to appear comfortable about objects borrowed without permission is not just an adolescent attitude. Many people have little intrafamilial sense of the importance to others within the group of their own property or of the hostility that is produced by taking objects without permission. In families in which the concept of personal ownership is well developed, brothers and sisters who take each others things without permission become enraged with each other. Sometimes family groups, in particular, middle-class families, act inconsistently; at one time, it is acceptable to borrow without permission, at others, not. Those social-class groups whose poverty makes them live in great intimacy with each other may have either an intense sense of

personal possession or none at all. The concept of personal property is related to a need for privacy; people whose houses have
been robbed often feel as if they had been personally violated.

The victims of offenses against property often have a role in
its loss. The ambivalence of individuals towards personal possessions is shown by their failure to protect them. Automobiles are
left open with the starting key; people go on vacation and forget
to cancel newspapers; windows are left open in empty houses.
This carelessness has multiple meanings: It may be associated
with a disinclination to be envied by others or with guilt about
possessing things in a poverty-stricken world. A disregard for the
importance of objects may be present either because they have
never been owned or because the individual has had so much that
things mean nothing. Sometimes careless behavior is rationalized
by alleging that objects are insured anyway. Adolescents who
steal often produce the same justification; no individual will be
hurt since the organization is large and can afford it or the insur-
ance company pays.

Theft is a typical way in which young people can engage in
aggressive self-assertion. The personality development of individuals in relationship to objects makes the act comprehensible.

Children develop the concept of objects apart from themselves initially as they perceive themselves as separate from their
mothers and then as they begin to recognize parts of their own
body. At about six weeks of age, a baby's smile implies a recognition that objects exist outside of its own body. Mother is seen
as separate but always available. Under stress the howl of a six-
month-old baby shows how enraged it feels at not having immediate succor and solace. The routine of living in which mothers do
not wait with bottle or breast poised to provide immediate satisfaction makes it possible for children to begin to learn to tolerate
frustrations. The awareness that the world is not automatically
their oyster is a precursor of the ability to recognize that some
objects belong to others and that greed must be automatically
contained.

Overanxious mothers, who cannot bear to hear their children cry, may have children who never learn to handle frustration, who find it difficult to accept that everything does not belong to them by right. They feel entitled to swallow the world and may become thieves who are unable to stop the practice.

Human beings use objects both to comfort themselves and meet essential needs. The pangs of frustration are appeased by infants using parts of their own bodies; early spontaneous thumb sucking, which may occur while babies are in the womb, becomes a learned response that occurs with a need for comfort. Children then amuse themselves by playing with their own toes and other parts of their bodies: Boys discover their penis; girls may find the vaginal entrance. Some children suck the end of their blankets under stress; others are given soothers or pacifiers. All these are the first transitional objects (Winnicott, 1971) used as a substitute for mothering. Bright objects are visually offered infants as a distraction; mobiles are made to attach to baby carriages and cribs. Bright objects are also handled and cuddly toys played with. Food is used in some cultures to comfort children. In the north of England when a child is hurt, it is commonly comforted with a "sweet" (candy).

From early infancy onwards an association develops in the child's mind between comfort, bright objects, cuddly toys, or food. These are used both to ward off tension associated with frustration and to be pleasurable. Toys are also used to gain a feeling of mastery over the world. Children throw them out of their cribs to have them picked up and returned; thus, they take the first steps to dominate their environment, using objects that can disappear, be lost, and then magically return. The genesis of "theft" becomes clear.

The two-year-old with a strong sense of possession clings to toys, however they are acquired. When toys that belong to others are taken, adults take these away, reinforcing the child's concept that some things belong to him and others do not. It may also reinforce the idea that the issue is not theft, but to be bigger and better at it.

Children who suffer from feelings of emotional deprivation may take money or food without permission, and one or both of these actions may be considered stealing by adults. Family feelings about this tend to be mixed. Some parents have no concern about children taking food from the ice box; others insist that the child always ask. Many parents make no fuss about the child picking up a dime that has been left lying about; some regard both of these actions very seriously and see them as wrong. The first object commonly stolen by children are other children's toys and food; money left lying about is picked up, initially because it is bright and shiny, later because parents spend money and children use it to identify with father and mother.

Money is then picked up to spend, which is different from money acquired as a squirrel takes nuts. Stealing money that is left lying around may be an identification with parents; girls put it in their purse; boys wish to rattle it in their pockets.

Money taken from a mother's purse or a father's wallet has still a different meaning. This is not just a theft, it is also messing about in the private possessions of a parent. The need to investigate mother's property, which may also include going into drawers and looking through closets, indicates both a preoccupation with mother's person and an aggressive involvement with her objects. The comfortable development of a sense of property depends, in a child who is not otherwise deprived, on the parental reaction to theft. Amusement may imply that there is nothing wrong with the action. Punitive overanxiety may make a child overanxious. If money is taken to shop "just like Daddy," punishment may also mean that it is forbidden to want to be like father. If a theft is an angry act designed to spite parents and if the latter react with spite, the message is that the fault is to be weak.

The feelings of chronic deprivation associated with chronic illness may be relieved by objects.

When I was sick and lay abed,
I had two pillows at my head,
And all my toys around me lay,
To keep me happy through the day.
                                        (R. L. Stevenson)

The same applies to those who suffer from emotional deprivation due to isolation from other children or parental absence or loss. The collection of small items is a reaction to such deprivation: a "squirreling" or "thieving magpie" syndrome. Children from underprivileged families may steal many small items from other children in school. In highly deprived neighborhoods children of eight or nine are the principle shoplifters from stores and supermarkets.

An outbreak of shoplifting may be a reaction to an acute stress. Its success may ultimately reinforce all the infantile demands that led to the outbreak; if it continues over a long period of time, it becomes difficult to convince adolescents that crime does not pay, because they feel it does.

The difference between stealing at home on one or two occasions and chronic, long-term theft has greater significance than simply that they are socially different acts. It would be simple if the former could be looked on as more normative, the latter more disturbed. But an adolescent who becomes a chronic thief is not necessarily severely psychologically disturbed. The situation is not unlike that with chronic drug abuse; the severity of the symptom is not necessarily an arbiter of the severity of the emotional maladjustment. Theft as a part of a personality crisis, which may lead as well to other types of antisocial behavior, may be the result of a conflict with authority in which the latter is always felt as persecutory. Antisocial behavior is then justified.

A fifteen-year-old high school boy was very fond of his math teacher, a woman of about twenty-eight. She collected funds for a school outing and had the money in her desk. John felt that she had marked him unfairly in a test and had been overly critical of him. He stole the money, did not spend it, but took it home and had it in a drawer. One week later, he confessed to the school social worker.

Just as with other adolescent symptoms, delinquent behavior carries an implied request for help. Theft in school often represents a seeking of help with a conflict at home. Guilt-ridden adolescents may steal in such a way that they will be caught; their goal is to be punished and perhaps rescued.

> Kenneth, age fourteen, began to steal from other children at school following the death of his father in a car accident. He obviously made no real effort not to be caught, and only the ineptitude of the system allowed him to get away with so much for so long. When he was apprehended, his immediate question was whether he could be tried as an adult and if he would be sent to the state prison.

Adolescent stealing from other children in school or from teachers is typical evidence of difficulty in developing a sense of self. This is particularly likely when the adolescent is always caught. The theft appears to be an attempt to establish a relationship with a stable extraparental adult, and young people do very well, providing they are given the opportunity to have this without theft as an intermediary. Such a relationship must often last for up to three years. When it is with a psychotherapist, the latter will often comment that his role is only to be interested. If such a relationship is terminated too soon, the adolescent will almost certainly return to theft. There is a striking inconsistency in the way these adolescents are treated by court social workers. Often they are seen regularly by the youngster during episodes of stealing; as soon as these stop, the frequency of contact is reduced. If these thefts are an attempt to obtain an adult relationship, such behavior reinforces antisocial rather than social conduct.

Until the advent of the drug scene, this syndrome was very evident. Today, adolescents may replace contact with adults with the regressive experience of drugs. There are three main psychological causes for theft:

1. *It may be due to a failure to develop an adequate conscience. The adolescent may feel entitled to steal and temporarily abstain normally only for fear of the consequences. Such an adolescent requires a prolonged and intensive period of help, which may have to be in some type of therapeutic setting.*

2. *It may be due to a transient psychological disturbance associated with an imbalance between the strength of the personality and the pressures put upon it by society or the conflicts of puberty. Auto theft is a typical example. Often boys who engage in this are unsure of their own masculinity and need to prove to others how powerful they are. If the lack of certainty is developmental, the chances of a boy becoming honest, whatever is done, clinically appears excellent.*

3. *Finally, theft may be due to feelings of profound deprivation of love and affection (Aichorn, 1935). This type of theft appears common among girls and is often associated with sexual promiscuity. These are symptoms of a failure of personality development, and recovery is unlikely without highly competent assistance.*

An inadequate approach on the part of society to the treatment of theft is possible, because most adolescents who engage in such activity spontaneously desist. Probably, of all caught delinquent acts, for every action taken by society, half the children will never reappear, at any rate until the stage of institutionalization is reached. This applies to everything from warnings by policemen to probation with a court social worker. Good therapeutic settings for delinquent adolescents should have an 80 percent recovery rate; most have an 80 percent recidivist rate. This is more a measure of institutional inadequacy than of a psychological disturbance in most of the adolescents.

Automobile Stealing, Burglary and Assault

Repetitious automobile stealing, burglary, and assault patently indicate a disturbed youth in a disturbed environment. But

such very disturbed behavior does not necessarily indicate an
equally disturbed personality, although this is not true when
serious assaults are made on others. Relatively minor conflicts
may be covered by repeated auto theft, for example, but quite
trivial antisocial behavior may be hidden by a profound personality difficulty:

> Paul was seen by a psychiatrist because his teachers felt that his
> inability to hand in homework on time, although he came from
> an apparently happy home, might indicate some hidden difficulty.
> The boy told his psychiatrist that he spent a lot of time riding
> around the neighborhood on his bicycle. It emerged that he was
> carrying a knife on these trips. Finally, it became clear that he
> was hunting a boy about two years younger than himself in
> order to stab him.

The Adolescent Runaway

A typical American symptom of adolescent and sometimes
child disturbance is running away from home, but this type of
behavior is extremely rare among adolescents elsewhere. The
etiology of this symptom, which is clearly culturally determined,
is the conflict between dependence and emancipation, and it is
socially reinforced in a variety of ways; novels and movies glorify
runaways, houses that are set up to shelter runaway adolescents
often may unwittingly encourage the activity. Historically, running away seems to be related to the concept of the open frontier,
but the mobility of the nuclear family in which all special roots
are left behind is, to an extent, mimicked by adolescents. The
fact that parents are often the only available adults to adolescents
arouses intense conflict over dependent feelings that have to be
denied. Physical withdrawal is a common way of trying to prove
that parenting is not needed. Drug-related and promiscuous behavior is common among runaway adolescents. They deal with
conflicts about dependence that are enhanced by the stress of

isolation of the nuclear family by a regressive dependent experience.

Often when adolescents have run away they leave a trail that clearly indicates where they have gone. Unfortunately, adults are not as perceptive and omnipotent as the runaway unconsciously would seem to wish. Sometimes young adults or other adolescents sexually exploit the runaway. Because of the intense wish for dependence of runaway adolescents, they are particularly vulnerable to this type of exploitation, as they seek the reassurance of physical contact.

Like all other syndromes of adolescence there are a multiplicity of personality difficulties behind an episode of running away. Furthermore, some adolescents who are legally described as runaways have gone to stay at the house of a friend; others have moved thousands of miles from home. In the late summer time certain towns and areas of the country seem to act as magnets for runaway adolescents, and numerous centers have properly been created to help these young pople. The usual goal is to provide help in the crisis and return the adolescents to their home base for further help.

In dealing with runaway adolescents the maturational age of the individual is always significant. Early adolescents need to understand that their behavior is inappropriate and a failure to take them to task for this self-destructive and antisocial behavior is an insult to a developing sense of autonomy. Only to be empathic may be to infantize. Furthermore, there should never be agreement that the child has bad parents and bargaining about a return home is not helpful. As with many other delinquent symptoms (Johnson, 1955) running away is often unconsciously encouraged by parents.

At the beginning of the middle stage of adolescence, running away may be related to anxiety about testing out new biological roles. A failure of identity formation is associated with feeling of bored emptiness and the excitment of running at this stage provides a special feeling of being alive. In middle-stage adolescents, who may appear with a pseudomaturity due, in particular, to early sexuality, the temptation is often to agree that these young people should live away from home.

The implication of reinforcing poor contact with parents, may be to destroy the possibility of a good adult relationship with their parents when the adolescents are older. Such reinforcement should then only be done if, after an adequate assessment, it is clear that family relationships are damaged beyond reasonable chance of repair.

Treatment Techniques

The problem with any type of antisocial activity is to reject the behavior without rejecting the individual. Apart from the importance of an adolescent not enjoying the fruits of ill-gotten gains, a treatment principle that is often ignored is the necessity to make reparation.

Punishment

Punishment, which has value in family situations, is frequently used to control antisocial behavior. It allows parents to relieve feelings of anger and frustration; it is an important way of showing a boy or girl that they are not emotionally helpless and can influence their parents' feelings. Punishment may convey to an adolescent boy that he is seen as manly and tough enough to take it.

The reasons for parental punishment may become blurred; sometimes in punishing their children, parents punish the bad part of themselves. Antisocial behavior is more often a request for external control than for punishment: An adolescent may have made no real effort not to be caught, yet when confronted he tells a series of blatant lies. A boy may steal because he feels his parents are giving him more responsibility than he can handle.

Punishment applied by loving parents may have a deterrent and controlling function. This certainly seems to be the case in emotionally healthy people, although the punitive repetition of such actions by parents is likely to produce emotionally immature adults. Children identify with such parental attitudes; they either become self-punitive or punish others, beating themselves as their parents did, or behaving toward others as their parents behaved.

Punishment that may be reasonable within a family has no value when applied by society in the treatment of delinquents as a technique of revenge (Menninger, 1969). It is used sometimes instead of necessary external controls, may be a substitute for reparation, and is related to a fantasy of deterrence. Punishment applied to adolescents by adults who do not love them is valueless. Such behavior deters only those people whose reality testing is good, and these individuals rarely appear in the courts of law. Reparation and control are adequate manifestations of society's disapproval.

Symptomatic Control and Therapy

The treatment of disturbed adolescents who engage in antisocial behavior requires the containment of symptoms, so that behavior is not socially reinforced, and an overall diagnostic assessment considering all the etiological factors, so that therapeutic efforts may be adequately applied. Adolescents need not be institutionalized in the service of rehabilitation or diagnosis unless the adolescent is a danger to himself or others, cannot be adequately contained while the diagnostic and therapeutic process is under way, or is getting so much emotional or reality gain from antisocial behavior that no motivation to change is possible. Large institutions are almost always destructive in that they are unable to meet the emotional, imaginative, social, creative, and vocational needs of the young people in their charge. Inevitably they institutionalize and create an "emotional deficiency disease" on the one hand, and a whole string of institutional reactions, on the other. Highly disturbed personalities with a distorted capacity for giving and receiving affection and with a tenuous control of aggressive impulses are thus created. Such individuals, unable to make an adjustment in the community-at-large, enter a vicious cycle of antisocial behavior, repression, and further antisocial behavior.

Adolescents who are dangerous require treatment in sophisticated settings that are aware of emotional needs and that do not institutionalize. Those who are not dangerous, if they cannot live at home, require either good boarding school placement, group homes, or excellent vocational training centers. Psychotherapy may be a necessary adjunct to treatment in either situation, but its type and quality need to be properly prescribed; therapy prescribed in any other way is likely to be valueless. Vocational training is essential. Without the capacity to be productive in a socially valued way, the development of identity is not possible (Miller, 1966).

When young people are starved of imaginative and creative outlets and when they are alienated from their own productive capacity, they are likely to become more destructive and rebellious The angry frustration that is so commonly created with underprivileged and working-class youth may lead to delinquent activity. This situation is so chronic that it is now hardly a subject for comment, except where there is a variation in its incidence. The help offered such youngsters in penal settings parodies their earlier experience. A constant shifting of human relationships, activities that offer them hardly any outlet for their imaginative and creative abilities, and dull, ugly, sterile surroundings means that there is little chance that efforts can be made to help them get in touch with themselves and be more responsive and responsible citizens. After attempting to be understanding, but not sufficiently imaginative to offer such young people appropriate help, society becomes repressive. The germ of rebellious antisocial activity is laid down long before the act takes place. Its repressive inhibition, without a change in the causes of the discontents, merely means that the next bout is likely to be more destructive.

More than any other syndrome, delinquency demonstrates the particular problems for the adults who are trying to be helpful to adolescents. Attempts to be useful, because they often arouse the primitive emotional greed of disturbed and delinquent adolescents, are likely to be met with manipulative compliance, sullen hostility, or withdrawal. The helping adult must not only bear the frustration his client may inflict upon him, he must tolerate, as has the adolescent, the frustration of living in a world in which individual integrity is often not respected. Sometimes parents cannot see a problem, but little can be done for younger adolescents without their parents' cooperation. Sometimes adolescents do not appear for help until their parents have lost all control over the situation.

It is difficult for the psychotherapist to compete with the short-term gratification that adolescents who are "into sex, drugs, or delinquency," can obtain. Such adolescents are tempted to fly from the treatment situation because therapy does not offer magic and no one contains them in the therapeutic situation.

In the psychotherapy of delinquent adolescents who suffer from severe personality difficulties a certain basic initial stance is necessary to make therapy possible:

1. The therapist must not allow himself to be corrupted in the eyes of the patient. The patient attempts to do this by getting the therapist to collude in an unwilling way in antisocial behavior.

An eighteen-year-old boy, in a burst of honesty told his doctor that he had on him many packs of cigarettes that he had stolen from a local supermarket. He told his doctor that he intended to sell them at 25¢ each to some of the doctor's other patients. The psychiatrist made interpretations about the patient's aggression but did not insist that the stolen goods be returned.

The patient in action thus made his doctor an accessory after the fact.

2. Delinquent character problem adolescents tell a therapist part of the truth to fob off investigation into the depth of their aggressive activity. If the therapist accepts a part truth, the patient feels only contempt and acting up increases because of enhanced anxiety.

A group of adolescent boys on a psychiatric ward were about to go on a camping trip. They were tense and restless and the staff felt there was something wrong. However, nothing was done and the boys left for camp. The first day there they were obviously smoking marijuana and the staff confiscated a cap of marijuana. They accepted the boys' statement that there was no more. The staff called one of the ward therapists who accepted this statement. The boys continued to behave in a disturbed way, and two days later a large cache of the drug was discovered.

3. Communication with therapist about delinquent activity commonly takes place with action rather than words. A failure to perceive the significance of the communication means that therapy flounders. The reverse, with appropriate counter action, may assist growth.

A seventeen-year-old English boy, on parole from a school for delinquent boys on condition he had psychotherapy, appeared for his third session dressed in a magnificent red velvet-lined black cloak. He was known to be jobless. After a short time the therapist asked him when the "rip off" had taken place. The boy reddened and described how he had robbed a well-known department store. There was a long discussion about what a poor crook the boy was. The therapist regretted that he could not agree that he could join with the boy in his actions because he had too much to lose and the boy was not good enough a criminal. At this the boy boasted of his numerous delinquencies about which the therapist was scornful. Finally, he told the boy that if the therapy was to continue the boy would have to return the cloak to the local police station.

The boy continued to come for his therapy, in many ways he acted out his conflicts but he remained out of trouble and ultimately abandoned his delinquent stance.

4. The therapist has to reinforce the patient's narcissism and to some extent the instinctual gratification obtained by the delinquent act has to be possible in the therapeutic session. The therapist should not be judgmental in a stereotyped way and should accept the communications of his patient and understand them.

5. Providing the patient is not acting destructively the therapist should look on all communications as significant and need not be preoccupied with whether the patient is telling the truth or not; a lie is an interpretable communication.

This type of approach allows the patient initially to perceive the therapist as an extension of himself, personality strengths are reinforced and sometimes therapeutic work with the underlying conflicts is possible. On other occasions the delinquent adolescent makes a firm identification with his therapist and either sustains himself thereafter, or returns to therapy as a young adult.

Society rarely provides helpful resources for the adequate treatment of disturbed delinquents. So, too, there is a temptation for helping adults to give up in despair. Many start to treat delinquents but give up because they feel the adolescent will not use the therapist's knowledge or skill. The treatment of these young people requires that therapists should be able to tolerate their own helplessness and be sufficiently in touch with their own delinquency so that they can see that that exists in their patient.

With all the difficulties of this period of life, adolescence provides the optimum time for therapeutic intervention. When the social systems of society value the integrity of the youth, the prognosis for their disturbances and the enhancement of maturation becomes excellent.

References

Erikson, E. H. (1959), Identity and the Life Cycle. *Biol. Issues,* 1: 1–171.

Jersild, A. T. (1957), *The Psychology of Adolescence.* New York: Macmillan.

Johnson, A. M. (1955), Sanctions for super-ego lacunae in adolescents. In *Searchlights on Delinquency,* ed. K. R. Eissler, 225–245. New York: International Universities Press.

Menninger, K. A. (1969), *The Crime of Punishment.* New York: Viking.

Miller, D. (1965), *Growth to Freedom, The Psycho-Social Treatment of Delinquent Youth.* Bloomington: Indiana University Press.

———— (1966), A model of an institution for treating delinquent adolescent boys. In *Changing Concepts of Crime and Its Treatment,* ed. H. Klare, 97–117. Oxford: Pergamon Press.

Offer, D. (1969), *The Psychological World of the Teenager.* New York: Basic Books.

Redl, F. (1955), The phenomena of contagion and shock effect in group therapy. In *Searchlights on Delinquency,* ed. K. R. Eissler, 315–329, New York: International Universities Press.

Sutherland, E. H., and Cressey, R. (1955), *Principles of Criminology.* Philadelphia: Lippincott.

Szurek, S. (1942), Genesis of psychopathic personality traits. *Psychiatry,* 5: 1–15.

Winnicott, D. W. (1971), Adolescence, struggling through the doldrums. In *Adolescent Psychiatry,* ed. S. C. Feinstein, A. Miller, P. Giovacchini, 48–59. New York: Basic Books.

Index

Index